W9-BVQ-478

*Rocky Mountain
Spotted Fever*

*The Henry E. Sigerist Series
in the History of Medicine*

Sponsored by The American Association for the History
of Medicine and The Johns Hopkins University Press

The Development of American Physiology
Scientific Medicine in the Nineteenth Century
by W. Bruce Fye

Save the Babies
American Public Health Reform and the
Prevention of Infant Mortality, 1850–1929
by Richard A. Meckel

*Politics and Public Health in Revolutionary
Russia, 1890–1918*
by John F. Hutchinson

Rocky Mountain Spotted Fever
History of a Twentieth-Century Disease
by Victoria A. Harden

Rocky Mountain Spotted Fever

History of a Twentieth-Century Disease

Victoria A. Harden

The Johns Hopkins University Press
Baltimore and London

The text for this book was prepared in the main part as
an intramural project of the National Institute of Allergy
and Infectious Diseases, National Institutes of Health.

Foreword © 1990 The Johns Hopkins University Press

Printed in the United States of America

The Johns Hopkins University Press
701 West 40th Street
Baltimore, Maryland 21211
The Johns Hopkins Press Ltd., London

The paper used in this publication meets the minimum requirements of American National Standard for Information Sciences—Permanence of Paper for
Printed Library Materials, ANSI Z39.48-1984.

Library of Congress Cataloging-in-Publication Data

Harden, Victoria Angela.
   Rocky Mountain spotted fever: history of a twentieth-century
   disease / Victoria A. Harden.
      p.   cm. — (The Henry E. Sigerist series in the history of
   medicine)
   Includes bibliographical references.
   ISBN 0-8018-3905-X (alk. paper)
   1. Rocky Mountain spotted fever—History. I. Title. II. Series.
RC182.R6H37   1990
616.9'223—dc20   89-48033
                                                      CIP

To the memory of
John R. Seal
who envisioned this history
and to
William L. Jellison
who preserved so many of the documents on
which it is based

Contents

Illustrations

Foreword

One of the factors that attracted me to Rocky Mountain spotted fever was the rich historic lore of the subject. Years of collecting and studying the literature of the field confirmed my opinion that the stories expressed the emergence of science from the Western frontier. In this book, Victoria Harden conveys the history with the vividness of the traditional storyteller and the care of the professional historian. What develops is the picture of the maturation of biomedical science in the United States. Scientists in the disciplines of entomology, microbiology, pathology, medicine, and immunology have elucidated a novel infectious agent that normally resides in ticks. They began with a prevalent public opinion that this dreaded plague was caused by drinking water from melted snow and over the years reached a more accurate state of knowledge. Because of the dramatic severity of the clinical illness, work on these difficult organisms has continued. Rickettsiology has now overcome many of the technical obstacles that for so long inhibited progress. By employing molecular methods, the field has accelerated its pace and is now in the mainstream of microbiology. Genes have been cloned for important rickettsial components and specific functions. The power of science to make significant advances in rickettsiology has never been greater.

Yet the number of institutions with research laboratories that are engaged in the investigation of *Rickettsia rickettsii* and its relatives are remarkably few. The medical importance of rickettsiae alone justifies considerably more effort. Rocky Mountain spotted fever is still a life-threatening disease for healthy persons who are engaged in outdoor activities. There are major pitfalls and deficiencies in both the clinical and laboratory diagnoses of Rocky Mountain spotted fever. The etiologic agent is firmly entrenched in nature and cannot yet be eradicated. Related rickettsiae frequently cause undiagnosed infections in southern Europe, Africa, and Asia. No effective vaccines are available. Medical treatment given late in the course of illness because of delayed diagnosis often fails to save the patient's life.

In addition to the practical problems, there are many interesting scientific questions about rickettsiae that could lead to better understanding of intracellular parasitism, pathobiology and immunobiology of intracellular bacteria, and endothelial pathophysiology. Numerous basic questions remain unanswered: How are rickettsiae maintained in nature? Is rickettsial infection pathogenic for the tick? What has prevented pathogenic *R. rickettsii* from occupying a greater proportion of the ecologic niche in ticks (less than 0.1 percent of the members of the major vector species of ticks contain disease-causing *R. rickettsii*)? How do the more prevalent nonpathogenic rickettsiae interfere with establishment of their pathogenic relatives? Why does the incidence and geographic distribution of disease appear to change during a period of time? What components of the immune system must be stimulated in order for it to resist infection or reinfection? How does the immune system rid the human host of an established infection? What is the composition of rickettsiae (e.g., what is the composition of the outer layer, putatively a slime layer?)? How do the rickettsial structural components mediate the various functions of the organism? How is virulence reactivated from its dormant state in ticks? How do host factors such as older age, male sex, the genetic condition of glucose-6-phosphate dehydrogenase deficiency, and possibly hemolysis lead to increased severity of illness? How do the rickettsiae cause human cell and tissue damage and disease syndromes? Do so-called nonpathogenic rickettsiae such as *R. parkeri* and *R. rhipicephali* infect humans, causing unrecognized syndromes?

The number of fruitful lines of inquiry rapidly overwhelms the corps of rickettsiologists, whose ranks are already thin. The specialized cadre of scientists who know and understand rickettsiae must be expanded by educating more young scientists, and more funding is required for significant scientific progress. Rickettsiology has for years been viewed as archaic even as it has quietly opened new avenues of knowledge. Rickettsiologists have delved into topics such as the pathogenic roles of phospholipase and protease or the role of interferon-gamma in immunity to intracellular pathogens. They have solved such riddles as the cause of Legionnaires' disease, Lyme disease, and Potomac horse fever. During the next decade, rickettsiologists must continue to do basic laboratory investigation, teach others the science and historic lore, reach out to collaborate with colleagues abroad on the prevalent infections in Asia, Africa, and Europe. It is hoped that in the process, important new scientific advances will answer questions remaining from the early days of studies in the Bitterroot Valley of western Montana. It is even reasonable to expect better approaches to prevention, diagnosis, and treatment. The pace of progress may be expected to reflect the support provided by public and private agencies.

David H. Walker, M.D.

Preface

In 1984 I was invited to write a history of Rocky Mountain spotted fever for the National Institute of Allergy and Infectious Diseases (NIAID), the component of the National Institutes of Health (NIH) that traces its roots to 1887, when federally sponsored medical research began. Since 1902, NIAID and its antecedent laboratories in the U.S. Public Health Service have supported research on Rocky Mountain spotted fever. The late John R. Seal, in 1984 deputy director and formerly director of intramural research, was the project's initial sponsor within the institute. He believed that a history of this disease would contribute to the understanding of twentieth-century medicine and medical research. The project gained the support of NIAID director Richard M. Krause and of his successor, Anthony S. Fauci, and was placed within the NIH intramural research program. I began the work under Kenneth W. Sell, intramural director, who framed the assignment in broad terms and provided support services for the research. His successor, John I. Gallin, continued these policies and graciously extended my deadline so that I might participate in preparations for the NIH centennial observance.

Although the U.S. Public Health Service was not the only agency that contributed to the diagnosis, prevention, and cure of Rocky Mountain spotted fever, it has played a key role throughout this century. Because spotted fever occurs only in the western hemisphere—but not exclusively in the Rocky Mountain region, as its name implies—it held particular interest for investigators in the United States from the time it was first differentiated from other fevers. During the early decades of the twentieth century, much of the work on spotted fever was conducted at laboratories in the Bitterroot Valley of western Montana, where the disease was particularly virulent. A laboratory building initially constructed in 1928 by the state of Montana subsequently became the Rocky Mountain Laboratory (RML) of NIAID. Fortunately for the historian, many of the investigators at the RML kept meticulous records and saved their correspondence. In conjunction with documents at other institutions and with the published scientific literature, these records provided a rich archival source for the preparation of this history. During the course of the project, many state and federal records at the RML were transferred to institutions where they will be preserved and made available to other scholars. The disposition of these records is discussed in the Note on Sources.

During the years of research for and writing of this book, I have incurred debts to many people, especially in Montana and at the NIH in Bethesda, Maryland. These included scientists, administrators, laboratory support staff, archivists, librarians, other historians, and lay persons whose lives have been touched by Rocky Mountain spotted fever. Many of these people are acknowledged in the Note on Sources, but doubtless I have not listed every one. I am grateful to all who took time from their schedules to enhance my understanding of this disease.

Special thanks are due to Carolyn Brown's staff at the NIH library, who filled an astronomical number of requests for copies of papers and interlibrary loan books. Betty Murgolo, especially, went to great lengths to locate obscure but key sources. John Parascandola, chief of the History of Medicine Division, National Library of Medicine, and his staff, especially the curator of modern manuscripts, Peter Hirtle, also proved most helpful in suggesting relevant documents from their rich manuscript collections. Lois South in the Judicial, Fiscal, and Social Branch of the National Archives and Records Administration provided knowledgeable guidance to records in the collections of the U.S. Public Health Service and of the NIH. Archivists and librarians at the Montana State Archives in Helena, Montana, and at the Renne Library of Montana State University in Bozeman, Montana, facilitated my search through their holdings. Archivist Richard Popp in the Department of Special Collections, Joseph Regenstein Library, University of Chicago, kindly assisted me in obtaining copies of the Howard Taylor Ricketts Papers. Carolyn Kopp, university archivist at the Rockefeller University, similarly provided key materials from the Hideyo Noguchi Papers. Citations from these collections are used by permission of the University of Chicago and of the Rockefeller University.

Because of the key role of the Rocky Mountain Laboratory in spotted fever research throughout the twentieth century, I made extensive use of materials held at the RML library and at the Ravalli County Historical Society. Many people in the Bitterroot Valley told me of their experiences and suggested other sources of information, but four people in Hamilton extended extraordinary assistance. Erma Owings, archivist at the Ravalli County Historical Society, helped in numerous ways as I researched this remarkable collection of county documents. William L. Jellison, a retired entomologist from the laboratory, active local historian, and curator of spotted fever artifacts, led me to records he had preserved from destruction, showed me historically important sites in the valley, introduced me to many long-term residents who remembered the early days of spotted fever, and made helpful suggestions for improving the manuscript. Robert N. Philip, a former epidemiologist at the laboratory, offered me his encyclopedic knowledge of western Montana and the fruits of his own extensive research on spotted fever. His criticism of the manuscript proved invaluable. Finally, Leza S. Hamby, librarian at the laboratory, not only filled my every request for information but also made arrangements for me to see firsthand a dipping vat used to combat spotted fever early in the century. In addition, she always extended warm hospitality during my research trips to the valley.

Among the numerous scientists and physicians to whom I accrued debts, special thanks must go to all whom I interviewed. Named in the Note on Sources, these people often became my patient teachers as I struggled to master a portion of the intricacies of microbiology, entomology, and immunology. Another dimension was added to my research when David H. Walker, then in the Department of Pathology at the University of North Carolina, School of Medicine at Chapel Hill, and now chairman of the Pathology Department at the University of Texas Medical Branch at Galveston, introduced me to the group of researchers in Palermo, Sicily, who are investigating Rocky Mountain spotted fever's rickettsial relative, boutonneuse fever. During a trip I made to Italy for a related research project, Serafino Mansueto, Giuseppe Tringali, and Vittorio Scaffidi extended hospitality, recounted their research strategies, and made it possible for me to observe a case of boutonneuse fever.

Once written, the manuscript received critical review from a variety of scientists and historians. Willy Burgdorfer, Eugene P. Campbell, James A. Cassedy, Alan M. Cheever, Robert Edelman, William Jordan, Richard A. Ormsbee, Margaret Pittman, Norman H. Topping, David H. Walker, and Charles L. Wisseman, Jr., read one or more chapters. Saul Benison, William L. Jellison, David B. Lackman, Robert N. Philip, and James Harvey Young read the entire manuscript. I am greatly indebted to each of them, whose suggestions significantly improved the accuracy and clarity of the book. Any errors that remain are mine alone.

I must also gratefully acknowledge many other members of the NIAID and NIH staffs in Bethesda who extended themselves to assist me in various ways. Mary Ann Guerra provided essential administrative support throughout the project. Patricia Randall and her associates in the NIAID Public Information Office, especially Karen Leighty and Judy Murphy, proved most knowledgeable about recent institute history and directed my attention to many internal files and pictures. Rurik Fredrickson, Harriet R. Greenwald, and Rhoda Laskin provided technical assistance during the course of the project. Rochelle Howard prepared computerized files of NIAID rickettsial grants and of a collection of photographs relating to this project. Joanie Shariat vetted the manuscript with skill and tact.

Once in production, the book received careful attention from several members of the staff at Johns Hopkins University Press. Particularly I would like to thank executive editor Henry Y. K. Tom for his support and patience in bringing this manuscript to publication.

Finally, I am grateful to my family, who never failed in their encouragement of this project, even when my research files and draft manuscripts threatened to engulf the house. My husband, Robert L. Berger, proved to be an excellent research assistant as well as my first critical reader and a continuous source of moral support.

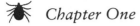

Chapter One

A Twentieth-Century Disease of Nature

The unwritten history of the investigational work in connection with Rocky Mountain spotted fever, if written, would read like a romance.
William Forlong Cogswell, ca. 1930

Some diseases have been known to human beings for eons. Epilepsy, for example, was well recognized by the ancients, who called it the falling sickness because of its sudden seizures. Other diseases are quite new, acquired immunodeficiency syndrome, or AIDS, being perhaps the most recent example. Many diseases have come into or gone out of existence according to conceptual models that guided the medical communities of specific societies. Dropsy was a recognized clinical entity in the eighteenth century, but today it no longer exists as a distinct disease, its swelling of the tissues being viewed rather as a symptom of several different pathological conditions. Rocky Mountain spotted fever, the subject of this book, may thus be termed a twentieth-century disease. It was not recognized as a distinct clinical entity until just before the turn of the century, and nearly all of the efforts to understand and combat it have been made within this century.

Rocky Mountain spotted fever is one of a group of maladies known as diseases of nature. The pathogenic organisms that cause these illnesses normally inhabit ticks, mites, fleas, mosquitoes, small rodents, and other wild animals. Malaria and bubonic plague are two other well-known members of this group. Human beings are usually accidental intruders into the natural cycles of these organisms that otherwise exist silently in nature. Because human beings are not a part of the organisms' biosystems, moreover, they often suffer more severely from infections of this group than do arthropod and mammalian hosts.

One subgroup of the diseases of nature is known today as the rickettsial diseases. They are caused by extremely small bacteria that have the peculiar characteristic of conducting their life processes inside the cells of their hosts—a property more generally associated with viruses. Measured in microns, a unit equal to one ten-thousandth of

a centimeter, rickettsiae take on three primary forms: spheres about
0.3 microns in diameter; short rods 0.3 by 1.0 microns long; and thin
rods about 2.0 microns long. In contrast, the cholera vibrio measures
1.5–5 microns long, and the rods of the anthrax bacillus, the first
pathogenic bacterium identified because of its large size, are 5–10
microns long.[1] The rickettsiae of spotted fever normally inhabit ticks,
those of murine typhus live in fleas, and the agents of rickettsialpox
and tsutsugamushi are found in mites. Only one of the rickettsial
diseases, in fact, has adapted to human beings as its hosts, and it is
transmitted from one infected person to another via the body louse.
This disease is classic, epidemic typhus, which is also noteworthy as
the only rickettsial disease recognized in the western world long before
the twentieth century.[2]

As the rickettsial diseases were differentiated, they were divided into
three groups: the typhus group, the spotted fever group, and the tsutsugamushi group, the last being a single disease limited to Asia and the
Pacific islands. In addition, diseases known as Q fever and trench fever
have generally been associated with the rickettsial diseases, but each
has exhibited sufficient differences from the other rickettsial diseases
to be classified in a separate genus. Members of the spotted fever
group, which includes *Rickettsia rickettsii*, the organism that causes
Rocky Mountain spotted fever, are responsible for similar but not
identical diseases scattered across the world. All are transmitted by
ticks, except for the rickettsia that causes rickettsialpox, a mild, mite-
borne disease that was initially confused with chickenpox. Each spotted
fever group rickettsia, moreover, seems to have evolved its distinc-
tiveness as have many animals and plants—through geographical isolation—for these organisms are found in "islands" of infection in
particular locations. As one early researcher noted, "spotted fever is
a 'place' disease, being definitely limited to a certain locality."[3]

In widespread areas of Africa, in India and Southeast Asia, and in
regions of Europe and the Middle East adjacent to the Mediterranean,
Black, and Caspian sea basins, close relatives of *R. rickettsii*, most
commonly *Rickettsia conorii*, cause relatively benign diseases similar
to spotted fever. The names given these diseases also reflect the localities
where they are known: Marseilles fever, South African tick typhus,
Kenya tick typhus, and Indian tick typhus. Another member of the
group, *Rickettsia sibirica*, produces a similarly mild disease, usually
known as North Asian tick typhus or Siberian tick typhus. Its habitats
are Siberia and many of the Asiatic republics of the Soviet Union,
various islands of the Sea of Japan, Mongolia, Pakistan, and possibly
Czechoslovakia. One other geographic area in which a closely related

disease is known to exist is the Queensland area of Australia. Caused by *Rickettsia australis*, this type of spotted fever is known as Queensland tick typhus.

Rocky Mountain spotted fever itself may be said to be an all-American disease, because its causative organism is found only in the western hemisphere—North, South, and Central America. Transmitted by several different ticks that flourish in each ecological area, *R. rickettsii* causes a disease that has been known by the local names São Paulo typhus, Tobia petechial fever, Choix fever, American spotted fever, and New World spotted fever. Because it was first identified in the Rocky Mountain region of North America, however, its oldest appellation was Rocky Mountain spotted fever. Later, when it was recognized in other areas of the hemisphere, many scientists argued that such a provincial designation should be replaced with a more precise name, such as tick-borne typhus, but their proposals came too late. The name of the disease had become fixed in both public and medical minds, despite the unfortunate consequence that the risk of infection outside the Rocky Mountain region was thus masked. Recognized in the United States, western Canada, western and central Mexico, Brazil, Colombia, Panama, and Costa Rica, spotted fever varies in virulence from place to place. The reason for this variation remains unknown. Spotted fever may exact a mortality as high as 70 percent or as low as 5 percent. On an average, if left untreated, it will kill just over 20 percent of its victims. Of all infectious diseases, spotted fever is one of the most severe, and it ranks as the most perilous of all rickettsial infections in the United States.[4]

Victims of Rocky Mountain spotted fever display variations of a closely related set of symptoms. A week or two after the patient has been bitten by a tick, the disease begins to manifest itself. The onset may be sudden or may be preceded by a few days of general malaise, after which the symptoms become more dramatic. The first sign is often a splitting headache—frequently described as the worst ever encountered by the victim—accompanied by pains in the back, joints, and legs. Light is painful to the eyes, and a stiff neck sometimes leads physicians to suspect meningitis. The spotted fever victim's temperature rises rapidly to 102° to 104° F. The patient is usually restless, cannot sleep well, and frequently suffers from periods of delirium. Occasionally, the initial symptoms of spotted fever may mimic appendicitis or the common cold, making diagnosis difficult.

As the infection progresses, the rickettsial organisms multiply within the endothelial cells that line the victim's capillaries. These cells eventually swell, some burst, and by the third or fourth day of recognizable

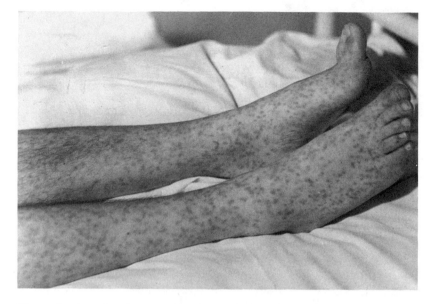

The rash of Rocky Mountain spotted fever covers the entire body, including the palms of the hands and the soles of the feet. Because so few diseases exhibit such an extensive rash, it is considered diagnostic in conjunction with high fever and history of exposure to ticks. (Courtesy of Eugene P. Campbell and used by permission of Norman H. Topping.)

illness, blood begins to seep through tiny holes in the capillary walls. These hemorrhages cause the characteristic spots of the disease, which often look like the rash of measles and can be felt as slightly raised areas under the skin. They appear first on the wrists and ankles, spreading later to the limbs, the trunk and the face. Unlike the rash of some other rickettsial diseases, the spots of Rocky Mountain spotted fever often appear on the palms of the hands and the soles of the feet. Since only a few diseases produce this symptom, it is often considered a definitive diagnostic sign.

If left untreated, most patients will recover from their illness within two weeks. Just over 20 percent, however, especially people over forty years old and those with existing medical problems, will die from their infections. In a few cases, the disease is fulminant, killing its victim within a few days of onset, often before the characteristic rash has appeared.

That *Rickettsia rickettsii* is so well adapted to life in its tick host indicates a symbiotic relationship that has evolved over eons. This suggests that spotted fever probably struck human victims long before it was distinguished as a separate disease. Recently, in fact, William D. Tigertt has argued that a 1759 epidemic in North Carolina was probably caused by Rocky Mountain spotted fever.[5] Civil War diaries also contain some references to afflictions that may have been spotted fever, such as seasonal occurrences of "black measles" chronicled by a nurse stationed near Cairo, Illinois.[6] Because Rocky Mountain spotted fever remained undifferentiated from other fevers identified by similar names and symptoms until the late nineteenth century, however, historical inquiry into earlier periods is limited to speculation. The story of Rocky Mountain spotted fever may thus be said to begin with the description of a peculiar affliction recorded by pioneers traversing the trails across the North American west. Research on the disease certainly had its origins in a single place, the Bitterroot Valley of Montana.

Although Rocky Mountain spotted fever was not identified until just before the twentieth century began, its louse-borne relative, epidemic typhus fever, had plagued European populations for centuries. Almost always linked to conditions of human misery, typhus was known to accompany prisoners, sailors, armies, and refugees—populations who, during cold weather, were likely to wear the same clothing day and night for weeks on end because of poor hygienic conditions. Because a widespread body rash, which does not spread to the face, also accompanies typhus, it, too, was often called spotted fever. In this book, however, I employ that term only as a synonym for Rocky Mountain spotted fever.

Before I commence the story of Rocky Mountain spotted fever, a brief digression to review the history of epidemic typhus fever may be helpful, especially in understanding why spotted fever was not identified as a distinct disease until the end of the nineteenth century. Hippocrates applied the word *typhus*, from the Greek word meaning "smoky" or "hazy," to confused or stuporous states of mind frequently associated with high fevers. Accounts of ancient plagues, however, do not differentiate typhus from other epidemic fevers. The first descriptions of a disease that closely resembled typhus appeared near the end of the fifteenth century. In 1489–90, during the civil wars of Granada, Spanish physicians described a typhus-like disease that killed seventeen thousand Spanish soldiers—six times the number killed in combat with the Moors. In the early sixteenth century, a similar malady appeared among armies arrayed in Italy and in the Balkans. In 1546, Girolamo Fracastoro (Fracastorius), who had observed the Italian epidemics, published the first clear description of what he termed a "lenticular or punctate or petechial" fever also characterized by headache and general malaise. Toward the end of the sixteenth century, typhus was also recorded in the Mexican highlands, where it killed more than two million Indians. It remains unclear, however, whether the disease was brought to the New World by Spanish explorers or, as some evidence indicates, was known to the Aztecs and some pre-Columbian Indians in Mexico.[7]

Typhus rose dramatically in early nineteenth-century Europe. In 1812, Napoleon's catastrophic expedition to Russia was plagued by typhus. Between 1816 and 1819 a great epidemic of the disease struck seven hundred thousand people in Ireland, whose population was only six million. For several more decades, however, medical understanding of the disease remained confused. By the late eighteenth century, the medical nosologist Boissier de Sauvages had begun using the word *typhus* to describe the neurological symptoms of a particular disease, but few attempts were made to distinguish pathologically between typhus and typhoid fever, which also displayed a red rash. Even into the twentieth century, the link between typhoid and typhus was perpetuated in nomenclature. In many European countries, the former was known as *typhus abdominalis* and the latter as *typhus exanthematicus*.[8]

During the first half of the nineteenth century, researchers centered in the clinical schools of Paris, London, Dublin, and Vienna compiled detailed histories of diseases, which were correlated with gross pathological lesions at autopsy. By this method they were able to distinguish more precisely among afflictions sharing similar symptoms, such as the many types of fevers from which people suffered.[9] In 1837 a Philadelphia physician, William Wood Gerhard, who had studied the distinctive intestinal lesions of typhoid as a student of Pierre Louis in Paris, noted their absence in victims of typhus fever, which had been epidemic in Philadelphia the previous year. Gerhard's work, however, was not immediately embraced by physicians who clung to older theories of the unity of fevers. It was not until mid century that additional pathological and epidemiological research, especially by William Jenner and Austin Flint, convinced most American physicians that indeed typhus and typhoid were distinct disease entities.[10]

The European revolutions of 1848 spawned typhus epidemics in Eastern Europe, as did African warfare in Ethiopia. During a particularly severe outbreak of typhus in Upper Silesia, the German physician and politician Rudolf Virchow published a radical assessment of the epidemic that subsequently cost him his government post. Observing that the disease afflicted the poor, the uneducated, and the unclean,

Virchow called for democracy, education, and public health measures as the proper "treatment" of the epidemic.[11] Although Virchow argued strongly for social reform as a means to benefit health, he also was in the vanguard of German scientists who believed that medicine would benefit from laboratory investigations. In research aided by improved microscopes, Virchow and other scientists focused on pathological changes in the tissues and cells to study the disease process.[12]

During the last quarter of the nineteenth century, such laboratory research culminated in the work of French chemist Louis Pasteur, German physician Robert Koch, and their associates, who identified specific microorganisms as the causes of particular infectious diseases. This new germ theory, when linked with the pathological changes documented for particular diseases, revolutionized the way physicians conceptualized infectious diseases. It also provided a framework in which rapid advances could be made in understanding afflictions such as typhus. Corollaries of the germ theory, which explained how microorganisms were transmitted, provided a basis for active intervention programs to prevent diseases. Purifying water supplies reduced the incidence of waterborne diseases, for example. Crusades against insect vectors were also mounted to control such diseases as malaria and yellow fever.

Rocky Mountain spotted fever was identified as a disease with symptoms and a clinical course distinct from other fevers just as the germ theory was making its way across the Atlantic from Europe. Even though many American physicians and lay persons remained skeptical about the new theory, their response to diseases such as spotted fever was informed, if not initially guided, by its constructs. During ensuing decades, the germ theory transformed medical practice, fostered the growth of an international medical research establishment with its own professional dynamic, and established principles on which investigational efforts were conducted. Furthermore, it furnished a context for lay persons to think about infectious diseases and altered their views of the role of governments in medical matters. In approaching the history of Rocky Mountain spotted fever, one must seek to understand the interactions between these broad trends and the experience of society with a single disease. What role did the professionalization of science throughout the world play in strategies to understand and combat this disease? What can the experience with spotted fever tell us about the process of scientific discovery and application? How did communities respond to the presence of this disease in their midst? What role did they expect their governments to play, and how effective was political action against the disease?

The history of Rocky Mountain spotted fever may thus serve as a lens through which we can view twentieth-century thought regarding infectious diseases and the application of new concepts to research, diagnosis, prevention, and treatment. One of the early Montana leaders in the effort to combat spotted fever, quoted in the epigraph to this chapter, asserted that the story of research on spotted fever should read like a romance. In the following pages, I hope that some of the romance may be evident as well as an increased understanding of how science, medicine, and society in the twentieth century have responded to one particular disease of nature.

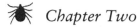 *Chapter Two*

A Blight on the Bitterroot

Charles Draper, 25 years, of Kendall's lumber camp on the westside died at the Sisters Hospital on April 4 of that dread disease spotted fever, after a few days' illness.

Obituary, *Northwest Tribune*, 1901

The curved western border of the state of Montana somewhat resembles the profile of an Indian brave. Thrusting into the Idaho panhandle like the nose of that brave is the spectacular Bitterroot Valley.[1] Protected from the full force of winter storms by the rugged Bitterroot Mountains on the west and the more gentle Sapphire range to the east, the valley's flat bottomlands are the remains of an ancient lake whose beaches remain visible as bench lands on either side. Through the valley, which stretches approximately one hundred miles long and from eight to ten miles wide at an average elevation of thirty-five hundred feet above sea level, the Bitterroot River flows from south to north into the Clark's Fork of the Columbia River near Missoula. Not far away is the so-called Yellowstone hot spot, where the earth's molten interior rises close to the surface, producing geysers, hot springs, and boiling mud. Although less geologically active than Yellowstone, the Bitterroot Valley became known as a medical hot spot just before the twentieth century began. It was here that a mysterious disease, virulent Rocky Mountain spotted fever, claimed many lives and challenged researchers seeking to solve its riddle to formulate new concepts about the nature of infectious diseases.

Until the last quarter of the nineteenth century, there were no accounts of any unusual disease in the Bitterroot, whose invigorating climate attracted first Indian and later white inhabitants.[2] The Salish, or Flathead, Indians, who lived in the valley and ate the bitter roots of a pink spring wildflower from which the valley took its name, reported no special local affliction. Like most primitive peoples, the

9

Salish interpreted disease as a magicoreligious process, in which a malevolent spirit, acting on its own or at the behest of an enemy of the sick person, brought suffering.[3] The Indians did not make detailed diagnostic observations that could be used later as medical evidence, and their oral tradition precluded written records in any case.

Before the arrival of whites, the Salish, like most other American Indians, were remarkably healthy. They were free from most diseases caused by airborne microorganisms because the cold, dry air of Montana was inimical to airborne bacteria. Contagious diseases such as smallpox, diphtheria, scarlet fever, measles, and venereal ailments, which ravaged European cities, did not touch them. Since accidents and wounds sustained in warfare were common, however, the Salish had developed competency in setting fractures. Intestinal problems and rheumatic complaints, of which there were many, were usually treated by sweat baths or plunges into icy streams; sometimes a combination of these methods was used. Among Salish traditions was a general spring warning against entering certain canyons in the Bitterroot said to be inhabited by evil spirits. After the identification of virulent spotted fever, this admonition suggested that the Salish might have been familiar with the disease, but later Indian testimony failed to confirm this. One of the earliest reports on spotted fever noted that "no authentic information" could be obtained linking the Indian superstition to the disease, "though many old residents, including Indians, white trappers, traders, and Catholic priests were consulted."[4]

Accounts of the periodic visits of non-Indians in the valley during the early nineteenth century, furthermore, are notable for the absence of any mention of a deadly disease. The most famous early visitors were members of the Lewis and Clark expedition, who traversed the valley in September 1805. Before embarking on their journey, Meriwether Lewis and William Clark had been given medical instruction by respected physicians, including the distinguished Benjamin Rush. The explorers were advised to pay special attention to the health of the Indians they encountered.[5] They recorded the presence of trachoma among the Columbia River Indians and the "calamity of blindness" that had resulted from this disease.[6] When they traveled through the Bitterroot, however, camping near the later towns of Grantsdale and Stevensville, the explorers did not record the presence of any feared local malady. In September the wood ticks that carry spotted fever are in estivation, or "summer hibernation," hence Lewis and Clark were not at great risk. On the return trip of the expedition the following year, Clark revisited the Bitterroot in early July—a time during which some ticks would probably still be active—while Lewis returned to

Saint Louis across northern Montana. Clark's path wound through the section of the Bitterroot where spotted fever was later shown to be most prevalent, yet he reported no unusual occurrences. The experiences of Lewis and Clark in the Bitterroot suggest three alternative scenarios with regard to spotted fever in the early nineteenth century: first, at this time virulent spotted fever was not widely spread through the Bitterroot; second, the disease existed, but its tick vectors were in estivation during both visits; and third, Lewis and Clark were simply lucky not to encounter the deadly fever.

For several decades after Lewis and Clark's expedition, few other white visitors came to the Bitterroot. The number of travelers to other western areas was stimulated by the Mormon immigration to Utah in 1847 and the discovery of the California goldfields two years later. Many of these mid-century settlers and prospectors commented on various fevers encountered on the Oregon Trail in Wyoming, northern Utah, and southern Idaho. Bull fever, mountain fever, typho-malaria fever of the Rocky Mountains, black fever, blue disease, and spotted fever were all names reported. Although these diseases are difficult to diagnose retrospectively, some may have been cases of Rocky Mountain spotted fever. Most early observers, including U.S. Army physicians stationed at outposts in the region, described the diseases they encountered in terms of those with which they were familiar in the east. They assumed that these diseases had been "altered by climate and altitude," changes that explained unusual clinical pictures.[7]

The first whites to live continuously in the Bitterroot Valley were neither prospectors nor settlers but rather Jesuit priests, who arrived in 1841 at the request of the Salish. This unusual attraction of the Indians to white religion had developed through the Salish's contact with Canadian Indians. In the 1820s a band of Iroquois had left their homes on the Saint Lawrence River and migrated across the continent to the Bitterroot. The Salish welcomed the Iroquois as friends, eventually intermarried with them, and rapidly adopted the Roman Catholic doctrines that the Iroquois had learned from French Catholic priests in Canada. During the 1830s, "a desire to have some 'Black Robes,' in their midst" took possession of the Salish. Between 1831 and 1836, they dispatched three envoys to Saint Louis to petition the church for a priest to be sent to their tribe. This request was granted in 1840, and the following year two Jesuit missionaries, Gregory Mengarini and Pierre-Jean DeSmet, arrived to found Saint Mary's Mission in the north end of the valley, near the later site of the town of Stevensville. In 1845 a medically trained Jesuit, Anthony Ravalli, was sent to serve the Indians at Saint Mary's. He remained for five years until Saint Mary's was closed in 1850 because of a threatened attack from hostile Indian tribes. In 1867, the year after the mission was reopened, Ravalli returned and expanded his medical practice to include white settlers who had migrated to the valley after the Civil War. Father Ravalli, after whom was named the county in which most of the Bitterroot Valley lies, was one of very few physicians available to valley residents until the mid 1880s. Many stories recount Ravalli's self-sacrificing medical practice, but none specifically mentions spotted fever as a problem with which he dealt.[8]

During the sixteen years that the Jesuits were absent from the valley between 1850 and 1866, white settlement commenced. As the priests departed, John Owen, a former army sutler and self-styled major, leased mission property for the construction of a trading post, which was quickly dubbed Fort Owen because of the walled stockade surrounding it. In the early 1860s, when gold was discovered in Montana, Owen profited from the sale of vegetables and flour to the mining camps. The gold rush also brought new settlers into Montana and the Bitterroot. In 1864 the brothers Harry and James Cohen settled in the valley with their wives, who became the first white women to establish residency in the Bitterroot.[9] During the next decade many other families arrived and helped found towns along the river that resembled pearls on a string. Stevensville and Corvallis were established in 1864 and 1868, respectively, and by 1880 there were more than a thousand white settlers living in the valley.[10] Many new residents were probably seeking to avoid the social upheavals caused by the Civil War and Reconstruction, for a significant portion of them came from Kentucky, Georgia, and the Carolinas. Others migrated from Missouri, Quebec, and New Brunswick. These early settlers produced grain, engaged in lumbering on a small scale, and experimented with fruit orchards, especially apples. The first fruit trees were apparently planted in 1866, and after 1870, under the leadership of the brothers W. E. and D. C. Bass, apples became a commercial crop.[11]

The increasing use of land in the Bitterroot for these economic pursuits eventually produced discord with the hunting-gathering way of life of the Salish. In 1871, President Ulysses S. Grant ordered that the Salish, along with the Nez Percé Indians who migrated annually through the valley, be removed to the Jocko Reservation in northern Montana. The following year, General James A. Garfield negotiated a treaty to this effect with two of the three Salish chiefs. Chief Charlot, son of Victor, for whom one of the valley towns was named, refused to sign. He won the right to remain in the Bitterroot until his death, but he and his followers were expected to live on small grants of land

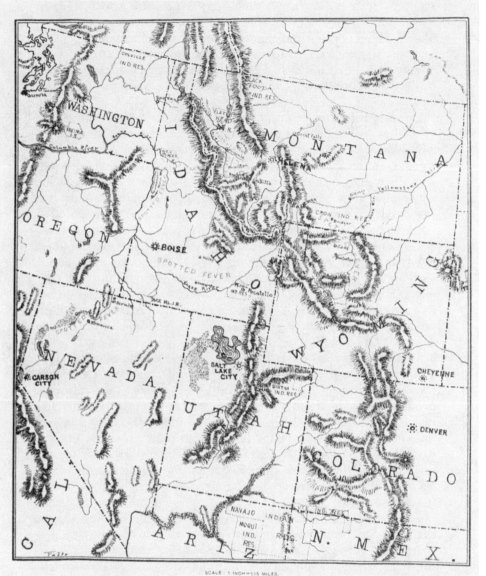

Retrospective studies in the early twentieth century revealed that spotted fever had been encountered throughout the West during the late nineteenth century by prospectors and settlers. This map shows its known distribution about 1900. (Courtesy of the Rocky Mountain Laboratories, NIAID.)

like white settlers. The Indians were not successful as farmers, hence in 1891, Charlot decided to abandon the valley. Accompanied by a hundred other Salish who had remained in the valley, Charlot moved to the reservation, leaving the Bitterroot Valley wholly in the hands of whites.[12]

During this transition period, the white population of the Bitterroot swelled as construction of the Northern Pacific Railroad approached Missoula. After 1880, sawmills sprang up to supply railroad ties, sheep were grazed on the east side of the valley, and, when quartz deposits were discovered, an interest in mining developed. The Northern Pacific was completed to Missoula in 1883, and five years later a branch line was constructed up the Bitterroot as far as Grantsdale. As opposed to the rough wagon road along the river in 1870, the railroad provided businessmen in the valley an efficient conduit for transporting their goods to market. By 1890 there were eight sawmills in constant operation; two flour mills; more than thirty-three thousand sheep producing wool for shipment to commercial markets; a growing number of quartz, silver, and copper mines; and more than one-hundred thousand fruit trees, which came to make the valley known as the apple center of Montana.[13]

Lumbering operations were especially active during this period. In 1887, for instance, one lumber mill near Lake Como was cutting ten thousand feet of lumber per day, and by 1890, one near Grantsdale produced forty thousand feet each day.[14] This was just the beginning of the boom, however, because railroads, mines, and other markets had an insatiable appetite for lumber. Sawmills provided jobs for hundreds of valley residents, and the bountiful forests of the Bitterroot seemed to offer an endless supply of trees. By 1896 lumbering operations in the valley produced some sixty to seventy million feet of lumber each year.[15]

Much of this massive deforestation took place on the west side of the valley, the site where virulent spotted fever was contracted. In recent years researchers have speculated about a relationship between the denuding of the valley's trees and the advent of virulent spotted fever. Robert N. Philip, an epidemiologist formerly at the Rocky Mountain Laboratory, has compiled extensive records about the history of the valley and the occurrence of the disease. He points out that the incidence of spotted fever "was vitally related to timber harvest and the opening of the west side woodlands to grazing and unwanted small mammal and tick infestation."[16] The scrub vegetation that replaced the forests was an ideal habitat for small rodents and their tick parasites. Humans entering this area consequently ran an increased risk of encountering infected ticks. This hypothesis offers a logical explanation for the apparently sudden appearance of the disease at the end of the century. Speculation about why spotted fever was more deadly in the Bitterroot than across the mountains in Idaho, on the other hand, focuses on a possible genetic mutation in the organism but remains a mystery.

In 1889, Montana was granted statehood, and expansion in the Bitterroot continued unabated. Marcus Daly, the copper magnate of the Anaconda Mining Company, bought acreage in the valley for breeding his celebrated race horses. In 1890, Daly established a sawmill near his property and founded a town named after one of his agents, James W. Hamilton, for the mill hands.[17] Three years later most of the Bitterroot Valley was split off from Missoula County and named Ravalli County after the venerated physician-priest. In 1898 the Ravalli County seat was moved from its original site in Stevensville to Hamilton.

As the population of the Bitterroot increased during these two decades of expansion, so did its need for medical attention. Some physicians had moved into the valley after 1870, but with under a thousand people scattered over its one-hundred-mile length, few stayed for very long, because a doctor had to engage in other pursuits as well as medicine to make a living.[18] In 1880, for example, the *Weekly Missoulian* published this advertisement: "A good physician is much needed up the Bitter Root Valley. There are probably a thousand people on the Bitter Root, and, save the venerable Father Ravalli, there is no medical advisor the whole length of the Valley. It strikes us that a man who is willing to do a little farming or stock-raising in connection with his medical practice could reap a harvest in this locality. He should be a young man and willing to make hard rides occasionally."[19]

In spite of the difficult conditions, this call for help was answered. By 1882 two physicians had accepted the challenge and established practices in the Bitterroot. One of them, R. A. Wells, was immediately charged with managing a smallpox epidemic.[20] In 1884, Father Ravalli died, and the new doctors who took his place assumed the arduous task of dealing with the common infectious diseases against which no successful therapy was then available. In 1885, for example, a diphtheria epidemic claimed six lives of its eight reported victims. Between 1883 and 1885, fifty-four Indians were buried, many of them young people, apparently victims of tuberculosis.[21] Typhoid was a recurring problem, primarily because of contaminated water at sawmills and mines. Smallpox epidemics flared annually because many people were not vaccinated, even though an efficacious vaccine was available.

During this period of settlement and growth, there were few reports of spotted fever cases. Before 1895 newspapers cited fifteen illnesses that might be construed as spotted fever, and a later official survey noted twenty-three cases certified by local physicians.[22] A retrospective diagnosis made after the turn of the century marked 1873 as the year in which the first definite case of the disease was evident. The victim, identified only as "J.W.," lived near Woodside and died in May 1873. Since the attending doctor, who may have been John B. Buker, an Indian agent and a physician, had died by the time this inquiry was made, diagnosis was on the basis of testimony from the stricken man's relatives and neighbors who had seen later cases of the disease.[23] Reports of spotted fever deaths first appeared in local newspapers in 1882 and 1883. Diagnoses in these cases were never confirmed, however, and they may in fact have been some other disease.[24]

Since there was no hospital in the Bitterroot until 1895, valley physicians transported their severely ill patients to Missoula. In 1873 a French Canadian order of Roman Catholic nuns, the Sisters of Charity of Providence, established the first hospital in Missoula, which was officially named Saint Patrick's Hospital but commonly called Sisters Hospital. Until 1889 it consisted of only one room. With the coming of the railroad, however, the Northern Pacific Beneficial Association, Western Division, Relief Fund was organized in 1882 with headquarters in Missoula. This organization, to which all Montana employees of the Northern Pacific belonged, erected the Northern Pacific Hospital in Missoula in 1884. Destroyed by fire in 1892, the hospital was rebuilt in 1893 and expanded in 1901.[25] As spotted fever cases increased toward the end of the century, both hospitals cared for its victims.

Many of the early physicians in the Bitterroot had studied medicine at respected schools in the midwest and east, including the Saint Louis Medical School, Jefferson Medical College in Philadelphia, Bellevue Hospital Medical College in New York, and the University of Virginia Medical School.[26] Some of these doctors made a special effort to stay abreast of the latest developments in medicine in order to incorporate the new techniques into their practices. Keeping up with new medical discoveries was no easy task in the 1880s, for during this decade the concept of infectious diseases was being revolutionized. In the mid 1870s, Louis Pasteur, a French chemist, and Robert Koch, a German physician, had demonstrated that bacteria caused anthrax, and their findings launched a heady period of searching for other microorganisms that might be the cause of dread epidemics. During the 1880s bacteria were identified as the culprits in typhoid fever, leprosy, tuberculosis, diphtheria, tetanus, pneumonia, and bubonic plague, among others.

Once bacteria had been demonstrated as the causes of particular diseases, scientists also sought to understand how they were transmitted from one sick person to another. By the end of the century, water, milk, insects, and human carriers had been implicated as potential routes for the spread of disease.[27] Some diseases, moreover, responded to treatment with the blood serum of recovered victims, and others were found to be preventable by vaccines made from killed or attenuated organisms. It was, in short, a period during which discoveries piled quickly on top of one another and the tree of knowledge was ripe for picking. For young physicians and scientists, medical research offered challenging intellectual problems, an opportunity to contribute directly to the welfare of the world, and even the possibility of great celebrity for themselves.

The bacteriological discoveries also provided new inspiration to the public health or sanitary movement that had evolved in the United States primarily since the Civil War. This movement had been divided philosophically between those who attributed the cause of infectious diseases to specific agents and others who believed that poisonous vapors, known as miasmas, rose from contaminated earth to bring disease. The former group, called contagionists, had long advocated quarantine when disease was present, while the latter, known as anticontagionists, called for strict sanitary measures designed to remove the contamination that gave rise to miasmas.[28] With the advent of bacteriology, these two views could be reconciled, and it appeared that public health programs based on scientific principles might indeed rid the cities of the world of recurring plagues.

In the United States, state and local public health boards, which had evolved since the Civil War in urban eastern areas, began to multiply in other areas of the country. By 1887 the town of Missoula had created a board of health, and in March 1896 the Ravalli County Board of Health was established in the Bitterroot Valley, with Samuel W. Minshall as first chairman.[29] In 1902, moreover, the U.S. Congress also fostered the development of public health by providing for an annual meeting of state and territorial health officers with the surgeon general of the U.S. Public Health and Marine Hospital Service.[30] It was hoped that the exchange of information at this meeting would enhance the attack on disease throughout the nation.

On 15 March 1901, Governor Joseph K. Toole signed an act passed by the Legislative Assembly creating a board of health for the state of Montana. As in other states, the Montana State Board of Health's charge was broad. It was to investigate epidemics; to suppress nuisances (that is, to see that unpleasant surroundings were cleaned up); to attempt to determine the influence of locality, climate, employments, and habits on the health of the people; and to cooperate with local boards of health. Unfortunately, the budget allocated for this work was only two thousand dollars a year, its small size another characteristic shared with many other state boards of health. William Treacy of Helena was elected president, and Albert F. Longeway of Great Falls, having just completed a year as president of the Montana Medical Association, was named secretary, the officer charged with enforcing the board's policies. Other members of the board were two physicians, James L. Belcher of Townsend and H. J. Loebinger of Butte; J. M. Robertson, a civil engineer from Bozeman; and the governor and attorney general as ex officio members.[31]

It was during this period, when medicine and public health looked forward optimistically to becoming truly scientific, that the problem of Rocky Mountain spotted fever was first addressed. Although the number of cases was increasing, paralleling the growth of the Bitterroot's population, only gradually was the disease given the uniform designation *spotted fever*. Many early cases were called black measles, probably because measles was widely known as an early childhood affliction, and spotted fever, with a similar rash, seemed to be a malignant form of it. The designations *black typhus fever* and *blue disease* occasionally appeared, and often the disease was called black fever or simply fever.[32] Physicians reporting on it frequently called it typhoid pneumonia, measles, and cerebrospinal meningitis, because of the symptoms it shared in common with these better-known maladies — a stiff neck, headache, high fever, and rash.[33] Known to occur in the spring, the affliction most frequently struck residents or visitors on the west side of the Bitterroot River and was most often reported in the northern section of the valley, which overlapped Ravalli and Missoula counties.

Spotted fever was not confined to the Bitterroot Valley alone, but it was known to be considerably milder in other locations.[34] The first published report on the disease, in fact, was made in 1896 by Major Marshall W. Wood, a U.S. Army physician stationed in Boise, Idaho.[35] A native of Watertown, New York, who had studied medicine at Rush Medical College in Chicago, Wood mentioned in one of his monthly reports the "prevalence of spotted fever in civil settlements in the neighborhood of his post."[36] When the surgeon general of the army requested particulars, Wood compiled reports from prominent Idaho physicians because, although he suffered a bout of the disease later, he had not at that time seen any cases.[37] Their comments on spotted fever, published in the surgeon general's annual report, revealed well-honed powers of clinical observation but also reflected the endurance of the older miasma theory of disease causation, especially when speculative bacteriological explanations did not correlate with epidemiological findings.

C. L. Sweet, president of the Idaho State Medical Society, clearly described the rash, the "breakbone pains," and the low fatality of Idaho spotted fever. He advised symptomatic treatment for the pain and fever, noting that for mild cases he primarily prescribed placebos. Acknowledging that there were "indications which seem to point out this peculiar affection as a water-borne disease," Sweet nevertheless was uncomfortable with this theory. "Frequently several cases occur in a household," he noted, while at other times "only the single case." This epidemiological picture militated against infection from a common water supply. Instead, Sweet leaned toward "other circumstances" that favored spotted fever's similarity to malaria, a disease whose transmission by mosquitoes had not in 1896 been demonstrated. Spotted fever was frequently seen, Sweet noted, "in persons who have been living in the vicinity of newly broken ground, post holes, plowed ground, and in those who have drunk seepage water from worked soil, etc." In a similar analysis, L. C. Bowers speculated that the true cause of the disease "was probably of a telluric character," that is, arising from the earth itself.[38] Ticks or tick bites were never mentioned as possible factors.

In October 1899, Edward E. Maxey, secretary of the Idaho State Medical Society, read a paper about spotted fever before the Oregon State Medical Society. Published in the Portland, Oregon, *Medical Sentinel*, a journal that had been adopted by many western state medical associations as an official organ, Maxey's paper was the first on the disease in a medical periodical. Maxey observed that spotted fever was "in all probability, caused by some peculiar organism, possibly a miasm," but that "no specific cause" had "yet been discovered." He pointed out that the disease invariably occurred during the spring months and was primarily contracted "while residing, or sojourning, in or near the foot-hills of the mountains." Aware of the discoveries about contaminated water and infectious diseases, Maxey noted that while in the foothills of the mountains, victims had no other water supply than that which came from the melting snow. "In other words," he said, "they drank the snow water and became sick, therefore there must be, in my opinion, some specific cause for this disease, either in the soil over which the water runs, or in the snow itself."[39]

Maxey also differentiated between spotted fever and other diseases with which it had previously been identified. "After once seeing and

recognizing spotted fever, the diagnosis is easy. . . . Even the laity
recognize it on sight." Noting, however, that physicians had variously
called it " 'dengue fever,' cerebro-spinal meningitis, typhoid, rheumatic
purpura, typhus and measles," Maxey pointed out the seasonal, geographic, or symptomatic differences between each of these diseases
and spotted fever. He reiterated the optimistic prognosis for the disease
as known in Idaho, and he did not mention the virulent form of spotted
fever known in the Bitterroot Valley.[40]

Although there were no published reports on this disease from other
states at this time, in retrospect it is clear that spotted fever had been
recognized during the last quarter of the nineteenth century throughout
the northwest states. In Colorado a later survey noted that the disease,
which exacted about a 23 percent mortality, had been known since
1885. In Oregon spotted fever was reported to be well known to early
physicians, "considered by them a mysterious disease with considerable
mortality." Later statistics showed that the death rate in Oregon was
"much less than in Montana" yet "somewhat higher than in Idaho."
Spotted fever was reported most frequently in the central part of eastern
Oregon, and, as was the case in Idaho and Montana, it seemed to be
contracted in or near the foothills of the mountains. No case was
known west of the Cascade Mountains.[41]

In Wyoming spotted fever apparently had been known by the names
mountain typhus, mountain sickness, mountain fever, and similar
terms. The Indians of Wyoming reputedly knew of the disease but did
not associate it with any particular region of the state. One old-time
prospector who had crossed the plains into Wyoming during the days
of the "bull trains" later told a Wyoming state health officer that
spotted fever was commonly called trail typhus by emigrants traveling
the Oregon Trail. It had plagued them particularly, he stated, from
"the point where the trail joined the Sweetwater River about at In-
dependence Rock" until they crossed the Green River. This description
coincided with the central and north-central location of the majority
of Wyoming cases. Like the situation in Oregon, moreover, mortality
in Wyoming seemed to be about 15–20 percent—higher than in Idaho
but lower than in the Bitterroot Valley.[42]

Other studies also concluded that spotted fever had been present
from an early period in Washington, Nevada, Utah, and California.[43]
Because the mortality in these states was relatively low, however, state
authorities had not initiated investigations. The Montana State Board
of Health, on the other hand, was confronted with the virulent spotted
fever problem at the first meeting it held after being organized. The
issue was raised by the Montana labor commissioner, Judson A. Fer-

guson, who had been pressed to take action on the problem by Bitterroot lumbermen, among whose ranks many victims of the disease were numbered. Ferguson had accordingly sent a questionnaire to Missoula and Bitterroot Valley physicians asking for as much information as possible about spotted fever. He presented the replies at the meeting of the state board on 9 May 1901.[44]

Although the board was principally concerned at this meeting with a smallpox epidemic in the state and with establishing rules for licensing undertakers, the members listened to Ferguson's report and expressed willingness "to call a special meeting at any time to consider the matter" of spotted fever. Desiring more scientific information, the board authorized Emil Starz, who was appointed state bacteriologist later that summer, to make a bacteriological investigation of the disease. Accompanied by Ferguson, Starz visited the valley, took water and soil specimens, and obtained "cultures" from one spotted fever patient, which he inoculated with negative results into two rabbits.[45] On the basis of his research, Starz hypothesized that the disease was really "cerebrospinal meningitis combined with one or the other of pneumonia or typhoid fever," but he also called for further investigation.[46]

Physicians and laymen who had more direct experience with spotted fever disagreed sharply with Starz. "While he may be able to peep through a microscope and see things," wrote one Missoula doctor, "he doesn't know what he is talking about in this instance."[47] Although no one else had any additional scientific evidence to offer about the disease, many theories were advanced. Melted snow water as the source of the disease was the most popular theory with Missoula physicians, but one Bitterroot Valley doctor asserted that spotted fever was generated by miasmas arising from north winds, which blew over decaying spring vegetation in swampland on the west side of the valley.[48] A layman from the Woodside area of the valley scoffed at this thesis. Edward Burrows noted that he had lived for twelve to fourteen years in the swampy area on the west side when it was virtually covered with timber, yet no spotted fever had then been known. "The land was cleared in the last six to seven years," he said, "and spotted fever began." Burrows did not suggest that the extensive lumbering operations in the valley might be the cause of the disease but believed instead that miasmas from "dooryard filth" were the cause.[49]

There were more than a dozen cases of spotted fever during the spring of 1901—one official count noted fourteen cases with ten deaths.[50] When compared with the number of deaths in Montana from smallpox, diphtheria, and typhoid, virulent spotted fever was not a widespread menace to public health. Like the infrequent visitations of cholera and yellow fever, however, the few spring cases of spotted fever each year struck fear in valley inhabitants. The dramatic symptoms of the disease—the blue-black rash, high fever, and delirium—and the high mortality rate, especially among the healthy young adults who were among its most frequent victims, produced anxiety about an early and horrible death. Furthermore, this dread disease seemed a particularly cruel blight on the future development of one of the most beautiful valleys in the western United States. Proposals for attracting new residents who wished to grow apples on irrigated farms were already being discussed, and the west side of the valley was prime land for this purpose. If a deadly infection lurked in the west side canyons, however, prospective land buyers would be understandably reluctant to place themselves in jeopardy. Economic aspirations of valley residents thus fueled a desire to "do something" about spotted fever. Decisions made by the Montana State Board of Health in the spring of 1902 addressed this demand and, in so doing, launched twentieth-century research efforts to understand, prevent, and treat this mysterious disease.

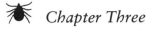 *Chapter Three*

The Beginning of Scientific Investigations

The great tragedy of Science—the staying of a beautiful hypothesis by an ugly fact.

Thomas Huxley, *Collected Essays*

In 1902 scientific experts began a decades-long search to elucidate the etiology, prevention, and treatment of the mysterious spotted fever of the Rocky Mountains. During the first two seasons of this work, in 1902 and 1903, it seemed that the etiology of spotted fever might quickly be explained, for the evidence indicated that the disease was caused by a protozoan organism transmitted by the Rocky Mountain wood tick. In 1904, however, this theory was called into question by other scientific specialists. For the inhabitants of the Bitterroot continually at risk of contracting the disease, each new finding seemed only to make it clear that their strange disease was more complex than anyone had previously envisioned.

Placing spotted fever investigations on a scientific basis began at the February 1902 meeting of the Montana State Board of Health. Since cases of the malady rarely appeared before mid March, the board could do little at the time, but it agreed unanimously to pursue the problem "as soon as the occasion arose." In early April spotted fever struck near Florence, a well-known infected area. By the end of the month there had been five cases in the valley, three of which were from the Hamilton area, south of the Florence—Lo Lo spotted fever district, and concern was voiced that the disease was spreading.[1]

The Ravalli County Board of Health met on 28 April to discuss the problem. Local physicians affirmed that this disease was neither typhus nor cerebrospinal meningitis, the two "spotted fevers" discussed in medical textbooks. They called for the state board of health to employ an expert pathologist to study the problem scientifically.[2] The Montana state labor commissioner, Judson A. Ferguson, who had initially

brought the spotted fever question to the attention of the state board
in 1901, also pressed the board for "decisive measures" to suppress
the disease that attacked many of the lumbermen who were his constituents.[3]

Responding to this outcry, members of the state board of health
visited the valley in early May. The board's secretary, Albert F. Longeway, brought along Earle Strain, a medical colleague from Great Falls
who had studied bacteriology in Europe. When Strain noticed a tick
in the hair around the genitals of a spotted fever victim, he reportedly
recalled a lecture given by John Guiteras at the University of Pennsylvania on mosquitoes as the vector of yellow fever. He suggested to
Longeway that the tick might have a similar connection with spotted
fever.[4]

On the whole, however, Longeway was disappointed that little was
accomplished by this visit "aside from obtaining information about
past illnesses and specimens of water and soil for laboratory study,"
but he decided that the services of a scientific expert were indeed
needed. He wired Governor Joseph K. Toole, who was in Washington,
D.C., attending a family funeral, for permission to act. Toole's reply
instructed Longeway "to employ the best skill that money could secure
and carry to conclusion a most thorough investigation."[5]

Armed with the governor's approval, Longeway consulted H. M.
Bracken, secretary of the Minnesota State Board of Health, who, along
with Frank F. Wesbrook, director of that board's bacteriological laboratory, suggested two young pathologists on their staff as potential
investigators. The two, whose services Longeway promptly engaged,
were Louis B. Wilson, an assistant bacteriologist with the state board
and senior demonstrator in pathology at the University of Minnesota,
and William M. Chowning, a junior demonstrator in pathology at the
university and staff pathologist to Saint Mary's Hospital and the Minneapolis City Hospital. Born in 1866, Wilson had studied with Wesbrook as a medical student at the University of Minnesota, after which
he spent a period at Harvard with Frank Burr Mallory, who developed
many of the tissue stains widely used in histologic pathology.[6] Wilson's
resulting laboratory expertise earned him second author status in 1900
on a distinguished Wesbrook paper concerning the varieties of the
diphtheria bacillus.[7] Wilson's associate, twenty-nine-year-old William
M. Chowning, had taken undergraduate degrees at Knox College and
Johns Hopkins University and had just completed his M.D. in 1901
at the University of Minnesota Medical School.[8] The Montana State
Board of Health hoped that Wilson and Chowning, with their expertise

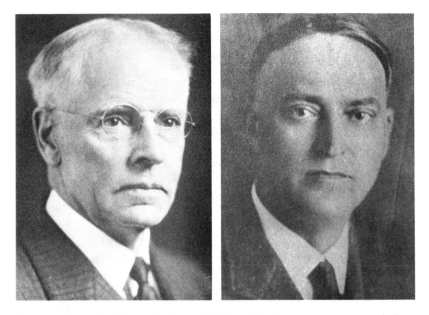

In 1902, Louis B. Wilson (left) and William M. Chowning, young patholo-gists from the University of Minnesota, launched scientific investigations into Rocky Mountain spotted fever. Wilson later pursued a distinguished career at the Mayo Clinic in Rochester, Minnesota. Chowning returned to the private practice of medicine. (Courtesy of the Rocky Mountain Labora-tories, NIAID.)

in pathology and bacteriology, would be able to shed light on the Bitterroot's strange blight.

Because the spotted fever season was so short each year, the two pathologists began work almost immediately. Arriving in Missoula on 16 May, Wilson was joined by Chowning on 26 May. With apparatus and media brought from Minnesota, they established a laboratory in a Northern Pacific Hospital room made available for the work. The railroad company was eager to assist in the spotted fever investigations, because the expansion of its rail lines into Idaho was jeopardized by the disease, as was its supply of lumber for ties from the Bitterroot. The physicians who administered the hospital, J. J. Buckley and E. W. Spottswood, cooperated fully with the visiting investigators, loaning the two men additional equipment. The arrival of Wilson and Chown-ing marked the beginning of scientific research into Rocky Mountain spotted fever.[9]

The investigation was broad: data were gathered from epidemiological, clinical, pathological, and laboratory studies. Within the first ten days, the two pathologists conducted three autopsies; subsequently they conducted five more. Victims of spotted fever, they observed, showed an enlarged spleen and small hemorrhages in the kidneys and at the base of the left ventricle of the heart. Most other organ systems appeared normal. Employing staining techniques by which the minute changes in tissues could be seen under the microscope, Wilson and Chowning found that the capillaries of the skin were distended and that many blood cells had escaped into the surrounding tissue. This, of course, explained the presence of the "spots."[10]

To gather epidemiological evidence, Wilson wrote each physician in the Bitterroot and Missoula, asking for detailed case histories on spotted fever patients. He enclosed a blueprint map of the valley on which the suspected point at which victims contracted the disease was to be marked with "a pen dipped in a strong solution of common baking soda." The response was satisfying—all but one physician responded, providing information from their records on 114 cases.[11]

Data from the blueprint maps were combined on a master map that showed definitively the sharp localization of spotted fever on the western side of the Bitterroot Valley. Two other foci were also identified outside the valley in western Montana.[12] In the Bitterroot, furthermore, the infected district did not include the entire west side of the valley. A later observer noted:

The boundary of the endemic area is not formed by the river but by the margin of the "bench" or foothills. People living in the river bottom, even on the west side, feel secure. . . . Exposure or residence on the "bench" might for some reason be more dangerous than in other near places because of the difference in the development. The east side of the valley is cleared thoroughly, highly cultivated, well settled and in thrift and prosperity resembles a fat Pennsylvania or Ohio Valley. The west side, especially the "bench," is not nearly so advanced. Much of it is not cleared at all, very little is well cultivated. The houses as a rule, are poor and there is a difference of many years in the advancement of the two sides.[13]

Other information from Wilson and Chowning's epidemiological study revealed that the earliest recorded case began on 17 March and the latest about 20 July, with most cases occurring between 15 May and 15 June. An analysis of the sex and age of victims revealed that although the disease had occurred in both sexes and in all age groups, the highest incidence was in males between 20 and 40 years old—a total of 41 cases in this group—and in females between 10 and 20 years old or between 30 and 40—there were 11 cases in each of these

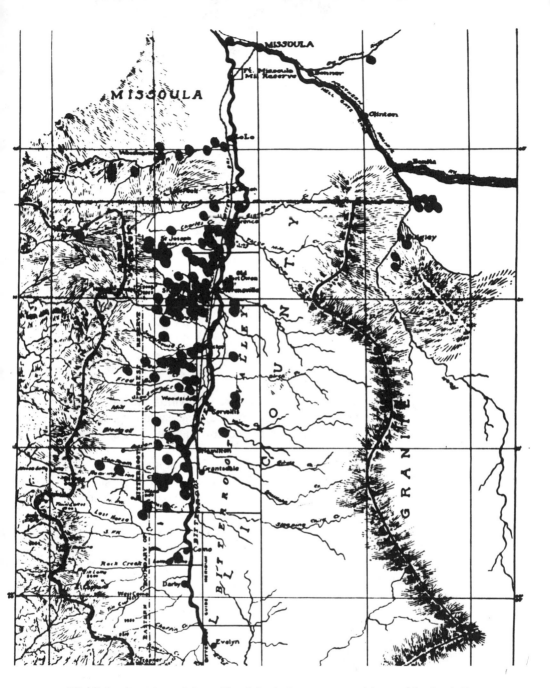

Highlighted version of the epidemiological map prepared in 1902 by Louis B.
Wilson and William M. Chowning during their study of spotted fever in the Bitterroot Valley. The horizontal line near the top marks the political division between Missoula and Ravalli counties. The dots representing cases clearly show
the concentration of the disease on the benchlands and in the canyons west of the
Bitterroot River. (From Louis B. Wilson and William M. Chowning, "Studies in
Pyroplasmosis Hominis: ['Spotted Fever' or 'Tick Fever' of the Rocky Moun-
tains]," *Journal of Infectious Diseases* 1 [1904]: 31–57.)

TABLE I. *Wilson and Chowning's Record of Spotted Fever Cases by Age and Sex of Patients*

Age	Males Cases	Males Deaths	Females Cases	Females Deaths	Total Cases
Under 5	8	4	5	5	13
5–10	6	5	7	4	13
10–20	8	5	11	5	19
20–30	17	13	7	3	24
30–40	24	19	11	7	35
40–50	8	6	2	1	10
50–60	3	2	2	1	5
60–80	4	4	2	2	6
Not stated	1	1	0	0	1
TOTAL	79	59	47	28	126

SOURCE: This table is adapted from Louis B. Wilson and William M. Chowning, "Studies in Pyroplasmosis Hominis" ('Spotted Fever' or 'Tick Fever' of the Rocky Mountains)," *Journal of Infectious Diseases* 1 (1904): 36. It includes information on cases studied in 1903 in addition to the 114 cases on which records were compiled in 1902.

two age groups (see Table 1). Wilson and Chowning attributed the higher infection rate in these groups to the "increased exposure to infection through their occupation or pleasure taking them outdoors in the foothills and mountains in the spring of the year." From clinical histories of the cases, moreover, Wilson and Chowning noted that the "general health of the patient" had "little part in determining susceptibility to the disease." In general, victims of spotted fever were healthy before the disease struck them down.[14]

Wilson and Chowning determined that between 1895 and 1902, the years during which spotted fever had become a fearsome presence in the valley, there had been 88 cases with 64 deaths, producing an average mortality of 72.7 percent. Their records correlated closely with newspaper reports during these same years, the newspapers recording 92 probable cases with 64 deaths, a mortality rate of 69.56 percent (see Table 2).[15] As a part of their examination of the "topography, meteorology and water and food supply," moreover, they found that "in no instance have two or more persons with the same food or water supply been simultaneously stricken with the disease." This finding cast doubt on melted snow water as the source of the infection. Neither was spotted fever contagious. "There is not even a suspicion," they wrote, that the disease had ever been "transferred directly from one human being to another, except in one instance, in

TABLE 2. *Cases and Deaths from Rocky Mountain Spotted Fever, 1895–1902*

Year	Wilson and Chowning		Newspapers	
	Cases	Deaths	Cases	Deaths
1895	3	3	6	6
1896	6	6	9	7
1987	6	5	12	9
1898	3	2	11	8
1899	23	14	10	3
1900	12	9	14	11
1901	14	10	17	10
1902	21	15	13	10
TOTAL	88	64	92	64
Average mortality		72.73%		69.57%

SOURCE: Louis B. Wilson and William M. Chowning, Report, Montana State Board of Health, *First Biennial Report, 1901–1902,* 32–41; idem, "Studies in Pyroplasmosis Hominis," 33; local newspapers as cited in Robert N. Philip, "A Journalistic View of Western Montana, 1870–1910: Some Newspaper Items Relevant to the Development of the Bitter Root Valley and the Occurrence of Rocky Mountain Spotted Fever," manuscript, 1984, passim.

which an infant born while the mother was suffering from the disease" also developed spotted fever. What they found instead—in every case they personally examined—were "small wounds of the skin, said to have been made by the bites of ticks." Working from this epidemiological picture, Wilson and Chowning began a series of laboratory experiments to elucidate the microscopic etiology of spotted fever.[16]

The intellectual milieu in which the two pathologists launched their laboratory studies was strongly influenced by recent discoveries relating to microorganisms and their potential vectors. Epidemiological data from earlier periods, for example, such as those gathered in the 1848–49 London cholera epidemic by John Snow, had suggested that contaminated water might be one vector by which bacteria were transmitted. This theory was confirmed in 1884 when Robert Koch discovered the comma-shaped bacillus of cholera, and subsequently water was suspect whenever a new disease was investigated. That the lay population of the Bitterroot was familiar with the concept of waterborne disease is evident in the popularity of the theory that held melted snow water to be the source of spotted fever.

Another recently discovered route by which bacterial diseases were spread was insects, such as flies and mosquitoes, and other arthropods such as ticks and mites. Transmission of bacterial diseases by insects

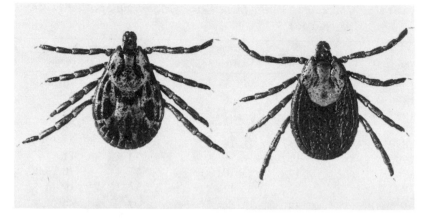

The Rocky Mountain wood tick, male and female *Dermacentor andersoni*, the first tick identified as a vector of Rocky Mountain spotted fever. (Courtesy of the Rocky Mountain Laboratories, NIAID.)

was believed to be a mechanical process: the insect accidentally picked up bacteria on its wings, feet, or mouth parts and carried them to food or other items contacted by a human or animal host. The Spanish-American War of 1898 had produced a convincing and well-publicized indictment of one insect, the house fly, in connection with the mechanical transmission of typhoid fever. An official investigation of the typhoid epidemic in U.S. camps documented the proximity of open latrines to cooking tents, noted the swarms of flies with access to both, and concluded that authorities concentrating on the purity of the water supplies had neglected to address the threat of transmission of typhoid by flies.[17]

A second line of inquiry about arthropods and disease had grown out of research in helminthology, the study of parasitic worms.[18] In 1878, Patrick Manson, a British medical officer studying the life cycle of *Filaria bancrofti*, the worm that causes the tropical disease filariasis, discovered that a portion of the worm's life cycle was spent in the body of a mosquito.[19] Manson's research inspired Ronald Ross, another British medical officer, to complete experiments that in 1898 demonstrated the presence of the malaria parasite, a protozoan rather than bacterial organism, in the mid guts of *Anopheles* mosquitoes. Although credit for this discovery was shared with Italian investigator Giovanni Battista Grassi and his collaborators, Ross reaped high honors. Fellowship in the Royal Society, a Nobel prize, and knighthood followed the realization that mosquito control measures might rid the world of the scourge of malaria and improve the habitability of Europe's tropical colonies.[20]

Five years before Ross's achievement, Theobald Smith and Fred Lucius Kilbourne, a physician and a veterinarian working in the Bureau of Animal Industry of the U.S. Department of Agriculture, published the results of their experiments on Texas cattle fever. They proved conclusively that this disease, which resulted in a significant economic loss to owners, was caused by the presence in the blood of a protozoan organism transmitted to the cattle by the bite of an infected tick. Moreover, they demonstrated that dipping cattle to kill ticks would effectively prevent the disease.[21]

The disease organisms of filariasis, malaria, and Texas cattle fever spent some portion of their life cycles developing in the body of an intermediate arthropod host, which passed them on to humans or animals through direct inoculation by biting. This developmental phenomenon, not shared by bacteria, defined initially the concept of biological transmission of disease by arthropods. Pathogenic helminths and protozoa, moreover, could not be cultured as bacteria were. The discovery that microorganisms other than bacteria could be sources of disease offered an explanation for a major problem besetting bacteriologists. Robert Koch had included as one of his postulates for demonstrating bacterial etiology of disease the isolation and culture on an artificial medium of the suspected organism.[22] Attempts to culture the organisms of yellow fever, rabies, and several other diseases had proven fruitless, but after the discoveries of Manson, Ross, and Smith and Kilbourne, many researchers suspected that the elusive organisms of a number of dread diseases were pathogenic protozoa or helminths. When the U.S. Yellow Fever Commission in Cuba demonstrated that Yellow Jack was a mosquito-borne disease, this suspicion became a working hypothesis.[23]

At the time these discoveries were made, moreover, the concept of the virus as a distinct pathologic entity did not exist. The term *virus* was used only in the general sense, like the word *germ*, to mean "infectious agent." As such, it was applied to bacterial, protozoan, and unknown pathogens. A few physical scientists argued that the so-called filterable viruses might be nonliving substances, but most medical and bacteriological researchers, who were advocates of the germ theory, supported the idea that ultramicroscopic agents were tiny, living microbes.[24]

The intellectual concepts that emerged from these findings linked bacterial diseases to mechanical transmission of diseases by arthropod vectors and protozoan diseases to biological transmission. Most researchers never concluded that these relationships were rigid, but in the face of no conflicting evidence, they often came to assume them as truth. In 1899, for example, George H. F. Nuttall, founder of the journal *Parasitology*, published the first exhaustive study of arthropod vectors. Simply by focusing on known information and adopting a skeptical attitude about alternative hypotheses, Nuttall reinforced such assumptions. In his section on ticks, he discounted the likelihood that they carried any sort of bacterial infection biologically, but he discussed at length tick transmission of protozoan diseases, especially Texas cattle fever.[25]

This model of how nature operated was powerful in suggesting what sort of disease to suspect given a known insect vector. House flies, for example, were known to carry bacterial diseases, but ticks and mosquitoes should be suspected of carrying protozoan diseases. Conversely, if a disease were of known bacterial origin, accidental transmission by an insect should be investigated, while if a protozoan or helminth had been identified, an arthropod that transmitted the disease biologically might be the likely culprit. During the first three decades of the twentieth century, the elegant logic of these concepts exerted a powerful influence on researchers in infectious diseases, including Wilson and Chowning and subsequent investigators of Rocky Mountain spotted fever.

All of the patients Wilson and Chowning examined had been bitten by wood ticks from two to eight days before the onset of the disease, hence they suspected the tick as the likely vector. Local citizens, moreover, may also have suggested the possibility of tick transmission, for ticks had occasionally been associated with "blood poisoning."[26] By analogy with known diseases transmitted by ticks, Wilson and Chowning doubtless theorized that a protozoan organism might be the infectious agent. To rule out possible bacterial causation, however, they examined fresh blood from patients and also attempted to culture bacteria from blood in a variety of media. All of these studies were negative, so they concluded that the disease was not caused by a bacterium. In the blood of eight patients, however, they believed that they saw "ovoidal bodies" that exhibited "amoeboid movements." Their studies convinced them that these bodies were a hitherto undescribed "hematozoan," a protozoan parasite that lived all or a part of its life cycle in the circulating blood of its host.[27] They announced their findings to the local press June 7.

We find the disease to be a disease of the blood. It is due to a parasite which infests the red blood cells. This parasite . . . resembles the parasite which causes malaria. The parasite apparently does not gain access to the body by way of the nose or mouth; that is, it is not carried by the air, drinking water or food, but is injected into the blood by some biting insect or animal. . . . All the facts point to some kind of a tick as carrying the disease to man by its bite. All of the above facts are circumstantial though not positive evidence that the parasite of spotted fever is conveyed to man through the bite of some small slowly moving animal or insect which is found early in the spring and disappears about July and only a few individuals of which are infested with the parasite. The tick answers to this description, though much work may yet be needed to determine its exact relationship to conveyance of the disease.[28]

Wilson and Chowning identified the hematozoan organism as a *Pyroplasma*, other species of which were known to cause Texas cattle fever and similar blood diseases in horses and dogs. They proposed that the organism be named *Pyroplasma hominis*, or "the pyroplasma of humans." Shortly after they published their findings regarding this organism, it should be noted, their spelling was corrected to *Piroplasma* to conform with accepted zoological nomenclature. They described three stages in which they found the organism, which they said varied in size from one to three microns in thickness and from two to five microns in length.[29] This piroplasma, they stated, resembled "in its smaller form very markedly the Pyrosoma bigeminum of Texas fever, yet [it] differs from that organism in being larger, and in its larger forms exhibiting active ameboid movements with the projection of pseudo-podia. The absence of pigment from the organism of 'spotted fever' would apparently separate it from the malarial group and place it with that of Texas fever."[30]

Although they admitted that this newly described organism was not always easy to find in blood, many protozoan organisms were similarly difficult to locate. What doubtless convinced them that the elusive organism was indeed the cause of spotted fever were the other elements in the paradigm under which they operated. The disease was most prevalent during the spring of the year, the time when ticks were plentiful. All of the cases of the disease they observed had shown evidence of tick bite before the symptoms appeared. The local ground squirrel, *Citellus columbianus*, moreover, existed in large numbers in the valley, and it was presumed that this mammal served as the natural reservoir of the disease, from which the infected ticks contracted it. It was known, moreover, and pointed out by a later observer, that the ground squirrel would not cross water except under extraordinary circumstances. "This being true, it would give the necessary explanation why the disease was confined" to the western side of the valley.[31]

Regarding the relationship between the parasite and the tick, Wilson and Chowning noted: "All hematozoa of warm-blooded animals, of which the life cycle is now known, pass at least one phase of their development within the body of some host (usually an insect or arachnid) other than the one whose blood cells they invade. This is probably also true of the hematozoan of 'spotted fever.' " They also noted that in both malaria and Texas fever, only one species of mosquito or tick carried the organism and not all members of the species were infected. This comment was offered to explain the low incidence of infection in the Bitterroot, because, as the local people noted, it was impossible to escape being bitten during "tick season" each spring.[32]

The *Piroplasma*-tick-ground squirrel theory of spotted fever contained all the elements of an elegant solution to a scientific mystery, and it was, as a later writer noted, "in the line of some of the most fashionable thought" of the time.[33] It conformed to prevailing beliefs about the relationship between protozoan organisms and biological transmission of disease; it identified a common mammal as probable host in nature; and it squared with the epidemiological data on the disease. Furthermore, this theory also gained currency from immediate experience. On 14 June, a week after Wilson and Chowning had announced their findings, Dan McDonald, a lumberman who worked on the west side of the valley near Victor, discovered a tick attached to his body. As he took it off, he remarked, "Now we shall see whether this gives me the spotted fever or not." Fourteen days later he died of the disease.[34]

While Wilson and Chowning were conducting their research in the Bitterroot, Montana Congressman Caldwell Edwards had been discussing the spotted fever situation with Walter Wyman, surgeon general of the U.S. Public Health and Marine Hospital Service. In 1901 this Service, founded to serve the medical needs of merchant seamen, received congressional authorization to investigate "infectious and contagious diseases and matters pertaining to the public health." Edwards or others had indicated to Wyman that spotted fever was "highly communicable and, therefore, a matter of importance to the public health of the country." The presumed contagious nature of the disease placed it within the Service's purview, hence on 23 June, Wyman telegraphed one of his commissioned officers, Surgeon Julius O. Cobb, to proceed to Montana to investigate the disease.[35]

The thirty-nine-year old Cobb, a fourteen-year veteran of the Service from South Carolina, had considerable experience investigating outbreaks of disease. Having contracted yellow fever in 1897, moreover, he doubtless had a keen appreciation of the new information regarding the biological transmission of disease by arthropods. Cobb reviewed the findings of Wilson and Chowning and agreed with their conclusions. In his report to Surgeon General Wyman, Cobb stated that he omitted "many interesting facts" because they had been published already by Wilson and Chowning as a preliminary note in the *Journal of the American Medical Association*. He summarized the findings of the two Minnesota pathologists and, from his own investigation, was satisfied that they had indeed found a hematozoon in the blood of spotted fever victims that was probably transmitted to humans by the wood tick from a natural reservoir in the local ground squirrel. Assured that the investigations were on the right track, Cobb noted that the original fear of contagion was "altogether groundless," and commented that "the alarm caused by newspaper reports" was "unjustifiable."[36]

At the end of the 1902 spotted fever season, Wilson and Chowning submitted to the Montana State Board of Health a bill for $1,466, which, in light of the board's annual budget of $2,000, starkly revealed the high cost of scientific research. For this sum, the investigators had produced a logical but unproven theory regarding the cause of spotted fever. They had not, however, developed any method to prevent or to cure the malady. At the meeting of the state board during which the expenses were allowed, there was considerable discussion about the investigation of spotted fever and about the state's authority for undertaking it. The board concluded that no more state money would be spent on spotted fever in 1902, and that the county commissioners of Missoula and Ravalli counties, where the disease was localized, should endeavor to raise the funds needed for further research in 1903.[37]

Faced with the possibility of no further state support for their medical crisis, the commissioners of Ravalli County appropriated $400 in April 1903 for continued investigations. They added a caveat, however, stipulating that Missoula County must raise a matching amount. The commissioners of Missoula County balked, according to newspaper accounts, because they believed that spotted fever was "more than a two county problem." It was also widely believed that the Montana congressional delegation could persuade the U.S. Public Health and Marine Hospital Service to fund and conduct the investigation.[38]

With its sparse population, Montana was allocated only one seat in the U.S. House of Representatives and, of course, two Senate seats. This three-man delegation, comprised of Congressman Joseph M. Dixon, who later became governor of the state, and Senators William

A. Clark and Paris Gibson, actively pressed the case and did indeed persuade Surgeon General Walter Wyman to continue federally sponsored research into spotted fever. The Service officer Wyman chose to study spotted fever in 1903 was Passed Assistant Surgeon John F. Anderson, who had demonstrated such competence in research that in 1902, at age twenty-nine, he had been named assistant director of the Service's Hygienic Laboratory. A Virginian, Anderson, after completing medical school, had done graduate work in bacteriology in Europe, including a period at the School of Tropical Medicine in Liverpool, where he studied protozoan organisms similar to the presumed agent of spotted fever.[39]

Anderson left Washington on 24 April, stopping in Great Falls, Montana, to confer with the secretary of the Montana State Board of Health, A. F. Longeway; then he continued on to Missoula, where he was offered the use of laboratories at the University of Montana and at the Northern Pacific Hospital. He decided to make his headquarters at the Northern Pacific in order to work closely with Wilson and Chowning, who had returned for an additional month's work in 1903. The Minnesota researchers shared their data with Anderson and studied five new cases of spotted fever, performing one autopsy. Anderson, whom they taught to stain the slides of blood in order to see the organism they had described, believed he saw two of the three forms Wilson and Chowning had described. "I was unable to find the paired form in stained preparations," he later wrote, "though Drs. Wilson and Chowning informed me that they had no difficulty in doing so." Anderson also collected specimens of the ticks suspected of being infected with spotted fever and sent them to the Hygienic Laboratory for identification by Charles Wardell Stiles, director of the laboratory's Division of Zoology.[40]

Like Cobb before him, Anderson was convinced that Wilson and Chowning had identified the spotted fever organism and that their theory of tick transmission was correct. Upon returning to Washington, Anderson published a lengthy report on spotted fever in a *Bulletin* of the Hygienic Laboratory. It recapitulated Wilson and Chowning's work and included their case histories and maps.[41] Anderson also inserted photographs and drawings of the eruption of the disease, which he proposed be called tick fever instead of spotted fever because the latter name was frequently identified with typhus and cerebrospinal meningitis. The only point on which Anderson disagreed with Wilson and Chowning had to do with the ground squirrel as the probable host in nature. Knowing that the *Piroplasma* of Texas cattle fever would not infect sheep nor would the *Piroplasma* of dogs infect cats, Anderson doubted that a *Piroplasma* of ground squirrels would easily infect humans. Because of his skepticism about this hypothesis, Anderson omitted any mention of the ground squirrel from his report.[42]

Satisfied that their 1903 investigation had confirmed the work of 1902, however, Wilson and Chowning also collaborated on a detailed scientific article, published in 1904 in the premiere issue of the *Journal of Infectious Diseases*. Entitled "Studies in Pyroplasmosis Hominis ('Spotted Fever' or 'Tick Fever' of the Rocky Mountains)," the paper included drawings of the presumed protozoan organism of spotted fever as well as epidemiological, pathological, microscopic, and clinical evidence supporting the tick transmission theory.

Most inhabitants of the Bitterroot Valley accepted the scientific experts' verdict that the tick was the culprit in transmitting spotted fever. Because ticks were so pervasive during the spring, however, implicating them as vectors of a dread disease had immediate economic consequences, especially for property owners and sawmill operators on the west side of the valley where the infection was localized. One observer noted:

Economically, I think it safe to say that the tick theory has been more disastrous to the infected region than the disease itself. Ticks are so common it is nearly impossible for a man working out of doors to avoid their bites, while at the same time they, if causing the disease, constitute a cause so tangible and real that the dissemination of this hypothesis excited a fear closely akin to terror. Land values were affected, probably a majority of the people on the west bank of the Bitter Root River desiring to sell and nobody willing to buy. Saw mills have been unable to procure a sufficiency of hands, and some families have sacrificed their property in order to get away as soon as possible. People who formerly frequented that region for business or pleasure could in most instances not now be induced to go there, except on most urgent business, during the tick season.[43]

As the implications of this natural calamity became manifest, civic leaders attempted to ameliorate the situation with pragmatic action. Taking stock of what was known about the disease, its tick vector, and the ground squirrel—or gopher as it was commonly known— which presumably served as a natural reservoir, they suggested that strong measures be taken to rid the valley of these threats. "It having been demonstrated that the woodtick is the cause of the so-called 'spotted fever,'" an editorial in the *Western News* counseled,

it would seem that the best preventive of the disease would be to put the venomous insect out of business. . . . The woodtick frequents localities only where there is much fallen and decayed timber. The abandoned settings of long-forgotten saw mills are its favorite haunts. These tick-infested localities should be scourged with flames. . . . If the gopher is an ally of the woodtick, aiding and abetting it in its death dealing mission, it too must be exterminated.[44]

By the following spring, preventive tactics were widespread. The *Western News* reported in April 1904 that "farmers in the vicinity of Stevensville and points throughout the valley are making a strong effort this year to rid the country of the gopher pest. A new preparation of poisoned wheat is being generally used," the article continued, "and farmers all through the valley have laid in a big supply. The big increase in the number of these destructive spermophiles has alarmed the ranchers to no little extent." Some farmers believed, so the reporter noted, that the state should offer a bounty of five cents "for the scalp of every one of the animals exterminated."[45] There was, however, one unfortunate side effect of the indiscriminate use of poisoned grain. Farmers who scattered it on the ground, hoping that the ground squirrels would eat it, often found that it killed game birds instead.[46]

Another approach to tick and gopher control was the burning of brush land. Reportedly done on the recommendation of John F. Anderson, a policy of spring burning was supported by the Forest Reserve office. "The great brooding [sic] places of the wood tick and gophers is in the old slash and cuttings along the foothills," reported the supervisor of the Bitterroot Forest Reserve, commenting also that "more spring burning this year has been done than during any three previous seasons."[47]

Although these efforts may have heartened valley residents by providing a means to strike back against a deadly enemy, it was impossible to exterminate all wood ticks. Careful and frequent examinations of the body to locate any ticks that had attached themselves thus became a ritual for many people. The *Western News* cautioned: "Should you be bitten by a woodtick, treat it as you would a snake bite. Be prompt in applying remedies to counteract the poison. Don't wait until the poison has permeated the entire system or you are likely to remain dead a long time."[48]

In response to this warning, many people, especially those who worked on the infected west side of the river, carried small bottles of carbolic acid for immediate application if a tick was found attached to them. Joseph Lister had popularized this chemical in the late nineteenth century by using it successfully to kill germs in the operating room. Since Bitterroot citizens applied the mouth of the bottles to their skin directly over the tick bite, however, many suffered "small round sores from undiluted acid." The *Ravalli Republican* even reported that on one occasion the cork had come out of a bottle in a man's pocket, "and the hot stuff burned him severely!"[49]

Every theory regarding the cause of spotted fever, moreover, was carefully followed and exploited by charlatans hoping to profit from the fear generated by the disease. During the heyday of the melted snow water theory, for instance, a number of people claiming to be scientists made a comfortable living testing drinking water for spotted fever infection. Within two weeks of Wilson and Chowning's announcement that a hematozoon had been found in the blood of victims, the promoters of King's sarsaparilla capitalized on the new scientific evidence to advertise their product as a treatment. "Spotted fever has been pronounced a blood disease," the advertisement asserted. "Use King's sarsaparilla and you are exempt not only from spotted fever, but a great many other diseases."[50] Two years later, a homeopathic physician in Missoula known only as Dr. Glasgow claimed that he had cured a sixteen-year-old boy of spotted fever within a few days by administering oral doses of "venom from a dagger-headed viper found in Brazil." Capitalizing on this *post hoc, ergo propter hoc* argument, Glasgow advertised in the *Daily Missoulian* that his unusual therapy was good not only for spotted fever but also in cases of "arthritis and spinal conditions." In this period of unrestrained enterprise, such exploitation was rampant. Not until 1906, with the enactment of the federal Pure Food and Drugs Act, were the worst abuses curbed.[51]

Quack treatments for spotted fever flourished, of course, because the orthodox medical profession could do little to treat the disease. After his investigation of spotted fever, for example, John F. Anderson suggested that physicians employ quinine therapy, "in large doses, preferably hypodermically," because of spotted fever's presumed similarity to malaria. Except for this strategy, which soon proved to have no beneficial effect and perhaps actually harmed patients, Anderson could only describe supportive therapies: strychnine, whisky, or other appropriate "cardiac stimulants" to support the heart; Dover's powders or morphine sulfate to relieve the severe headache; large quantities of water to flush out the kidneys; and warm sponge baths to reduce the fever and refresh the patient.[52]

At the conclusion of the 1903 tick season, it seemed even more probable than in 1902 that the wood tick was indeed the vector of spotted fever, but for all the monies and time expended, no effective cure or prevention had been found. The Montana State Board of Health was beleaguered by other public health problems, especially noncooperation from physicians who refused to report and enforce quar-

antines for designated infectious diseases, such as measles. Secretary
A. F. Longeway, moreover, seemed reluctant to enforce the board's
rules vigorously.[53] Possibly because of this, when the board met on 5
May 1903, Longeway was replaced as secretary by Thomas D. Tuttle.[54]

The thirty-three-year-old Tuttle was a Missouri native who had
migrated to Montana after completing his medical studies in 1892 at
the College of Physicians and Surgeons in New York.[55] His initial
activities and reports to the board revealed an energetic, no-nonsense
approach to public health.[56] Shortly after taking office, for example,
Tuttle sought out Anderson and Chowning in Missoula to gather
information on the spotted fever situation. "I visited the bacteriologists
investigating the 'Spotted Fever' in the Bitter Root Valley," Tuttle stated
in his July quarterly report, "but was unable to learn that they had
made any progress over the work accomplished last year." Realizing
how little state money would be available to continue investigations,
Tuttle wrote in early February 1904 to Senator Paris Gibson and
Congressman Joseph M. Dixon of Montana for assistance in persuading the U.S. Public Health and Marine Hospital Service to continue
researching the disease. On 15 February he received a wire from Dixon
stating that Anderson and another expert would be detailed to Montana in March. When neither researcher had appeared by mid April,
Tuttle again wrote Dixon, "asking him to hurry the matter along,"
since the spotted fever season had already begun and would end within
three months.[57]

Surgeon General Walter Wyman responded by sending Montana his
most experienced researcher in protozoan diseases, Charles Wardell
Stiles, who had joined the Hygienic Laboratory in 1902 as the first
director of the newly created Division of Zoology. Stiles had taken his
Ph.D. in zoology in 1890 with the distinguished Leipzig helminthologist
Rudolph Leuckart and from 1891 to 1902 had served as principal
zoologist for the Bureau of Animal Industry in the U.S. Department
of Agriculture, where he worked alongside Theobald Smith and F. L.
Kilbourne, discoverers of the Texas cattle fever piroplasma. Shortly
before joining the U.S. Public Health and Marine Hospital Service,
Stiles had won considerable fame by identifying a new species of
hookworm and correctly deducing that it rather than malaria caused
the anemia prevalent in the southern United States. For this work he
had been hailed as the discoverer of the "Germ of Laziness."[58] Surgeon
General Wyman hoped that Stiles would be able to trace the life cycle
of the parasite that caused spotted fever, study the tick that transmitted
it and the ground squirrels that harbored the disease in nature, and
arrive at a workable means of preventing the disease.[59]

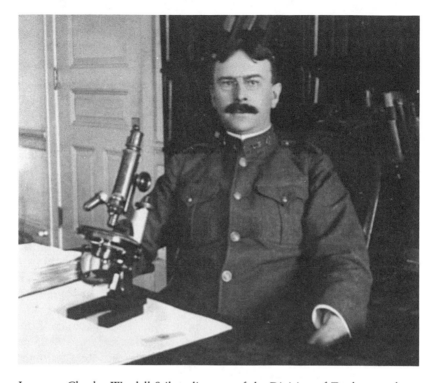

In 1904, Charles Wardell Stiles, director of the Division of Zoology at the Hygienic Laboratory of the U.S. Public Health and Marine Hospital Service, refuted Wilson and Chowning's assertion that a protozoan organism caused spotted fever. Because of widespread assumptions about microorganisms and their arthropod vectors, Stiles concluded that the disease was not transmitted by ticks. (Courtesy of the National Library of Medicine.)

With his strong background in zoological subjects, Stiles was predisposed to look favorably on the findings of Anderson and Wilson and Chowning. In fact, Stiles looked upon the biological transmission of protozoa by arthropods as a law of nature rather than a working hypothesis. In April 1901, when he had presented the annual Toner Lecture, which he titled, "Insects as Disseminators of Disease," at Georgetown University, Stiles had stated:

We may lay down two general biologic rules, which, I believe, are enunciated tonight for the first time: *The first rule, to which at present a few exceptions are known, is that diseases which are* accidentally *spread by insects are caused by parasitic* plants, *particularly bacteria. The second, to which no exceptions are as yet known, is that those diseases which are* dependent *upon insects or other arthropods for their dissemination and transmission are caused by parasitic* animals, *particularly by sporozoa and worms.*[60]

After working in the Bitterroot from 7 May to 6 July, however, during which time he saw ten patients, drew blood samples from nine, attended an autopsy on one, and conducted more than one hundred hours of work at the microscope, Stiles completely changed his mind about the earlier work.[61] He could find no trace of the reported organism in the blood of spotted fever victims. In his microscopic work, Stiles was joined by U.S. Army physician Percy M. Ashburn, who was investigating the disease under orders from the surgeon general of the army. The two men worked independently but met almost daily to compare notes. "I used daylight, lamplight and electric light," Stiles wrote, "dry and oil lenses of Zeiss, Spencer, Leitz, and Bausch & Lomb. The specimens were taken at regular and irregular intervals, day and night, from both fatal and non-fatal cases." Stiles and Ashburn then consulted with Chowning, who was in the Bitterroot Valley at that time, but Chowning was unable to demonstrate the *Piroplasma* in the blood.[62]

"Accordingly," wrote Stiles, "the work of 1904 has failed to confirm the conclusions of 1902 and 1903, and indications are not lacking that at least some of the stages of the supposed *Piroplasma hominis* consist in reality of vacuoles, blood platelets, blood dust, artifacts, and tertian malaria parasites."[63] Later in the year, another U.S. Army physician, Charles F. Craig, who had considerable experience investigating tropical diseases, reported in *American Medicine* the results of his own "most careful study of the subject." Confirming the findings of Ashburn and Stiles, Craig suggested that "Chowning, Wilson, and Anderson . . . have mistaken areas devoid of hemoglobin in the red cell . . . for a protozoan parasite."[64]

The evidence seemed overwhelming that no *Piroplasma* was present. Such organisms, however, were often difficult to find under the microscope, so Stiles attempted to determine the presence of the organism by indirect means—by comparing symptoms of spotted fever with symptoms of known piroplasmic maladies, especially Texas cattle fever. When he applied his wide knowledge of piroplasmic diseases in a comparison with spotted fever, however, he found few similarities. Most known piroplasmic diseases flourished in swampy valleys, but spotted fever occurred in the foothills of the Bitterroot Mountains. Piroplasmic diseases were also "apt to attack large numbers of patients at about the same time in the same locality," Stiles noted, and "if 'spotted fever' is a piroplasmosis, transmitted by a tick, we should expect a large number of cases to develop in any locality in which one case develops. This, however, is exactly what we do not find in 'spotted fever.' " This observation, he admitted, "was the first point to lead me to seriously doubt the tick hypothesis."[65]

Stiles continued, comparing one point after another about spotted fever and known piroplasmoses. No known protozoan disease was characterized by a rash, but in spotted fever the rash was the principal diagnostic sign. Victims of piroplasmosis normally became emaciated; victims of spotted fever appeared well nourished. In Texas fever the organism caused the blood to become "thin, watery, and pale," while the blood of spotted fever victims became "thick, molasses like, and dark." The bile in piroplasmosis became thickened, but in spotted fever the bile remained fluid.[66] Stiles concluded that the disease was not a piroplasmosis. The tick transmission theory and its corollary, the ground squirrel host, were totally dependent, in Stiles's thinking, on the presence of protozoan organisms. "An important point upon which I desire to place considerable stress," he stated, "is that the tick theory is a secondary hypothesis based upon the idea that 'spotted fever' is caused by a protozoon. If the *Piroplasma* theory is correct, the tick theory immediately receives a very strong argument in its favor, for other species of *Piroplasma* are known to have ticks as their intermediate host."[67]

From his work in 1904, Stiles concluded that the earlier investigators had been wrong about the causative organism, about the tick transmission theory, and about the ground squirrel host. His own investigation, however, yielded entirely negative results, for he produced "no new theories . . . regarding the cause, transmission, and origin of this disease."[68]

Although lacking evidence, Stiles offered some speculation about alternative causes that was, as he said, "in accord with the generally accepted view" regarding arthropods and disease. If spotted fever were not a protozoan disease, he reasoned, it must be a bacterial disease. If it were bacterial, it would probably be contagious. Supporting Stiles's contention, moreover, Percy M. Ashburn cited the cases of Mrs. Robert Allen, a twenty-eight-year-old housewife, and Miss Helen McConnon, a twenty-four-year-old schoolteacher, both of whom insisted that because of heightened awareness that ticks might spread the disease, they had meticulously examined their bodies daily and had not been bitten by ticks before the onset of spotted fever.[69] Such evidence suggested to Stiles and Ashburn that contagion might be present. "It seems to me," Stiles wrote, "that the possibility is by no means excluded that, despite the general experience regarding the noncontagiousness of the disease, such close intimacy as sleeping in the same bed might perhaps result in a transmission of the disease to a healthy individual."[70]

Stiles also attempted to explain the seasonal occurrence of spotted fever within the existing theoretical framework. "Practically all authors lay stress upon the fact that the affection under discussion is preeminently a disease of the spring months," Stiles did not, however, relate the emergence of ticks to spring warming, but he did note the connection between the coming of spring and a rise in the amount of water in streams from melted snow. In fact, he revived the old theory that melted snow water might be a source of infection. "Such as the data are," he said, "they tend to support rather than to negative [sic] the popular idea that the melting snow has some direct or indirect connection with the development of cases, or . . . that conditions which favor the melting of the snow also favor the appearance of cases of spotted fever."[71]

When he returned to Washington, Stiles published the most lengthy report on spotted fever yet produced. In addition to his scientific conclusions, he added an observation that would be used to question his integrity in later years. "The tick theory has caused serious financial loss to the Bitter Root Valley and has produced an effect which in a few cases had bordered on hysteria. In justice to the property interests of the valley and the peace of mind of the inhabitants, I think no time should be lost in publishing the statement that the results of study this year have absolutely and totally failed to confirm this hypothesis."[72] This statement inspired one author to suggest that Stiles succumbed, at least unconsciously, to pressure from Bitterroot residents who rejected the tick theory because of the damage it had already done to their property values.[73] Such an interpretation misses the clear intellectual motivation behind Stiles's rejection of the tick hypothesis and ignores the responsibilities of government scientists in the Progressive era.

Stiles, like other employees of government agencies, had to be responsive to the concerns of his employers—the taxpayers of the United States. As James H. Cassedy has noted in his analysis of Stiles's hookworm activities during this same period, such an awareness did not compromise a scientist's integrity, but it made him think twice before publishing findings that could have a potentially negative economic impact. Like most other government scientists during the Progressive era, Stiles was not doctrinaire on major political or social issues. For instance, in 1896 he strongly supported the extension of governmental authority to regulate filthy country slaughterhouses. He had also been willing, however, to apply his knowledge on behalf of U.S. pork producers in 1898, when German restrictions on pork allegedly contaminated with trichinosis threatened their livelihoods.[74] As a government-employed professional, Stiles could warn his colleagues that "diseases have an economic as well as an academic side," and caution them: "If it can be foreseen that a given working hypothesis is calculated to result in financial loss to an infected district, such hypothesis should be subjected to most searching criticism before it is published. And if it can be foreseen that any good to be accomplished by its announcement is far outweighed by its probable evil effects, its publication should be postponed until its correctness is demonstrated or is beyond reasonable doubt."[75] In a period when the status and authority of experts were increasing, it was the opinion of Stiles's zoological colleagues that mattered to him, but when he found no evidence of tick transmission of spotted fever, he felt duty bound to correct the economic hardship produced by the "premature" conclusions about ticks and the disease published by Wilson and Chowning.

The results of the work of Stiles, Ashburn, and Craig, coming at the end of two seasons of vigorous tick and gopher control efforts, left valley residents more mystified than ever about their strange disease. The elegance of the *Piroplasma*-tick-gopher hypothesis had seemingly been destroyed by the "ugly little fact" that no *Piroplasma* existed. The intellectual model that linked only protozoan organisms to arthropod transmission, moreover, held such control over the thinking of the research community that no one seems to have considered the possibility that some other organism might be transmitted by the ticks. No one even attempted to verify tick transmission of the disease as a separate experiment.[76] Doubtless the scientific stature of Stiles, of army surgeon Ashburn, and of Craig, who had distinguished himself in tropical diseases during the Spanish-American War, added considerable authority to their conclusions about spotted fever.

Although the spotted fever question was an intriguing intellectual problem for these men, they were not insensitive to the desire of valley residents for some means to combat the disease, which continued to claim victims each spring. In 1904 local newspapers reported fourteen cases of spotted fever and documented ten deaths. Among those who died was John Rankin, an early Missoula County pioneer whose daughter Jeanette later served as a congresswoman from Montana.[77] Percy M. Ashburn suggested a new approach to treatment, basing his notions on the presumption that a toxin-producing bacterium was possibly the cause of the disease. Employing an analogy with typhoid fever, Ashburn stated that "the grave symptoms" were probably produced by "a powerful toxin circulating in the blood; and the fact that we do not know the maker of the poison should not deter us from trying to eliminate it and to strengthen and sustain these parts and functions especially injured by it, until the organism has time to form the proper antibodies in sufficient amount to overcome the disease."[78]

What Ashburn suggested was the use of hydrotherapy, or water treatment, popularized by Simon Baruch and John Harvey Kellogg and recommended in 1892 as a treatment for typhus by the distinguished Johns Hopkins physician, William Osler.[79] Under the hydrotherapeutic regimen that Ashburn suggested, the patient was to be bathed in cold water at 70° F for ten to twenty minutes, while the attending nurse or physician constantly applied "hand friction to the body and limbs, with cold applications to the head." This procedure was to be repeated every three hours as long as the patient's temperature remained above 102.5° F. In difficult cases, ice water enemas, given while the patient drank alcohol or hot coffee—both considered stimulants—were said to increase the "efficiency of the bath and hasten the reaction." The theoretical basis of hydrotherapy rested on the observation that cold water and friction produced at first a contraction of the blood vessels followed by their dilation, which brought blood to the surface of the body where the heat of a fever might more readily be dispersed. "Quite possibly," Ashburn opined, "by so keeping up the tone of the peripheral vessels from the beginning of the disease they might be saved from the degeneration" that permitted hemmorrhages into the skin and caused "the darkening of the spots." Reportedly this cold water treatment was routinely employed in spotted fever cases by some Bitterroot physicians.[80]

In the space of three years, the seasons of 1902, 1903, and 1904, scientific investigations of spotted fever had been launched, but the inconclusive results revealed only that the disease remained an enigma. Noting the muddled picture that emerged from the investigations of Wilson and Chowning, Anderson, Stiles, and Ashburn, an editorial in the *Journal of the American Medical Association* deplored the fact that the cause "of this strange disease is as obscure as ever," and called for a continuation of the investigation. "Further investigation is of great importance, not only from a scientific view but also from an economic point of view. The tick theory of the disease seems to have reduced the inhabitants almost to a state of panic, and it is hoped that the disease will be reinvestigated . . . if only to reassure them and to render the development of this fertile valley practicable."[81]

Chapter Four

Dr. Ricketts's Discoveries

Most of the knowledge and much of the genius of the research worker lie behind his selection of what is worth observing. It is a crucial choice, often determining the success or failure of months of work, often differentiating the brilliant discoverer from the plodder.

Alan Gregg, *The Furtherance of Medical Research*

By 1905 advances in many fields of science and technology were making tangible changes in American life. X-rays, for example, discovered just before the turn of the century, were already revolutionizing the practice of medicine. Similarly, if more gradually, the advent of electric lights, telephones, automobiles, phonographs, and vacuum cleaners was altering the daily lives of thousands of citizens.[1] During this so-called Progressive era, optimism nourished by faith in the promise of science also spurred reform movements to improve industrial slum conditions, to conserve natural resources, and to curb the abuses of unbridled capitalism. In the Bitterroot Valley of Montana, however, boosters hoping to attract new residents may have harbored doubts about the efficacy, or at least the efficiency, of science. The results of three years' work by highly regarded scientific experts had failed to uncover the cause of the valley's terrifying affliction, spotted fever. Yet the stalemate produced by conflicting theories was not a defeat but an indication that a new approach was needed. Beginning in 1906, valley residents would witness rapid progress in spotted fever investigations as researchers, especially Howard Taylor Ricketts of the University of Chicago, studied past findings and explored the question from new directions.

In June 1904 the secretary of the Montana State Board of Health, Thomas D. Tuttle, attended the second annual meeting of state and territorial health officers with the surgeon general of the U.S. Public Health and Marine Hospital Service to lobby for continued investigations of spotted fever by the federal government. Noting enthusiastically in his report to the board the "hundreds of little points" regarding health work he obtained at the meeting, Tuttle related the considerable interest that Montana's "unknown" disease engendered in other delegates. Most importantly, Tuttle announced that he had convinced Surgeon General Wyman to continue supporting spotted fever research until the nature of the disease was positively determined. This commitment, Tuttle noted, was well worth the cost of his trip, since it might stem the plunge of property values in the Bitterroot.[2]

The confusion generated by the conflicting reports of Wilson and Chowning, Anderson, Stiles, and Ashburn about the germ of spotted fever, and especially about the tick as a vector of the disease, had indeed jeopardized property values on the west side of the valley. This threat appeared just as the Bitterroot launched a major effort to expand its economy by developing an irrigation system that would open the benchlands—the dry shores of the ancient lake bed—to cultivation. Since the mid 1890s, valley residents had sold their apples commercially, claiming that the climate in the Bitterroot was ideal for producing the tart, flavorful McIntosh Red apple. In a period before dry farming was employed, however, the waterless bench lay barren. In 1905 a group of Chicago financiers developed a scheme to irrigate west side benchlands, a plan that was soon expanded into an enormous irrigation project to bring water to the east side bench as well. Locally the proposed irrigation canal and flume were called the Big Ditch. Advertising in Chicago newspapers, the plan's promoters offered potential buyers a bearing orchard and a contract with Bitterroot citizens who, during the first five years of ownership, would tend, harvest, and market the apples for 10 percent of the net profit. By 1907 land in the Bitterroot was selling for $100–$150 an acre.[3]

Spotted fever represented a distinct menace to this enterprise, which was expected to swell the population of the Bitterroot nearly tenfold as new orchards came under cultivation. Since scientific research had produced no cure and much confusion, local Bitterroot boosters adopted the tactic of officially ignoring the disease's existence. Beginning in 1904, newspapers rarely mentioned spotted fever in obituaries, usually describing it as fever or a brief illness. Distinguishing spotted fever cases from other maladies in news accounts thus became much more difficult. Only the time of year and the duration of the disease provided clues. Because few states at this time monitored any but the most contagious diseases, the Bitterroot Valley suffered no official reprimand for such action. Spotted fever was not one of the reportable diseases—those, such as diphtheria, smallpox, and typhoid fever, that physicians were obligated to report to state health authorities. Vital statistics on births and deaths in the state were not even required to be collected until mid 1907, and Montana preceded many other states in that endeavor.[4]

Despite this vote of no confidence in science by local residents, in 1905 research into spotted fever reached a turning point. Montana Congressman Joseph M. Dixon and the State Board of Health secretary, Thomas D. Tuttle, held Surgeon General Walter Wyman to his promise to continue investigating the disease. Tuttle sent a written request and Dixon visited the surgeon general. At the beginning of May, Edward Francis, a Hygienic Laboratory physician who had contributed to the Service's study of yellow fever in Vera Cruz, Mexico, was detailed to Montana.[5] Fifteen years later, Francis would make a significant contribution to the understanding of tularemia, another disease of nature found in the Bitterroot and in other areas, but in 1905 his research on spotted fever produced no significant results. Although he corroborated Stiles's findings that no *Piroplasma* was present, Francis was unable to throw further light on the etiology of the disease and never published an account of his work.[6] These negative findings, however, indicated that the next spotted fever experiments must move in a different direction if they were to be productive.

In November 1904, Charles Wardell Stiles unwittingly fueled this fire when he delivered the Middleton Goldsmith Lecture, an address published in early 1905 in the highly respected and widely read scientific journal, *Proceedings of the New York Pathological Society*. Taking as his title, "Zoological Pitfalls for the Pathologist," Stiles cautioned pathologists to be careful about drawing zoological conclusions if they were not thoroughly trained in zoology. He held up the *Piroplasma* theory of Wilson and Chowning as a case in point, and his refutation of their theories "savored of scorn," as one observer noted.[7]

Stiles's pointed and uncharitable remarks stung Wilson and Chowning, but they also stimulated the interest of other investigators in the debate over this mysterious disease. Louis B. Wilson abandoned spotted fever research in 1905 when he accepted a position at the Mayo Clinic. There he pursued a distinguished career as a pathologist and administrator. William M. Chowning, however, continued spotted fever investigations while engaging in his newly established private surgical practice. He hoped to justify his earlier work and produce an antitoxin for spotted fever. In early 1906, Chowning corresponded with Howard Taylor Ricketts, a pathologist at the University of Chicago, who was interested in beginning his own investigation of spotted fever. Although Chowning had hoped that the two might work together despite Stiles's adverse criticism, Ricketts stipulated that his would be an independent study. "I may say," Ricketts wrote, "that it was exactly this criticism of Stiles which gave me the idea of going to Montana to study spotted fever. I was not at all pleased with the tone of his criticism as it was presented to the New York pathological society, and it occurred to me that this would be a good time for a third party to go into the field and repeat the ground covered by yourself and Wilson."[8]

Chowning also revealed that he had "experimentally reproduced" spotted fever in a human in Minneapolis and was presently "watching another similar inoculation." The material used "was a blood (defibrinated) culture from a Montana case (fatal)." The first experimental case was recovering; the second was too recent to predict. Ricketts made no comment to Chowning about the human experiments, and Chowning never published the results of this daring and ethically questionable investigation. Neither of them knew that Idaho physicians had also conducted tick transmission experiments on humans. The ticks used, however, were infected with the mild Idaho strain of the disease, not the fatal Bitterroot strain Chowning used. Although this study was not published until 1908, Lucien P. McCalla and his colleague H. A. Brereton had in May 1905 obtained permission from two patients, one male and one female, to attach to each a tick that had been affixed to a patient suffering from Idaho spotted fever. Both patients became ill with the disease and both recovered.[9]

Ricketts was undoubtedly interested in Chowning's proposed antitoxin against spotted fever, for this was an area in which Ricketts had just published a major textbook, *Infection, Immunity, and Serum Therapy*. This promising young researcher, born in Findley, Ohio, in 1871, had taken his undergraduate degree at the University of Nebraska, where he studied zoology with the distinguished animal parasitologist Henry B. Ward. In 1894 he had entered Northwestern University School of Medicine in Chicago as a member of the second-year class because of his solid undergraduate preparation, a criterion many of his classmates lacked.[10] Despite a nervous breakdown from overwork and constant financial problems—his family had lost its fortune in the panic of 1893—Ricketts had excelled and graduated in 1897, winning an internship at Cook County Hospital. In 1900 he became a fellow in pathology and cutaneous diseases at Rush Medical College in Chicago, where he accomplished his first important research, a study of blastomycosis, the first disease known to be produced by a yeast.

This work brought him to the attention of Ludvig Hektoen, who was shortly to become chairman of the Department of Pathology and Bacteriology at the University of Chicago and director of the John

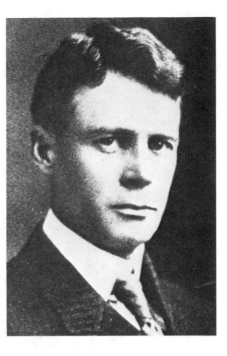

Howard Taylor Ricketts of the University of Chicago designed the experiment that first demonstrated tick transmission of Rocky Mountain spotted fever. Ricketts's contributions to the understanding of spotted fever, including identification of the causative organism, were later recognized when the microorganisms that cause spotted fever and related diseases were designated *Rickettsiae* in his honor. Ricketts died in 1910 during a study of epidemic typhus in Mexico. (Courtesy of the National Library of Medicine.)

Rockefeller McCormick Memorial Institute for Infectious Diseases. At Hektoen's suggestion, Ricketts spent a year abroad, in Berlin, Vienna, and Paris, where he perfected his laboratory technique and broadened his understanding of theoretical microbiology. Upon his return in 1902 he was appointed instructor in Hektoen's department at Chicago. With the publication of his book in 1906, Ricketts had established his reputation as a rising scientific star.

Since Montana had appropriated no additional monies in 1906 for spotted fever investigations, the three researchers who appeared in the field that year had to supply their own funds. Ricketts obtained a small grant from the Committee on Scientific Research of the American Medical Association (AMA) to defray his expenses. He arrived on 21 April at the Northern Pacific Hospital in Missoula and, at the invitation of the chief surgeon, E. W. Spottswood, erected laboratory and personal housing tents on the hospital grounds. William M. Chowning also worked in the field at his own expense, limiting his research to microscopic analysis of the blood of spotted fever victims. Having apparently abandoned the *Piroplasma* theory, Chowning focused instead on what he described as "a myriad of fantastic but highly deceptive forms," which he classified as fungi.[11]

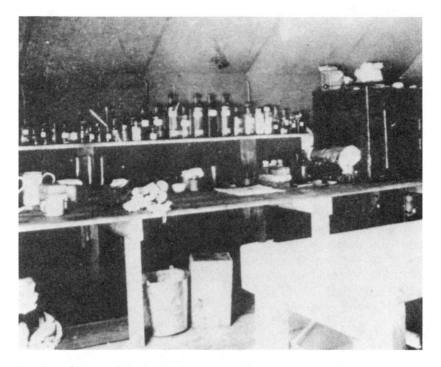

Interior of Howard Taylor Ricketts's tent laboratory, erected in 1906 in Missoula, Montana. (Used by permission of the Department of Special Collections, University of Chicago Library.)

Joining Ricketts and Chowning in late April was Walter W. King of the U.S. Public Health and Marine Hospital Service, who, fresh from five years' service as chief quarantine officer in Puerto Rico, had been sent by Surgeon General Wyman to continue the Service's investigation of spotted fever. In Puerto Rico, King and a U.S. Army physician, Bailey K. Ashford, had demonstrated that a severe anemia found on the island was caused by the American species of hookworm identified by Charles Wardell Stiles. As members of an anemia commission established in 1904, King and Ashford had worked with a Puerto Rican physician, Pedro Gutierrez, to develop a treatment program that reduced the death rate from 30 percent to less than 1 percent.[12]

Despite King's experience in public health work, Ricketts took control and directed the experimental work from the outset. King noted that Ricketts's "education for the work was very thorough," and that he "looked at things in a big way," always going "straight to the grist of the matter."[13] Ricketts's ability to conceptualize experiments that others could not, or had not, perhaps best reflects the impact of his training with leading European bacteriologists, for the actual techniques available to researchers were at that time quite simple. Pure strains of bacteria were obtained by culturing them on solid gelatin media. Experimental animals provided a means to isolate pathogenic bacteria from a sick animal as well as to show that a bacterial culture would produce a particular disease. In order to see microorganisms under the microscope—itself an indispensible bacteriological tool—common dyes and special stains were used on blood and tissue smeared on glass slides.[14]

A rudimentary knowledge of biochemical reactions facilitated the physiological study of bacterial metabolism, and theories of immunity informed attempts to produce vaccines, antisera, and diagnostic tests. The agglutination test, for example, was generally considered a reliable indicator of the presence of particular disease organisms. Blood was typically drawn from a person recently recovered from a disease, and a procedure known as defibrination was employed to speed clotting. After the clot was removed, the blood was centrifuged to separate the solid cells from the liquid. To the serum were added organisms suspected of causing the disease. The serum of the recovered patient contained antibodies, proteins produced by the body in response to the presence of foreign proteins, or antigens. Since antibodies bind to their complementary antigens, the serum would clump or agglutinate if the patient had suffered from the disease caused by the suspect organisms. Although exceptions were possible, such a reaction provided strong evidence for the presence of the disease under suspicion.

Skilled in such methods, Ricketts had already begun a microscopic study and culture experiments, and he was outlining future experiments by the time King arrived. Since Ricketts could find neither *Piroplasma* nor bacteria in the blood, and King's independent study confirmed that none was present, it seemed clear that the spotted fever organism was of a type that could be studied only in an experimental animal. Both Ricketts and King thus turned their energies to identifying an animal in which the disease could be easily recognized. Ricketts first attempted to inoculate rabbits with infected blood, but the results were inconclusive, two animals showing no signs of illness and a third only a slight fever.[15] If readily available rabbits were unacceptable models, funds would be needed to purchase other laboratory animals until a good model was identified. To this end, E. W. Spottswood addressed the Missoula Chamber of Commerce on 15 May, and nine days later the Missoula County commissioners appropriated one hundred dollars to fund the purchases. The Montana State Board of Health secretary, Thomas D. Tuttle, contributed an additional forty dollars from the board's appropriation.[16]

Ricketts and King worked independently, but they shared the small amount of blood available from spotted fever victims as they inoculated guinea pigs, monkeys, white rats, and mice purchased with the appropriated funds. Since the most favorable route for inoculation was unknown, the two men drew lots for subcutaneous and intraperitoneal injections. As it happened, both routes proved successful. Only the guinea pigs and monkeys, however, displayed a definitive feverish, or febrile, reaction. The less expensive guinea pig proved an ideal model of the disease in humans. It ran a marked fever, and the males displayed a swollen scrotum that became a characteristic sign of spotted fever infection. When Ricketts attempted to maintain the disease in guinea pigs, however, he had difficulty, but he was able to sustain the infection in animals by alternating injections in monkeys and guinea pigs. This achievement had far-reaching implications. It meant that he could study the disease year round, making research independent of the incidence of spotted fever cases. Identifying an acceptable, inexpensive experimental animal was, in Ricketts's evaluation, the most important work accomplished that spring.[17]

Once the reaction of guinea pigs was known to be a reliable indicator that the disease was present, Ricketts conducted experiments to determine whether the infectious agent was a microbe or a toxin and whether it was confined to the red blood cells of victims or was transmitted also by the serum of the blood. Short on blood from spotted fever victims, Ricketts discovered by chance on 11 June that a nine-year-old girl, Etta Bradley, was severely ill with the disease near Stevensville.[18] From her he obtained 60–70 cc of blood, some of which he centrifuged to separate the heavier red and white cells from the lighter serum. The solid cells were washed to remove any remaining serum, and samples of the serum and washed cells were injected into guinea pigs. Some of the serum, moreover, was passed through a ceramic Berkefield filter at low pressure. The small pores of such filters obstructed the passage of most microorganisms, but toxins and so-called filterable viruses passed through unimpeded. This filtered serum was also injected into a guinea pig.

All the guinea pigs suffered a fatal infection except for the one injected with filtered serum. This indicated that the infectious agent was not a toxin or filterable virus and that the microbe trapped by the filter should be large enough to be seen under a microscope. In addition, the infectiveness of both blood corpuscles and unfiltered serum demonstrated that the spotted fever microbe was not localized in one part of the body, as was true in tetanus, but rather circulated in the blood. The finding that serum was infective threw further doubt on Wilson and Chowning's *Piroplasma* theory, because those organisms were found almost exclusively in red blood cells.[19]

Ricketts sent a manuscript describing these experiments to the *Journal of the American Medical Association*, which published it in the issue of 7 July. Although these preliminary experiments were vital in making further work possible, they did not yet answer the question burning in everyone's mind: Was this spotted fever microbe transmitted by the bite of a tick? Both Ricketts and King began tick transmission experiments just as their stay in Montana ended. They fed ticks on infected guinea pigs and placed them on healthy guinea pigs. Both researchers got positive results from their experiments—thus demonstrating for the first time that a human disease in the United States could be transmitted by a tick. After returning to their laboratories in Chicago and Washington, Ricketts and King prepared papers on the experiment. King's paper, "Experimental Transmission of Rocky Mountain Spotted Fever by Means of the Tick," however, was published in the *Public Health Reports* eight days before Ricketts's paper on the subject appeared in the *Journal of the American Medical Association*.[20]

Having spent a good deal of his own money to finance the research as well as having conceived the experiment, Ricketts was annoyed at King's priority in publishing on this important question. "In view of the result which I had obtained," Ricketts wrote in his article, "I was not surprised to note the recent report of Dr. King, . . . who, starting with material which I had given him, accomplished transmission in the same manner."[21] Ricketts had already complained to the secretary of the Montana State Board of Health, Thomas D. Tuttle, about the necessity of several researchers sharing the limited quantity of available spotted fever blood. Admitting that it was "a little bit selfish on my part," Ricketts requested Tuttle to "limit the number of workers" on spotted fever in the Bitterroot the following season, a plea Tuttle had no power to enforce.[22] The incident with King caused Ricketts to exercise much more caution in sharing material or revealing the results of his research before publication.[23]

The results of the 1906 work infused new life into spotted fever investigations. In the same issue that announced the enactment of the first federal pure food and drugs law, the *Journal of the American Medical Association* commented editorially that Ricketts's and King's "extremely interesting and important work" would provide "a new impetus" to spotted fever research. Reflecting prevailing assumptions about arthropods and the types of organisms they might transmit, the editorial also observed that further experiments were necessary "to determine whether the infecting organism must undergo a cycle of development, as in the case with some organisms, notably the *Plasmodium malariae*."[24]

The secretary of the Montana State Board of Health was jubilant over Ricketts's discoveries but dismayed that the state legislature had not supported the undertaking financially. In his summary of the 1906 work, Tuttle remarked sarcastically that the "magnanimous" contribution of the state toward the purchase of experimental monkeys amounted to "the extravagant expenditure of forty dollars." To continue the work properly, he stated, the legislature should appropriate not less than fifteen hundred dollars, and preferably two thousand dollars. Ricketts had also urged the state to appoint a legislative study committee and to appropriate sufficient money to continue the investigation when he spoke in May 1906 at the Montana Medical Association.[25]

In his annual report, moreover, Tuttle broadened his crusade for increased funding to public health in general. He noted that the $2,000 budget of the state board of health was paltry compared to the generous increases given to other state boards—Massachusetts, for example, expended $96,500 per year; Minnesota, $20,000 per year; and even scantily populated Colorado, $5,000 per year. Raising the question of whether the legislature considered the life of a Montanan to be worth as much as that of a Bostonian, Tuttle challenged the lawmakers to increase funding for all public health measures, including spotted fever research. This emotional appeal apparently swayed state legislators, because they appropriated $2,000 for further work by Ricketts during 1907.[26]

The additional funds were certainly welcome, because the work of 1906 opened a promising new direction for spotted fever investigations that would require much additional research before the disease could be prevented or treated. The tick transmission experiments had to be repeated, since Ricketts and King had infected only a single guinea pig each. Furthermore, proof that the tick could transmit the disease in the laboratory did not demonstrate that infected ticks existed in nature. If such ticks did exist, virtually nothing was known about their life cycle or about the hosts from which they might contract the infection. In addition, although Ricketts had postulated that a visible microbe might cause the disease, no one had yet been able to locate it under the microscope or culture it in the laboratory.[27]

During the fall and winter of 1906–7, King and Ricketts continued their research on spotted fever in Washington and in Chicago. To enable their experiments to go forward, both needed a continuous supply of ticks. Each wrote to contacts in the Bitterroot, who enlisted local newspapers to advertise for people to collect ticks. Locating ticks after they disappeared in mid summer, however, was an almost impossible task. The *Western News,* believing that it was "worth something" to discover "where the ticks are in the winter," offered ten dollars in gold to the first person bringing "50 or more live, able-bodied ticks" to the newspaper office between 29 November and 15 December 1906. Even with this financial incentive, local tick sleuths were apparently baffled. No report announced that the gold had been claimed, and in mid December the paper advertised for ticks again, offering "two bits per head" for any number of able-bodied ticks.[28]

With the few ticks he was able to obtain, Ricketts continued his experiments in Chicago, where he was promoted to assistant professor in the Department of Pathology and Bacteriology.[29] Using a wire mesh collar he had designed to hold ticks in place on the guinea pigs, Ricketts conducted experiments to demonstrate that male as well as female ticks could transmit the disease. He had also hoped to settle the question of whether female ticks transmitted the spotted fever organism to their offspring. Unfortunately, the ticks failed to breed, so the experiment was postponed until the following spring. One major success crowned Ricketts's efforts during the cold Chicago winter: he solved the problem of how to preserve the spotted fever strain in guinea pigs alone. He had, of course, already managed to maintain the infection by alternating inoculations between guinea pigs and monkeys, but monkeys were expensive. In his first attempts with guinea pigs, Ricketts had taken blood from a dead or dying pig and inoculated it into a fresh one. The infectious agent, he discovered by repeated experiments, was most virulent during the height of the disease. With this information he was able to perpetuate the infection in guinea pigs alone by utilizing blood from a sick but not moribund guinea pig.[30]

Ricketts began the new season's work with the strain of spotted fever he had successfully sustained in guinea pigs. This proved fortunate, for spotted fever cases occurred only sporadically, and the families of victims did not always welcome a doctor whose primary interest was research. In 1907 the first case of spotted fever did not appear until mid April. It struck a twenty-six-year-old lumberman,

Maurice J. Holden, who was secretary-treasurer at the Florence lodge of the International Workmen of the World. Ricketts visited the patient, but Holden's family "objected to a thorough examination" and refused to allow Ricketts to draw any blood. When Ricketts apprised Tuttle of this situation, the secretary of the state board of health prepared an official-looking document instructing local people to cooperate with the investigation. He admonished Ricketts, however, not to present the document "where people are liable to look into it too closely," because in truth "we have no authority" to issue it.[31]

Walter W. King also returned to the Bitterroot in the spring of 1907, as did William M. Chowning, who continued to study the variety of organisms he found in spotted fever blood.[32] Ricketts and King resumed their studies, jointly visiting cases and drawing blood. Wary of King's competition, however, Ricketts conducted his experiments alone. "King and I have had no difficulty so far," Ricketts wrote to Ludvig Hektoen, but he characterized King as having "many questions to ask in his smooth 'governmental' fashion."[33]

Ricketts worked intensely on the question of whether female ticks could transmit spotted fever to their offspring. He worried that King might again publish first on this important question. In a letter to Hektoen, Ricketts noted that King had "sent ripened females to Washington," where "doubtless" King's colleagues would soon be "at work on these points." Ricketts's assistants also collected ticks from known spotted fever locales for experiments to determine if infected ticks existed in nature. Describing this work to Hektoen as the most important of all, Ricketts emphasized that this experiment in particular was the one he wanted "to get into print as soon as possible." Although King appeared to be conducting only small-scale research on this problem, Ricketts feared that it might be "just his luck" for King to get the answer first.[34]

For all Ricketts's foreboding, however, King's 1907 work resulted in no publications, and shortly after King returned to Washington, D.C., he was detached from the Hygienic Laboratory and ordered to San Francisco for duty. Since the laboratory director, Milton J. Rosenau, retained only the Service's most promising research scientists on his staff, it is possible that King's failure at least to match Ricketts's achievements indicated to Rosenau that King was more suited for other types of work. After leaving spotted fever investigations, King returned to his work as a quarantine officer, serving at San Francisco, Ellis Island, and Naples, Italy.[35]

After the 1907 spotted fever season, Ricketts had the field virtually to himself. His research was conducted on a variety of fronts, including efforts to identify the spotted fever organism and experiments with a potential antiserum and a vaccine against spotted fever. Realizing that effective therapeutic measures might take a number of years to develop, Ricketts devoted much of his time in 1907 and 1908 to understanding the relationship between spotted fever and the tick. Such knowledge, he hoped, would provide the basis for developing a practical program for controlling the tick, thereby reducing the incidence of the disease.

The question of possible hereditary transmission of the spotted fever organism was of vital importance. With the assistance of two students, Paul G. Heinemann and Josiah J. Moore, Ricketts devised an experiment in which sixty female ticks were fed on infected guinea pigs and then allowed to breed. Of these, twenty-six produced eggs. The larvae produced by each female were then placed on a healthy guinea pig to see if spotted fever had been transmitted to them by their mothers. The results of this tedious process, which required meticulous handling and record-keeping at each stage, were somewhat surprising. Of the twenty-six groups of larvae, only two infected the guinea pigs on which they fed. "If this was the result in twenty-six laboratory experiments," Ricketts wrote, "it is fair to conclude that . . . only a small percentage of infected females passes the disease on to their young" in nature. When Ricketts and his part-time colleague Maria B. Maver repeated these experiments, they achieved somewhat higher percentages of transmission.[36] The results were clear, however: hereditary transmission did occur, but only in a minority of cases. This finding, coupled with additional research that showed the salivary glands of the tick also to be infective, led Ricketts to conclude that spotted fever was probably a generalized infection of tick tissues that was transmitted biologically by the tick through biting.[37]

Determining whether infected ticks existed in nature—the work that Ricketts had been so anxious to publish—was likewise a tedious process. Each year from 1907 to 1909, Ricketts collected ticks and watched to see if any guinea pigs on which they fed became ill. As in the hereditary experiments, Ricketts found that only a small number of ticks contained the virulent organism, because most of the guinea pigs remained healthy. Convinced at last that his work was definitive, Ricketts wrote to Tuttle that three years of experiments should be "enough to prove to the satisfaction of everyone that infected ticks do occur naturally" but in small numbers.[38]

Having determined that the Rocky Mountain wood tick carried spotted fever, Ricketts assigned Maver the task of determining whether other ticks could carry the infection as well. Initially, Maver demonstrated that the tick carrying the mild Idaho spotted fever could also transmit the virulent Bitterroot Valley strain and, conversely, that the tick found in the Bitterroot could transmit the mild Idaho strain of the disease. During the summer and fall of 1909, Maver began experiments with the dog tick common to the eastern United States, the "lone star" tick common on cattle from Missouri to Texas and Louisiana, and a rabbit tick from Utah. All three ticks transmitted spotted fever to guinea pigs. "From these experiments," Maver wrote, "it appears that . . . the disease might find favorable conditions for its existence in localities other than those to which it now is limited." At this time there was concern that spotted fever might spread within the western United States but no indication that it might exist in other parts of North America.[39]

The life cycle of the Rocky Mountain wood tick was another problem to be solved before tick control could be implemented. From his brief observations over a single year, Ricketts provided an initial description of how ticks reproduced. After fertilization, which occurred on large host animals such as cattle and horses:

the female continues to feed for several days . . . and during this time enlarges very rapidly, until she is finally transformed into the large gray or slate colored tick. On the other hand, the male, after prolonged feeding, undergoes no more enlargement than would be caused by the distension of a good feed. The enlargement of the female is due partly to the quantity of blood it has ingested, but, in addition, the change is to be looked on as sexual. The ovaries become greatly developed and hundreds or even thousands of minute eggs begin their rather slow formation.

When the female has reached its greatest degree of enlargement, it drops from the animal and, after a rest of about two weeks or longer in cold weather, begins to lay eggs. The eggs are withdrawn from the anterior end of the lower surface of the body, the head parts assisting in their extrusion, and they accumulate in small masses on the back of the head. As their bulk becomes heavy they fall off and are replaced gradually by a second mass. This process continues until all the eggs, which may number several hundred or even two or three thousand, lie in a heap before the tick. In the meantime the female becomes greatly flattened and wrinkled and, in a comparatively short time dies. A female which has laid eggs never again assumes the appearance of the young red female and her life is ended in one season.[40]

The newly hatched six-legged larvae, Ricketts believed, fed on small animals, molted into eight-legged nymphs, and fed again. The nymphs then molted into sexually mature adults. Ricketts could not determine precisely how long this process took but noted that it was possible to speed it up in the laboratory by using incubators and providing immediately available hosts for each stage. He believed, however, that eggs deposited one year became adults capable of reproducing during the following spring.[41]

Working from an assumed twelve-month life cycle, which later would be shown to be incorrect, Ricketts attempted to formulate a program for control of the tick. Other arthropod-borne diseases that served as models for this effort were malaria, yellow fever, and Texas cattle fever. Yellow fever control efforts had clearly demonstrated that the *Anopheles* mosquito needed only to be reduced to a certain level to control the disease; it did not have to be eliminated.[42] Since Ricketts had already demonstrated that the percentage of ticks in nature infected with spotted fever was small, diminishing the total tick population promised a significant reduction in spotted fever cases.

One key intervention strategy was preventing adult ticks from reaching the large animals on which they fed and mated. If this could be accomplished, subsequent generations of ticks would never be born. The Texas cattle fever tick had been virtually eliminated by this method. Because that tick remained through its entire life cycle on a single animal, it had been possible to create tick-free pastures simply by removing stock. Ticks remaining on the ground starved for lack of a host. Once a pasture had been purged of ticks, stock from which all ticks had been carefully removed could be safely returned. A few years of alternating pastures in this manner effectively eliminated the Texas cattle fever menace. A second approach to tick control consisted of oiling the bodies of stock by hand or by dipping them in large vats several times during tick season. Oil was repugnant to ticks, repelling unattached ticks and causing those already attached to lose their hold. According to the Bureau of Animal Industry, moreover, oiling produced no permanent injury to the cattle and horses.[43]

Ricketts corresponded about these methods with an entomologist at the University of Tennessee Agricultural Experiment Station, H. A. Morgan, who had a great deal of experience in the control of Texas cattle fever. Because the spotted fever tick had different hosts at each stage of its life cycle, Morgan doubted that alternating pasturage would be effective. In his report to the Montana State Board of Health, therefore, Ricketts recommended that the state undertake a program of oiling to reduce the tick population in settled areas. "Total extermination of the tick cannot be promised or expected," Ricketts wrote, since wild animals in the mountains would continue to act as hosts. "But this does not mean that the territory inhabited by the residents must continue to be infested with ticks."[44]

These preliminary recommendations, which included the admonition that citizens also rid their premises of the ground squirrels that served as hosts to immature states of the tick, were based on the scanty information about the life cycle of the tick that Ricketts was able to gain in a few months' time. He advised that additional observations should be carried out year round, and he recommended entomologists M. J. Elrod of the University of Montana and Robert A. Cooley of the Montana State College as potential candidates.[45] In 1908, Cooley, whose work will be discussed in chapter 5, took up the study.

The first of two reports Ricketts prepared was written in a popular style and widely disseminated because many people in the Bitterroot continued to doubt the tick theory of spotted fever transmission. "It is absolutely necessary," Ricketts noted, for Bitterroot residents "to know something about the life history of the tick and its bearing on the question if they are to accept the tick theory."[46] Thus, in addition to his formal recommendations, Ricketts included practical information on dealing with tick bites. Countering superstitions about how one must approach an attached tick, Ricketts stated: "The tick, if attached, should be removed immediately, not by attempting to 'unscrew' it as is so often recommended, but by grasping the body firmly and pulling gently and continuously. . . . A sudden jerk is likely to tear the body from the head, leaving the latter imbedded in the skin. A drop of kerosene oil will cause the animal to loosen its hold."[47]

He also advised those bitten not to apply carbolic acid with the stopper of the bottle or by inverting the bottle over the wound. Such a procedure, Ricketts warned, was "both inefficient and dangerous" because it burned an excessive area of the skin. The actual point at which the tick inserted its fine toothed proboscis into the skin and deposited the spotted fever organisms was small. "The proper method of applying the carbolic acid," therefore, was "to dip a sharp pointed toothpick or splinter of wood into the acid . . . and then to thrust the tip deeply into the point of the bite, twisting the wood as it penetrates." The first application was rather painful, Ricketts admitted, but the acid had a tendency to destroy the sense of pain, and the second and third applications immediately following would cause only "a small degree of discomfort."[48]

Even this recommended method, however, carried no guarantee since, as Ricketts observed, "we have, as yet, no experimental evidence to show just how effective cauterization of the tick wound with carbolic acid is in preventing spotted fever." He doubted that any treatment was effective if the tick remained attached for several hours. "The virus in a short time probably extends too far for the acid to have any effect on it," he stated. Later experiments by his student, Josiah J. Moore, indeed demonstrated that within two hours, an attached tick could inject enough spotted fever organisms to cause the disease.[49]

Opinion remained divided in the Bitterroot about the tick theory, but businessmen supported Ricketts and hoped his findings could be used to stabilize land prices. In June 1907 a "woodtick dance" at Florence raised funds for burning brush in which ticks were plentiful. Real estate salesmen promoting sweet and sour cherries as well as apples to Chicago clients sought to minimize the impact of spotted fever on land sales with tangible proof that the entire valley was not affected. A representative of the Bitter Root Valley Irrigation Company asked Tuttle, the secretary of the state board of health, if he and Ricketts would prepare a joint statement that the west side of the valley alone was infected. The company planned to publish this document "for the purpose of furthering the sales of land." Ricketts and Tuttle complied, with the stipulation that their names be used "with due modesty and discretion."[50]

Although his plan to control ticks was of paramount importance, Ricketts also pressed forward in a number of other areas. One was identifying the elusive spotted fever organism. From the beginning of his work, Ricketts had tried to culture a bacterium with no success, although his filtration experiments had convinced him that the germ must be large enough to see with a microscope. He tried various staining methods, including the Giemsa and Levaditi stains, considered best for revealing parasites in the blood. With the Giemsa stain—the world's standard diagnostic agent for malarial organisms—Ricketts consistently found "small spherical, ovoid and diplococcoid forms," which seemed to be bacteria. To prove bacterial causation according to Koch's postulates, however, Ricketts had to culture the organisms on artificial media. Despite repeated attempts, he had not been successful.[51]

Ricketts therefore declined to publish a claim that the diplococcoid bodies were the cause of spotted fever. Prevailing scientific opinion, moreover, continued to support the belief that arthropods transmitted only protozoan organisms biologically. In a 1908 article reviewing the state of knowledge of ticks and disease, W. A. Hooker of the U.S. Bureau of Entomology outlined the piroplasmic diseases carried by ticks. Although he noted that the spotted fever organism remained unidentified, Hooker's evidence lent credence to the hypothesis that spotted fever would probably also be a *Piroplasma* or *Spirilla*—organisms known to be transmitted by ticks. Two years later, Rennie W. Doane, an assistant professor of entomology at Leland Stanford, Jr., University, published a popular book entitled *Insects and Disease*, in which he argued that, among parasitologists, spotted fever was "quite generally believed" to be carried by some sort of protozoan organism.[52]

Nonetheless, by January 1909, Ricketts was convinced that he had indeed identified the spotted fever microbe. His published description of the bacillus was conservatively entitled "A Micro-Organism Which Apparently Has a Specific Relationship to Rocky Mountain Spotted Fever: A Preliminary Report." He characterized the organism as "a bipolar staining bacillus of minute size, approximating that of the influenza bacillus [sic], although definite measurements have not yet been made." Agglutination experiments with the bacillus in tick eggs produced no reaction with the blood of normal guinea pigs, but the blood of immune guinea pigs—those which had recovered from a bout with spotted fever—produced the "striking result" of complete agglutination in dilutions of up to 1 to 320. "In so far as I know," Ricketts wrote, "it would be an unheard-of circumstance to obtain such strong agglutination with an immune serum, in the presence of negative controls, unless there were a specific relationship between the organism and the disease."[53]

Noting that he had employed reliable staining methods in searching for presumed *Piroplasma* or *Spirilla*, moreover, Ricketts argued that the organism of spotted fever showed bacterial, not protozoan, characteristics. In addition, he reiterated Charles Wardell Stiles's clinical findings that clearly differentiated spotted fever from the piroplasmoses.[54] "That a bacillus may be the causative agent of a disease in which an insect carrier plays an obligate role under natural conditions may be looked at with suspicion in some quarters," he observed, anticipating the reaction his preliminary communication might bring. "Yet . . . it would seem to be unscientific," he admonished his colleagues, "to be tied to the more or less prevailing belief that all such diseases must, on the basis of several analogies, be caused by parasites which are protozoon in character."[55]

Ricketts was cautious in his published statements, but to his friends he revealed complete assurance. "Just a note to tell you that I have found the microorganism of spotted fever," Ricketts wrote to Tuttle just before the *JAMA* article was published. "The eggs of infected female ticks are loaded with them," he added, describing the organism as "similar to the plague bacillus" but smaller. A distinguished Michigan bacteriologist, F. G. Novy, who had corresponded with Ricketts about staining techniques during his research, congratulated Ricketts and observed that the tick-bacillus connection, if proven, would overturn existing beliefs about arthropod vectors: "If you can clinch the story it will be a fine one which will kind of upset some of our cocksure friends." William M. Chowning, still unforgiving about Stiles's ridicule of his earlier work, was "more than pleased" that Ricketts had "placed the problem where Stiles will be compelled to backwater again."[56]

Feeling certain that he had identified the spotted fever organism, but also knowing that scientific proof as yet eluded him, Ricketts commented on his dilemma to Tuttle: "I remind you that we have not yet been able to cultivate [the microbe], and thus meet one of Koch's great laws. This makes it necessary to bring all kinds of indirect evidence to bear showing that we have the real thing." He promised Tuttle that the cultivation work would be continued until success was achieved "or until we have satisfied ourselves that it cannot be done." Ricketts placed much of the responsibility for these studies on Eugene Franklin McCampbell, a professor of bacteriology at Ohio State University, who in 1909 was a visiting lecturer at the University of Chicago. Interested in the challenge presented by this stubborn organism, McCampbell seemed to make headway against it; in November he wrote Ricketts that he had isolated a culture of the small diplobacillus that corresponded morphologically "exactly with that seen in the tick eggs and in the blood." It was so virulent, McCampbell claimed, that injections of water condensation in the culture tubes killed guinea pigs in twenty-four to thirty-six hours. Unfortunately, McCampbell did not describe his method, nor did he publish his results.[57]

Ricketts also utilized his specialized knowledge of vaccines and serum therapy in attempts to produce a prophylactic vaccine and a curative serum. As early as 1907 he had optimistically commenced vaccination experiments, "à la Pasteur." In using this phrase, Ricketts was referring to Louis Pasteur's empirical attenuation of the rabies virus by drying infected spinal cords of animals over a period of time, for no one had isolated the rabies pathogen when Pasteur worked. Assisted by his student Liborio Gomez, Ricketts similarly endeavored to attenuate the spotted fever organism. They desiccated it "over sulphuric acid" and planned a series of injections that would use increasingly "smaller quantities of virus which had been dried for shorter periods, passing finally to minute amounts of fresh virus."[58] Unfortunately, this method did not work; the organisms were either killed outright or remained completely infective.

Having determined that the minimum pathogenic dose of blood infected with spotted fever was between 0.01 and 0.03 cc for guinea pigs, Ricketts and Gomez next attempted to produce immunity by allowing animals to build up resistance to extremely small doses of the organism. This idea was also quickly abandoned. "As a rule," they noted, a minute quantity [of infected blood] either produces frank infection or causes no disturbance whatever. . . . On account of the uncertainty as to what the virus will do when injected in quantities which approximate the minimum pathogenic dose, it is manifest that minute doses cannot be utilized for practical vaccination."[59]

More promising experiments resulted from mixing small quantities of infected blood with "immune" blood—that is, blood from an animal that had recovered from spotted fever. Since it was known that a single infection with the disease produced lasting immunity—which was also passed to the offspring of immune females—Ricketts hypothesized that the immune blood would neutralize the live organisms sufficiently to prevent a fatal case of the disease and, at the same time, produce immunity in the inoculated animal. Experiments with guinea pigs demonstrated that this "sero-vaccination" was efficacious. Ricketts was cautious, however, about generalizing the findings from guinea pigs to humans. Observing that "the unknown susceptibility of man in comparison with that of the monkey and guinea pig" was a serious stumbling block to direct application of the technique to humans, he suggested, "Only one method could possibly be advocated at the outset; namely, to use such proportions of virus and immune serum as would leave no question as to the safety of the procedure, assuming for the time that the virus has the greatest possible virulence for man."[60]

Before this method could be pursued further, Ricketts made a discovery that stimulated a completely different approach toward producing a spotted fever vaccine. While examining the tissues and eggs of noninfective ticks used as controls in his experiments, Ricketts was astonished to find that many contained bacilli morphologically identical to the virulent organisms in infective ticks. These bacilli, moreover, would also agglutinate immune serum but not normal serum. "I have come to the conclusion," he stated, "that avirulent strains of the spotted fever microbe are to be found in nature in the tick." He realized, of course, that this point must be proved "in order to have the microbe above reproach in the eyes of scientific critics," but he also viewed the avirulent organisms as potentially the "nucleus of a successful vaccine."[61]

Ricketts asked Eugene Franklin McCampbell to conduct experiments on the vaccinating power of noninfective tick eggs. A shortage of guinea pigs slowed the new work to some extent, but results of initial experiments were promising. "We have a few experiments," Ricketts wrote to Ludvig Hektoen, "which indicate that vaccination takes place when the eggs or organs of ticks which contain avirulent bacilli are injected into guinea pigs." Ricketts hoped to bring this series of experiments to a conclusion during the winter of 1909–10.[62]

At the same time, Ricketts also pursued the development of an antiserum for treating those already ill with the disease. Elie Metchnikoff had pioneered serum therapy by producing an antitoxin in horses that would dramatically halt the ravages of diphtheria. Hoping to produce a similarly effective product for spotted fever, Ricketts began by "hyperimmunizing" a small group of guinea pigs and horses.[63] This was accomplished by injecting an animal that had recovered from spotted fever—and thereby had achieved immunity to it—with additional doses of the organism. Over a period of time, the animal's blood built up massive amounts of antibody to the pathogen. This process rendered the animal "hyperimmune" and, potentially, made its serum valuable as a treatment against an active case of the disease.

By the spring of 1908, Ricketts had produced an antiserum that protected guinea pigs against spotted fever if given a short time after infection. It was impossible, of course, to judge whether it would have any effect on humans, especially since it would have to be given in relatively large amounts. Moreover, information about anaphylaxis— the life-threatening allergic response that struck some people injected more than once with the foreign proteins in horse serum—was just becoming widely known. Writing to Thomas D. Tuttle, Ricketts noted a recently published article in the *Journal of the American Medical Association* dealing with anaphylaxis, but he expressed the opinion that large doses of his antiserum would carry no significant risk. "I have known over 1000 cc of horse serum, in the shape of tetanus antitoxin, to be given subcutaneously, intravenously, and subdurally, without producing any serious damage."[64]

Because of the high mortality from spotted fever in the Bitterroot Valley, Ricketts concluded that it would do no harm to test the serum on victims of the disease. During the spring of 1908 he administered the serum to nine spotted fever patients. Six of them, all extremely ill, died in spite of the treatment. In each of the three recoveries, there were circumstances that threw doubt on the efficacy of the serum. The disease was exceptionally mild from the beginning in a seven-year-old boy, who received 138 cc of the serum, and in one adult male, whose physician failed to keep records on the amount of serum administered. In the case of the child, moreover, it was widely known that children were more likely to recover than adults. A more typical case treated that spring occurred in an adult male, who received 120 cc of the serum over three days. Although the man lived, his recovery took two weeks. Ricketts doubted that the serum caused the recovery, observing that "there would be less difficulty in recognizing a curative effect of the serum if its injection were followed by a sudden subsidence of symptoms, such as antitoxin causes in diphtheria."[65]

In contrast to Ricketts's own conclusions, the local press judged that the serum had indeed saved the victims' lives.[66] It was hardly surprising that the relatives of spotted fever patients grasped at the promise of the serum and rarely worried about its proven efficacy. Because of this, Ricketts received numerous appeals in the spring of 1909 for additional quantities of his serum. Financial constraints had prevented him from producing additional batches, but he sent what he had on hand, even though it was old and had probably lost, in his estimate, 20 percent of its curative value. Since the efficacy of the serum had not been disproved, Ricketts was reluctant to deny it to those who sought it. "From the humanitarian standpoint," he wrote to Tuttle, "it seems that the serum should be supplied until it has been shown to be worth something or nothing." Ricketts also noted that his student Paul G. Heinemann was attempting to concentrate the serum as was done with diphtheria antitoxin to make it more effective.[67]

All of these lines of research were suspended or slowed down in 1909 because of one insurmountable obstacle: money. In 1907 the Montana state legislature had appropriated two thousand dollars for Ricketts's work, but it was completely used up during that year. In 1908 Missoula and Ravalli counties appropriated five hundred dollars each, and the state board of health contributed five hundred dollars, a total of fifteen hundred dollars that was also rapidly consumed. Ricketts and Tuttle also appealed to Idaho authorities for financial support, noting that spotted fever afflicted their citizens as well. It was a futile request. Idaho apparently felt no obligation to appropriate funds for what was perceived as Montana's unique problem.[68]

In March 1909 the Montana state legislature committed itself to continuing Ricketts's work through a special bill appropriating six thousand dollars for two years' investigations. Ricketts was gratified, observing to Tuttle that it was "quite a remarkable thing for a state legislature to fall in with the plans of the State Board of Health so harmoniously in the interests of public health."[69] Unfortunately, the state legislature had voted to expend more monies than would be collected in revenues. Since the Montana state constitution required a balanced budget, the task of reconciling revenues with outlays was given to the State Board of Examiners, the body appointed to oversee the state's finances. In order to assure funding of the essential state projects, authorized by public bills, the examiners suspended appropriations for all special bills enacted in 1909 until revenue was increased to cover them. Funds for the spotted fever investigations were not the only ones withheld; those for the state agricultural experiment station, for example, were similarly impounded.[70]

The examiners' decision came just before the 1909 tick season in the Bitterroot Valley. Miles Romney, proprietor of the *Western News*, informed Tuttle about an early spotted fever death that spring and pleaded with the state board of health, "in the interest of common humanity," to allow Ricketts's work to proceed. No large local subscription drive or appropriation, however, was undertaken to replace the impounded state money. To demonstrate appreciation for Ricketts's work, the University of Montana, at the urging of the Montana Medical Association, conferred on him an honorary degree at its 1909 commencement.[71]

Although no one was able to budge the State Board of Examiners from its fiscal decision, members of the state board of health suggested to Ricketts that if he could obtain funds from a private source, such as the university or the associated John Rockefeller McCormick Memorial Institute for Infectious Diseases, the funds would eventually be released and the state would pay him back.[72] For those institutions, however, the probability that Montana would raise the needed revenues was too uncertain to convince them that this would be a wise course of action. Ricketts's spotted fever work had earned him a gold medal from the American Medical Association as well as several offers of professorships from universities, and it was difficult for the rising research star to stop productive investigations until money again became available.[73]

During the summer of 1909, Ludvig Hektoen urged Ricketts to consider working on tabardillo, the Mexican typhus fever named for the rash that resembled a red cloak on its victims. This disease, Hektoen noted, had many characteristics in common with spotted fever, and neither its cause nor its means of transmission was known. Later noting that he would have declined or postponed his work on typhus had he "known surely that . . . [Montana authorities] would come up with the money," Ricketts decided that he must go forward in some line of research. Hektoen arranged for the Mexican government, the University of Chicago, and the Memorial Institute to share the financing of the project. Since the annual epidemics of tabardillo usually started in late autumn, Ricketts left for Mexico City in December 1909.[74]

Only after arriving in Mexico did Ricketts learn that a French researcher, Charles Nicolle, working in Tunis, Africa, had recently demonstrated the body louse as the vector of typhus. In addition, Hygienic Laboratory researchers John F. Anderson, who had investigated spotted fever in 1903, and Joseph Goldberger, who suffered a bout with typhus while studying it, had confirmed Nicolle's findings and succeeded in directly inoculating the typhus pathogen into monkeys. Gamely proceeding with his work even though he had lost the chance to claim priority, Ricketts and his student Russell M. Wilder also confirmed these findings. More importantly, they described an organism similar to the spotted fever organism that was consistently found in the blood of patients, in the lice that fed on these patients, and in the feces of the infected lice.[75]

Shortly after the new year, Thomas D. Tuttle, secretary of the Montana State Board of Health, received word that the State Board of Examiners had released the funds for spotted fever work. A relieved Ricketts, who had recently accepted a professorship at the University of Pennsylvania and was preparing to leave Chicago, wrote Tuttle that he hoped the 1910 work—a "pretty heavy piece of work" on "the role of the small wild animals"—would conclude his spotted fever investigations. Ricketts projected that he would be able to leave Mexico City by 20 April and would be in Montana in mid May. Tuttle, however, urged him to come even sooner, assuring him that the state would fund all necessary expenses, including the salaries of his assistants. "Employ such men as you need," Tuttle wrote, but "for goodness' sake get them out as soon as possible, as the weather is getting very warm and the ticks are coming out."[76]

From his lodgings at the American Club in Mexico City, Ricketts wrote to his student Josiah J. Moore, instructing him to proceed to Montana, but Ricketts himself continued to work on tabardillo. The work was dangerous, for the tiny lice that had been implicated as the vectors of the disease were often difficult to detect. Ricketts avoided the hospital in which typhus patients were treated. The medical staff, he observed, were "very filthy in the care of their patients," and living lice could be found in the bed linens of victims "almost any day." Except for comments to trusted scientific colleagues, Ricketts said little of the peril in which he worked. "Mrs. Ricketts is more or less worried now," he confided to one friend, "and if she should learn about . . . [the hospital conditions], I think I should have to go home in order to quiet her fears."[77]

In mid April, Ricketts did become infected with typhus. Russell M. Wilder communicated this unfortunate turn of events to Tuttle but added optimistically, "I have every reason to believe that Dr. Ricketts will make a safe recovery from his illness." Ricketts was only thirty-nine and, like Goldberger before him, should probably have been able to fight off the disease. Throughout the fall of 1909, however, Ricketts referred to an unnamed illness that periodically plagued him and possibly lowered his resistance. On 3 May 1910 he succumbed to typhus in Mexico. In Montana the news was grimly received. "In the midst of his experiments," said the *Daily Missoulian*, "the man, beloved in Montana and honored in the world of learning, was stricken by the very ailment for which he sought a remedy."[78]

Ricketts's death brought spotted fever investigations to an abrupt halt. Tuttle wired Josiah J. Moore, who had already arrived in the Bitterroot and established a camp, to make up a statement of expenses and return to Chicago. Since the Montana state legislature had appropriated funds specifically for Ricketts's use, not even Moore—a Montana native of "exceptionable ability" who had worked with Ricketts for three years on spotted fever—was authorized to carry on the investigations.[79] A few experiments already underway were published, many in a memorial volume prepared by Ricketts's colleagues and students.[80] Tuttle corresponded in vain with several of Ricketts's associates, hoping that they might continue the work.[81] Without the leadership of the dynamic Ricketts, however, laboratory experimentation on spotted fever virtually ceased.

In the short space of three years, Howard Taylor Ricketts had redirected scientific thinking about Rocky Mountain spotted fever. Moving beyond the dogma surrounding arthropod transmission of disease, he demonstrated that spotted fever was indeed tick borne and that infected ticks existed in nature. His studies of the tick produced a plan for controlling the pests and their mammalian hosts. With relentless persistence, he pursued techniques for producing a vaccine and antiserum against the disease. Trusting his experimental observations, Ricketts refused to be discouraged by his inability to culture the spotted fever organism in accordance with Koch's postulates. Although his untimely death cut short further work, each line of research was productively followed by his successors in spotted fever work. Ricketts's contributions were recognized by his scientific peers when the group of diseases to which spotted fever and typhus belong was named *rickettsial* in his honor. For the people of the Bitterroot Valley, his expertise and imagination provided not only a hope, unfulfilled, for an effective antiserum, but also a focus, the tick, for efforts against the dread disease.

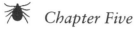 *Chapter Five*

Tick Eradication Efforts, 1911-1920

When the devil made the tick, he overlooked a bet in not giving it wings.
Bitterroot Valley rancher, 1919

If the first decade of spotted fever research in the Bitterroot Valley belonged to bacteriologists, the second decade clearly was dominated by entomological control methods. Since no effective medical preventive or therapy had been developed for spotted fever, an attack on the tick itself seemed the only immediate hope of ridding the valley of its scourge. Texas cattle fever was being controlled in the southern states with a rigorous vector control program, Major William Crawford Gorgas of the U.S. Army had dramatically demonstrated in Havana that yellow fever could be halted with mosquito control methods, and the U.S. Public Health and Marine Hospital Service had suppressed bubonic plague epidemics in San Francisco and New Orleans by attacking fleas and their host rats. These successful campaigns inspired hope that spotted fever could be eliminated in a similar manner.

It was not until the late nineteenth century that ticks were identified as carriers of pathogenic microorganisms, but they had been recognized as unwelcome parasites at least as early as 550 B.C., when Homer described the sufferings of an infested dog. The misery-causing potential of ticks was somewhat offset by allegedly therapeutic qualities for which they were valued. In ancient Chinese medicine white cattle ticks were ground with rice powder, formed into cakes, and administered to children as a preventive for smallpox. Galen and other authorities of late antiquity, whose medical opinions continued to dominate the thought of the Middle Ages, recommended the crushed bodies of ticks for a variety of medical problems. Used as a paste or taken in wine, ticks were employed as aphrodisiacs and used to clean ulcerations, to arrest menstruation, to prevent the regrowth of unwanted hair, and to treat anal fistula.[1]

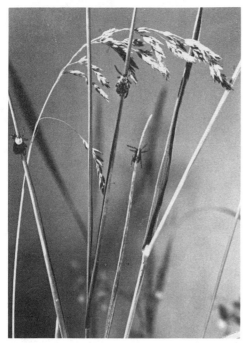

Ticks waiting on vegetation
for a host to pass by.
(Courtesy of the Rocky
Mountain Laboratories,
NIAID.)

From the Renaissance until the nineteenth century, ticks were rarely mentioned in medical treatises. By the time Theobald Smith and Fred L. Kilbourne discovered that the cattle tick transmitted a pathogenic protozoan organism, however, zoology had become a flourishing enterprise in universities, hence much was already known about ticks themselves. In zoological classification schemes ticks resided in the phylum *Arthropoda*, comprised of creatures having segmented bodies with paired jointed appendages and an exoskeleton. Containing more species than all other phyla combined, the arthropods encompassed insects, centipedes, crabs, lobsters, mites, and scorpions as well as ticks. Ticks, mites, and scorpions—arthropods having eight legs, no wings or antennae, simple eyes, if any, and a fused head and thorax—were further subdivided into the class *Arachnida*. Within this class, the order *Acarina* included ticks and mites but excluded scorpions. Ticks alone were placed into the superfamily *Ixodoidea*, which contained two families, the *Argasidae* and the *Ixodidae*. These were commonly known as soft ticks and hard ticks, respectively, because the latter possessed a shield or scutum that partially covered their backs.

Among the hard ticks, the *Dermacentor* genus was widespread in the United States and contained many species.[2]

When first suspected of transmitting Rocky Mountain spotted fever, ticks were generally described in nonspecific terms. In their initial 1902 report, Louis B. Wilson and William M. Chowning spoke of spotted fever as a disease carried by "a tick."[3] They sent specimens to zoologist Charles Wardell Stiles at the Hygienic Laboratory of the U.S. Public Health and Marine Hospital Service in Washington, D.C., for his expert determination, as did John F. Anderson the following year. Possibly influenced by Wilson and Chowning's claim that a *Piroplasma* was the cause of spotted fever, Stiles provisionally determined that the tick was *Dermacentor reticulatus*, the same tick that transmitted a piroplasmic disease to dogs. The zoologist stipulated, however, that further study was necessary for a definite determination because of certain differences he had observed between the Rocky Mountain wood tick and *D. reticulatus*.[4] When Stiles published the report of his own investigation into spotted fever, he called the tick *Dermacentor andersoni*. This new name, by which he honored his colleague John F. Anderson, implied that the tick was a separate species. Stiles mentioned the name only once, however, and he provided no description of uniqueness. Both Walter W. King and Howard Taylor Ricketts called the tick used in their transmission experiments *Dermacentor occidentalis*, which was actually a common California tick. Ricketts continued to use this name until 1909.[5]

In June 1908, Nathan Banks, a specialist on ticks with the U.S. Bureau of Entomology, seemed to resolve the confusing nomenclature when he published "A Revision of the Ixodoidea, or Ticks, of the United States," describing and defining the Rocky Mountain wood tick as *Dermacentor venustus* (Banks).[6] Less than a month later, however, Stiles refuted Banks's claim, maintaining that *D. venustus* was a Texas tick with different characteristics and that his 1905 designation, *D. andersoni* (Stiles), should be retained. In August 1910, Stiles published a detailed scientific study on the value of microscopic structural differences in choosing names for *Dermacentor* ticks. This new research, Stiles argued, proved his designation *D. andersoni* beyond doubt. Banks, in contrast, continued to support his claim that *D. venustus* was the identical tick and that his 1908 published description established priority.[7]

After 1910 the inconclusive war of names stalemated. Entomologists continued to call the tick *D. venustus*, and physicians from Stiles's agency, the U.S. Public Health and Marine Hospital Service, always referred to *D. andersoni*. Reports from the two groups appeared side by side in official Montana publications, utilizing the two different names without explanation or apology to the lay reader, who must have been somewhat confused if not familiar with the controversy.[8] In 1923 the question was submitted to the International Commission on Zoological Nomenclature, an official body created to resolve such disputes. Although a member, Stiles did not vote because of his personal involvement in the case. Declining to judge which tick carried the disease, the commission took a narrow approach to the types of specimens represented by Stiles's and Banks's names. The majority opinion declared that *Dermacentor venustus* belonged to a form with a Texas tick as a holotype and that *Dermacentor andersoni* belonged to a form with a tick from Woodman, Montana, as the holotype. Since spotted fever was unknown in Texas at that time, *D. andersoni* became the official name for the spotted fever tick.[9]

This taxonomic tempest embodied on a superficial level a deeper internecine rivalry between physicians and entomologists. Before the link between arthropods and disease had been established, each group's areas of expertise seemed clearly defined: physicians treated sick people; entomologists primarily assisted farmers in eliminating crop-destroying insects. A relatively new professional group, entomologists were still struggling to establish a separate identity from zoology, their older and broader parent discipline.[10]

During the earliest period of white settlement of North America, there had been no need for such specially trained scientists because indigenous insects rarely caused problems for farmers. After the American Revolution, however, the gradual normalization of trade led to the importation of foreign plants, some of which harbored injurious insects that multiplied rapidly. Individual states began to employ entomologists during the 1840s, and in 1854 the U.S. Patent Office employed a person to collect statistics on seeds, fruits, and insects. Specialists in entomology were few and the literature sparse throughout the 1860s, even though the 1862 act establishing the Department of Agriculture boosted the status of entomologists by authorizing their employment to provide useful information for farmers. The 1874–76 flight of locusts from Montana and the Dakotas as far south as Missouri focused additional attention on the devastation that insects could cause and led to the formation of a federal entomological commission to study the depredations of the locusts. In 1887, partly as a result of the commission's reports, Congress authorized the establishment of agricultural experiment stations that included specialists in entomology.[11]

The development of graduate programs in universities and the establishment of professional societies, such as the Association of Economic Entomologists, founded in 1889, also advanced entomology as a profession. Post–Civil War industrialization and urbanization enhanced this trend, altering traditional cultural patterns and fostering the development of expert knowledge in a variety of fields. The term *medical entomology* was coined in 1909 for the specific study of arthropods and disease, but actual professional differentiation remained far from rigid.[12] Zoologists interested in all forms of parasitism studied arthropods as well as worms, bacteria, and protozoa. With the discoveries in the 1890s that arthropods could transmit pathogenic microorganisms to animals and humans, veterinarians, physicians, and public health researchers also became interested in the field. As these groups pursued overlapping goals, professional rivalries often marred the more altruistic aim of selfless devotion to the advancement of science.

Physicians, who had a much longer professional history than most other groups and whose status was rising with each new bacteriological triumph, were often accused of ignoring or subordinating the contributions of other professions.[13] For human diseases, physicians countered such criticism with the observation that they alone were properly trained to apply specialized knowledge to a public health problem. Because Rocky Mountain spotted fever was transmitted by ticks, both physicians and entomologists were interested in its control. Unfortunately, a bitter power struggle developed between the two groups in Montana that reverberated to the federal level and retarded coordination of the effort.

Initially this struggle centered on two strong-willed men, Thomas D. Tuttle, secretary of the Montana State Board of Health, and Robert A. Cooley, the Montana state entomologist. Tuttle, who had fought for increased funding for public health and had vigorously enforced local health ordinances, assumed after the death of Howard Taylor Ricketts that the Montana State Board of Health would continue to direct the attack on Rocky Mountain spotted fever. In March 1911 he appealed to Surgeon General Walter Wyman of the U.S. Public Health and Marine Hospital Service to send a new researcher who could utilize state funds appropriated for spotted fever research. Wyman stalled, citing the heavy demands on Service officers. After continued appeals from Tuttle and Montana Senators Paris Gibson and Henry L. Myers, however, Wyman relented and in mid May detailed Passed Assistant Surgeon Thomas B. McClintic to Montana.[14]

A thirty-eight-year-old graduate of the University of Virginia Medical School and twelve-year veteran Service officer, McClintic had considerable experience in quarantine work, both in the United States and abroad, including "the usual tour of duty of officers in the tropics." During several periods when he was stationed at the Hygienic Laboratory, McClintic had been found to have a "special fitness for research work," and it was the combination of field experience and laboratory expertise that induced Wyman to select him as the officer who would tackle the mysterious spotted fever. During the summer of 1911, McClintic hoped to demonstrate the practicability of preventing spotted fever in the limited area around Victor, Montana, using tick control principles outlined by Ricketts.[15]

On his way to the Bitterroot, McClintic stopped in Bozeman, Montana, to consult with Cooley, the state entomologist, who had been researching the life cycle and habits of the tick. To his surprise, McClintic found that Cooley had already raised a subscription to construct an experimental dipping vat for tick control in the Florence area, about fifteen miles north of Victor. This project, Cooley noted, was actually funded and staffed by representatives of the U.S. Bureau of Entomology and the U.S. Bureau of Biological Survey. When McClintic and Tuttle arrived in Florence three days later to assess the situation, they were utterly astonished to discover Cooley in the field, supervising the project himself.[16]

Having known nothing about the experimental dipping vat and, perhaps more importantly, having expended great effort to persuade the U.S. Public Health and Marine Hospital Service to resume spotted fever work, Tuttle experienced embarrassment that rapidly turned to fury. It appeared clear to him that the entomologists were meddling in a public health matter.[17] Tuttle and other members of the Montana State Board of Health immediately undertook efforts to force the perceived interlopers out of spotted fever work, but Cooley proved as adamant as Tuttle, and the hostility between the two men intensified.

Robert A. Cooley, the focus of Tuttle's concern, was born on 27 June 1873 in Deerfield, Massachusetts. After receiving a B.S. degree in 1895 from Massachusetts Agricultural College, Cooley completed four additional years of graduate work in the pioneer entomological graduate school of that institution.[18] Before fulfilling all the requirements for his Ph.D., however, he accepted a position as professor of zoology and entomology at the Montana State College in Bozeman. Since the college housed the state agricultural experiment station, Cooley also assumed duties as the station entomologist. In 1903 he helped write legislation that conferred upon the agricultural station entomologist the additional title of Montana state entomologist. A man who inspired intense loyalty in his friends and students, Cooley, like

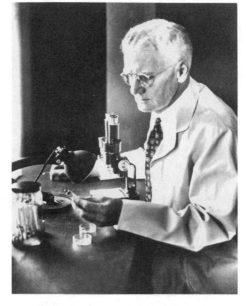

Robert A. Cooley, secretary of the Montana State Board of Entomology, championed livestock dipping to eliminate the spotted fever tick from the Bitterroot Valley. He hoped to repeat the success of southern entomologists who had controlled Texas cattle fever, another tick-borne disease, by this method. (Courtesy of the Rocky Mountain Laboratories, NIAID.)

Tuttle, had a stubborn streak that made him unwilling to compromise when facing someone he perceived as an adversary.

Cooley first entered spotted fever work as a result of Ricketts's recommendation that the Montana State Board of Health locate an entomologist to launch long-range, year-round studies of the spotted fever tick. Having no idea that conflict lay ahead, Tuttle logically sought assistance from the state entomologist. In 1908, Cooley and his student Willard V. King began to study Montana ticks in a noninfected area near Bozeman and formulated plans to repeat Ricketts's work on the tick's life cycle. Ricketts, who was not entirely pleased that Cooley chose to repeat these experiments, commented to Tuttle that Cooley seemed little inclined "to concede that the direction of his work should be guided by my results and conclusions." Cooley's efforts to raise a separate fund from Missoula and Ravalli counties for entomological work on spotted fever, Ricketts continued, also suggested that Cooley "was inclined to carry on his work independently." Tuttle had found Cooley unwilling to allow the report on his 1908 work to be incorporated in the state board of health's biennial report. Cooley preferred to publish it with his own report as state entomologist since the work had been done with funds from that office.[19]

During the winter of 1908–9, Cooley traveled to Washington, D.C., and consulted with representatives of the U.S. Bureau of Entomology, who had already sponsored a tick survey of the northwest states in which Willard V. King had participated. Since the range of the Rocky Mountain wood tick was found to extend from the northern edge of New Mexico to Canada and from California's Cascade range to the western Great Plains, plans were laid for a collaborative study between the U.S. Bureau of Entomology and the U.S. Bureau of Biological Survey, the federal agency charged with wildlife surveys and control of animal pests, to investigate further the hosts and habits of the disease-bearing tick.[20] During the spring of 1910, while the Montana State Board of Health awaited Ricketts's arrival only to be devastated by news of his death, Cooley established a field station in the Bitterroot Valley on Sweeney Creek, southwest of Florence, an area known to be infected with spotted fever. Calling the station Camp Venustus after Nathan Banks's designation of the spotted fever tick, Cooley assembled three representatives from federal agencies to conduct the study: Willard V. King from the U.S. Bureau of Entomology and Arthur H. Howell and Clarence Birdseye from the U.S. Bureau of Biological Survey. Birdseye, who later developed a technique for freezing foods and launched the company that bears his name, was embarking on his first practical research as a young college graduate. Howell, the group's senior member, returned east after a short time. Purportedly, King and Birdseye, seeking first-author privileges on the publications that were expected to result, employed an elaborate practical joke to scare Howell into believing that he had been bitten by a potentially infected tick.[21]

In order to protect themselves, King and Birdseye developed a number of methods that became standard procedure for field studies of spotted fever. They wore high-topped shoes to which were attached pieces of khaki cloth fastened by drawstrings higher up on the leg. To their cotton outer garments, they applied kerosene as a tick repellent, a measure that seemed to be useful, at least until the kerosene evaporated. At night they fumigated their clothing in an airtight closet with bisulphide of carbon. On the basis of Josiah J. Moore's research that an infected tick had to feed for nearly two hours in order to transmit spotted fever, the men regularly conducted rigorous examinations of their bodies within that time period. This regimen proved successful: although occasional bites occurred, neither of them contracted spotted fever.[22]

King and Birdseye sought to determine more precisely the life cycle of the tick and to identify its hosts in each stage. Using a white woolen or flannel cloth attached to a pole like a flag, King collected ticks from brush. Birdseye shot and trapped 717 small wild animals—thereby incurring the wrath of the game warden—and collected 4,495 addi-

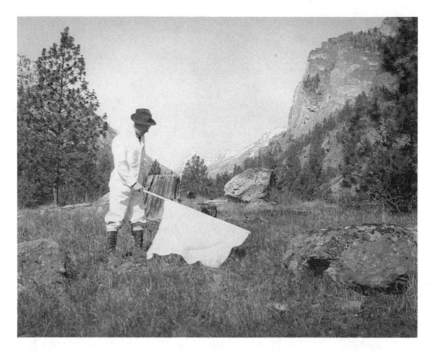

Flagging for ticks in the Bitterroot Valley. The flannel flags, dragged across brush vegetation favored by ticks, were used to obtain ticks for entomological studies and for spotted fever vaccine production. The collector protected himself by tucking his pants into his boots, by wearing long-sleeved clothing, and by inspecting his body at regular intervals. (Courtesy of the Rocky Mountain Laboratories, NIAID.)

tional ticks.[23] Samples of different species were sent to the Dallas, Texas, station of the U.S. Bureau of Entomology to be reared and identified. King's studies established that the spotted fever tick did not complete its life cycle in one year, as Ricketts believed, but instead had at least a two-year life cycle, spending the winter either as an adult or as a nymph. Birdseye determined that the immature stages of the tick fed on a variety of small animals while the adult ticks fed exclusively on large animals such as horses, cows, sheep, and goats. When he assessed these findings, Cooley concluded that the spotted fever tick might be eliminated like the Texas cattle fever tick—by preventing adults from reaching a host on which to feed and breed. Birdseye's observation that adult ticks fed only on large animals, moreover, suggested that destroying the small rodents that served as hosts to the larval and nymphal tick stages might be completely unnecessary.[24]

As this work was being completed, Tuttle was preparing the biennial report of the state board of health. Perhaps wishing to include some positive note on progress in spotted fever research to lessen the impact of Ricketts's death, Tuttle again invited Cooley to incorporate a full or summary report of the entomological work, or, at a minimum, a mention that cooperative work was taking place. On the advice of W. D. Hunter of the U.S. Bureau of Entomology, however, Cooley again chose to publish his findings separately.[25]

During the fall and winter of 1910, Cooley sought funds to implement a tick control program from Governor Edwin L. Norris and from W. E. McMurry, Ravalli County's representative to the Montana state legislature. Cooley asserted that the execution of his plan was "purely an Entomological matter" and asked for ten thousand dollars over two years either for the use of the state entomologist or for the state board of health with the specification that the money was for tick eradication under the direction of the state entomologist. Although neither state official seemed inclined to support this request, Cooley intimated to several people that Tuttle might be persuaded to turn over all or a portion of the two-thousand-dollar state board of health appropriation to him for tick eradication work. After the incident with McClintic, however, Tuttle would scarcely have allocated Cooley a dime.[26]

With no state money available, Cooley's 1911 program went forward under continued funding from the U.S. Bureaus of Entomology and Biological Survey. Stationed at an abandoned saloon in Florence, King conducted experiments to determine how long ticks could survive without feeding, and Birdseye, who maintained that rodent destruction was indeed necessary, developed an improved formula of poisoned rolled oats.[27] In King's longevity experiments, conducted outside Florence at the same cabin on Sweeney Creek used the year before, ticks were placed in tubes in the ground. A plug of earth in the bottom prevented their escape but ensured contact with ground moisture. Although a "man and animal proof fence" was built and a caretaker hired, the experiment was judged by Tuttle to constitute a menace to the surrounding citizenry, and Cooley, on the advice of his superior at the college, reluctantly removed them.[28]

In May 1911, just before McClintic arrived in the Bitterroot, Cooley published an outline for control of spotted fever based primarily on the 1910 investigations. His principal recommendation appeared in boldface type: "The key to the situation seems to be the destruction of ticks on domestic animals only." Montana newspapers did not miss the implication of this statement, and the headline of one paper pro-claimed, "Cooley Sounds the Key Note to Spotted Fever Eradication."[29]

For Tuttle the cumulative effects of Cooley's actions inspired outrage. The newspaper headlines indicated that Cooley was arrogating to himself the program outlined in 1908 by Ricketts, whom Tuttle ad-mired greatly. Cooley's longevity experiments implied disregard for public safety. When these offenses were added to Cooley's persistent attempts to establish and fund a separate entomological program for spotted fever eradication—not to mention the embarrassment over the incident when McClintic arrived—Tuttle and his colleagues on the state board of health determined that strong action was necessary. At its meeting on 5 June, the state board passed a resolution asking Cooley's employer, the state board of education, to instruct the en-tomologist that he should cooperate with the work of the state board of health already in progress.[30]

Apparently nothing came of this request and the situation escalated, for Tuttle called a special meeting of the board of health 24 July. He read a prepared statement outlining in detail Cooley's high crimes and misdemeanors. In addition to the other charges, Tuttle noted that in 1910, Cooley had conducted experiments in his laboratory at Montana State College with spotted fever–infected ticks. The four guinea pigs used in the investigation had died, but Cooley had not suspected spotted fever because their temperatures had not risen precipitously. Only when he examined the body of the last dead guinea pig did Cooley notice a rash and the characteristic hemorrhagic scrotum. Tuttle cited this incident as a dangerous venture into work that should have been done only by a physician. "Playing with dynamite on a platform where there are fireworks being discharged is a mild experiment compared with that of working with infected ticks in a school or college by one who is not able to detect such a fatal disease as spotted fever." The board, already incensed, resolved to raise the matter more strongly with the state board of education. "We must uphold Dr. McClintic in every way," asserted the board president, William Treacy, "and if necessary fire this man Cooley."[31]

The battle between Cooley and Tuttle, which was peppered with rumors of wildly intemperate remarks by both men, spilled over to the federal level when the Montana State Board of Health appealed to the U.S. Public Health and Marine Hospital Service and Cooley appealed to the U.S. Bureau of Entomology to clarify jurisdiction in spotted fever work. L. O. Howard, chief of the U.S. Bureau of En-tomology, contacted Surgeon General Walter Wyman, but to no avail. Commenting to Cooley that he had run "up against a stone wall,"

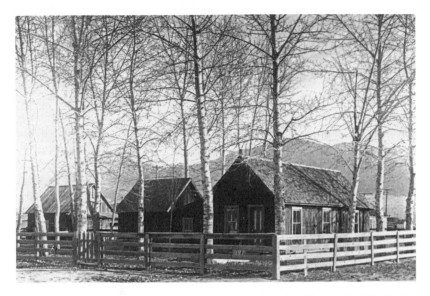

Buildings in Victor, Montana, used as a laboratory by Thomas B. McClintic and Lunsford D. Fricks of the U.S. Public Health Service from 1911–16. (Courtesy of the Rocky Mountain Laboratories, NIAID.)

Howard observed that the U.S. Public Health and Marine Hospital Service saw "no necessity for any cooperation whatever" and apparently felt "perfectly competent to handle the whole matter."[32] Having successfully employed insect and rodent control measures to suppress other arthropod-borne diseases, the Service doubtless believed that its officers had sufficient expertise to oversee the dipping of livestock and the destruction of small rodents in Montana. Moreover, since all officers were physicians, they could also employ bacteriological techniques in the study of the disease organism itself and offer medical assistance to the victims of spotted fever. As a result of this federal-level interchange, the U.S. Bureau of Entomology withdrew its support from Cooley's work at the end of the 1911 season. The animosity generated by the episode, however, remained.

While this political storm raged around him, Thomas B. McClintic initiated his own spotted fever research. Using funds appropriated by the Montana state legislature, McClintic hoped to test the feasibility of eradicating the tick in infected territories, to continue Ricketts's work of testing the susceptibility of the wild mammals to experimental inoculation with spotted fever, and to search for the infection among the wild mammals in nature. McClintic worked in a heavily infected district near Victor bounded on the north by Sweathouse Creek and on the south by Bear Creek. This was the territory in which Ricketts had found infected ticks in nature, and which, because of the presence of the disease, had become almost depopulated.[33]

Because McClintic did not arrive until the latter part of May, it was quite late in the season to begin the work. Nonetheless, he determined to proceed, hoping to continue the work on a broader scale the following year. In his plan for tick eradication, McClintic rejected the idea that dipping alone would accomplish tick eradication in the Bitterroot, because, he said, "both in point of numbers and variety of species the fauna of the valley is excelled by very few other localities of similar size in the United States, and most of the mammals, both wild and domestic, harbor the tick in one form or another."[34]

McClintic oversaw construction of a $520 concrete vat for dipping livestock, which was made according to plans published by the Department of Agriculture and was similar to the vat used in Florence by the U.S. Bureau of Entomology. Nine feet deep, about five feet wide, and thirty-eight feet long at the water line, it was filled with approximately twenty-five hundred gallons of arsenical dipping fluid to a depth of five and one-half feet. This sufficed to immerse all stock, except for exceptionally large horses.[35] Arriving at the vat, stock were herded into a corral and then driven individually up a ramp and onto a boiler-metal slide that sloped downward into the vat itself. After immersion, the stock were dried in dripping pens before being returned to pasture.

Because corralling and driving the stock into the vat could be difficult, a seasoned stock handler was essential. During the farmers' busy season, moreover, yet another person was needed to bring stock in from the surrounding farms. Most stock owners cooperated, McClintic observed, but a few, "as is usually the case in undertakings in the interest of the public health," objected to having anything done that caused "any inconvenience or work." By the middle of June the vat was completed, and dipping began under the supervision of McClintic and his assistant William Colby Rucker, who had recently arrived. Initially, 116 horses, 199 cattle, and 108 sheep were dipped. Two weeks later, on 3 July, redipping was begun, but "as the stock . . . was found to be practically free from ticks," only 38 horses, 57 cattle, and 60 sheep were dipped again.[36]

In addition to the dipping program and recommendations for clearing and cultivation of land, McClintic and Rucker launched a campaign to destroy the wild mammals on which the immature stages of the tick fed. The pine squirrel, yellow-bellied chipmunk, wood rat, woodchuck, weasel, and badger were all targeted in this program, but the local ground squirrel, *Citellus columbianus*, was believed to be by far the most significant pest in the valley. Of 3,465 animals shot or trapped during the 1911 season, 3,233 were ground squirrels. An uncounted number of other animals were killed with poisoned oats or with carbon bisulphide placed in their burrows, a method employed successfully against ground squirrels in the Service's antiplague campaign in California.[37]

McClintic and Rucker concluded their work in early August and moved their laboratory studies back to the Hygienic Laboratory in Washington, D.C. With the 1912 election approaching, they found politics as well as the weather heating up in the nation's capital. To the Democrats' delight, the split between President William Howard Taft and his predecessor Theodore Roosevelt was polarizing the Republican party. McClintic and Rucker's own agency was likewise embroiled in a political battle. A bill was before Congress to expand the authority of the U.S. Public Health and Marine Hospital Service, but another bill proposed to create a wholly separate department of public health. Surgeon General Wyman was busily promoting the Service's bill and maneuvering to thwart those who would challenge his agency's hegemony in the federal bureaucracy.[38]

In November the sixty-three-year-old Wyman died suddenly. Having served as surgeon general for twenty years, he was the only leader many Service officers could remember. McClintic interrupted his research to accompany Wyman's body to Saint Louis for burial. Ironically, Wyman's death breathed new life into a scaled-down version of his Service reform legislation. By the time McClintic and Rucker left for Montana in the spring of 1912, another bill was moving through Congress that proposed to shorten the name of the Service to the U.S. Public Health Service and to broaden its authority to conduct research.[39]

During the fall and winter of 1911–12, McClintic tested a number of drugs for their therapeutic properties against spotted fever. This work, which resulted in negative findings, will be examined more closely in chapter 10. The spring of 1912 held great promise for McClintic, both personally and professionally. On 2 March he married Theresa Drexel, and the following day the couple left for Montana to combine a honeymoon in the Bitterroot Valley with spotted fever research.[40] McClintic and Rucker continued the work begun in 1911, dipping livestock and killing small mammals. Their laboratory experiments were designed to study the natural history of the disease, the important work Ricketts had planned before his death from typhus.

The natural history experiments were tedious. Ground squirrels and most other small mammals showed no identifiable illness, hence an indirect method had to be employed. McClintic and Rucker would inoculate a wild animal with spotted fever, and after five days its blood was injected into a guinea pig. Another waiting period followed, during which the guinea pig was observed for symptoms of the disease. If it became ill, the original animal was judged to be susceptible to experimental inoculation with spotted fever. If the guinea pig remained well, a final test was made by inoculating it with virulent spotted fever blood. If the guinea pig again remained healthy, the experiment was inconclusive because it was judged to have been immune to spotted fever from the outset. If the guinea pig succumbed, however, the original mammal was declared to have acquired immunity from an earlier infection in nature.[41]

By this time-consuming method, McClintic determined that, in addition to ground squirrels, weasels, woodchucks, and mountain goats were susceptible to the disease. Many other animals were tested with negative results. Badgers, for example, could be experimentally infected, but infection was slight and infrequent. Since the spotted fever tick had never been observed feeding on a badger, moreover, the animal could practically be eliminated as a potential reservoir in nature.[42]

Locating immune ground squirrels in nature was one key to identifying them as a significant mammalian reservoir of the disease. During the 1911 season, McClintic had experimented with 21 ground squirrels from the heavily infected Victor area, but the results were inconclusive. In 1912 he expanded the experiments, using 194 ground squirrels. Of these, 34 again gave questionable results and had to be discarded. Among the 160 remaining ground squirrels, McClintic found 40 to be naturally immune. When the ground squirrels were grouped according to the locality from which they were collected, a higher percentage of immune squirrels was found in highly infected spotted fever areas.[43]

Another major line of research focused on a large-scale study of infective ticks in nature. McClintic collected nearly 2,000 ticks from different localities in the Bitterroot and from Bannock County, Idaho. His results were similar to those obtained by Ricketts, but, because of the large scale on which they had been conducted, they established more conclusively that infected ticks did indeed exist in nature.[44]

Early in August, McClintic completed the season's work and prepared his laboratory experiments once more for transfer to the Hygienic Laboratory. On 9 August, however, Service headquarters in Washington, D.C., received a wire from Thomas D. Tuttle that McClintic was

In 1911 and 1912 Thomas B. McClintic of the U.S. Public Health and Marine Hospital Service continued Howard Taylor Ricketts's studies of spotted fever in nature, providing more conclusive proof of Ricketts's tentative results. Near the end of his work in 1912, McClintic became infected with spotted fever and died—the first of many laboratory investigators who lost their lives in the study of the deadly disease. In 1914 the U.S. Congress recognized McClintic's death in the line of duty with a private act. (Courtesy of the National Library of Medicine.)

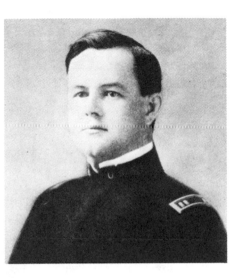

ill with an undiagnosed disease but proceeding east by train, where he planned to join his wife, who had returned earlier. By the time the train reached Chicago, it was clear to Karl H. Kellogg, a Stevensville physician who accompanied McClintic, that the young investigator had fallen victim to spotted fever. Determined to return home, however, McClintic rebuffed an offer of medical care in Chicago. Before the train reached Baltimore, McClintic had lost consciousness, and he died at Georgetown University Hospital on 13 August 1912, the evening of his arrival and the day before President Taft signed the act that shortened the Service's name to U.S. Public Health Service. In 1914 the U.S. Congress recognized McClintic's service and death in the line of duty in a private act. It provided a lump sum award of $5,760— an amount equal to two years' pay and allowances—to Theresa Drexel McClintic, who never remarried.[45]

Spotted fever had claimed its first victim among the researchers who probed its mysteries. McClintic's death cast the dangers of research in bold relief, but according to a newspaper in Washington, D.C., there was no question that the work would be resumed. Rupert Blue, the new surgeon general of the renamed U.S. Public Health Service, chose Lunsford Dickson Fricks to replace McClintic in spotted fever work.[46] The son of a physician in Rising Fawn, Georgia, Fricks was born on

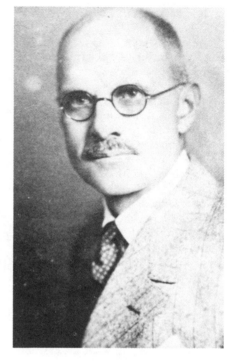

From 1913 to 1917, Lunsford D.
Fricks supervised the U.S. Public
Health Service program to rid
the Bitterroot Valley of spotted
fever. His proposals clashed with
those supported by the Montana
State Board of Entomology.
(Courtesy of the National
Library of Medicine.)

18 July 1873. After graduating first in the 1897 class of the Chattanooga (Tennessee) Medical College, he joined the Service as an intern
and by 1913 had progressed through the ranks to Surgeon. During
the Spanish-American War, Fricks monitored U.S. troops to prevent
the introduction of yellow fever into the United States. While on quarantine duty two years later, he suffered a bout with the infamous
Yellow Jack. From his medical school days, Fricks had been interested
in microscopical investigations. Like McClintic before him, Fricks arrived in Montana, in the spring of 1913, only to be surprised by new
political developments relating to spotted fever.

When the U.S. Bureau of Entomology had withdrawn from spotted
fever work, Robert A. Cooley had been unable to continue his own
tick eradication efforts. Taking a new approach, Cooley proposed to
F. B. Linfield, director of the Montana agricultural experiment station,
that a state entomological commission be established to supervise tick
eradication work in the Bitterroot. Linfield concurred and suggested
that the board be comprised of Cooley as state entomologist, Tuttle
as secretary of the state board of health, and—to serve as a buffer

between the two strong-willed men—W. J. Butler, the state veterinarian. State Senator Fred Whiteside agreed to sponsor the bill in the 1913 session of the Montana state legislature. Working with Whiteside, Cooley ensured that the bill was broadly worded, allowing the board to investigate other disease-carrying insects as well as the spotted fever tick. The new board was needed, Cooley stated, because there existed no official state agency "clothed with all the legal authority needed to prescribe and enforce the necessary rules and regulations" for the eradication of the spotted fever tick. Approved on 18 March 1913, the new law authorized a Montana State Board of Entomology to "take steps to eradicate and prevent the spread of Rocky Mountain tick fever, Infantile Paralysis and all other infections of communicable diseases that may be transmitted or carried by insects."[47]

Smooth functioning of the new state board was fostered by the resignation of Thomas D. Tuttle as secretary of the Montana State Board of Health. His term ended in December 1912, and when Governor Samuel V. Stewart offered him a position as first director of the Montana Tuberculosis Sanatorium, he accepted. For all of his efforts on behalf of public health, including a state food and drug law as well as the sanitorium, the Montana Medical Association awarded Tuttle its first Ricketts Memorial Medal, established to honor the revered research martyr.[48] Tuttle appeared happy to escape the continual battles with Cooley, which, he noted, had contributed to a chronic stomach ulcer. As his successor he recommended William Forlong Cogswell, a physician in Livingston, Montana, and a Canadian native trained at Dalhousie University Medical School in Halifax, Nova Scotia.[49] Cogswell was duly elected at a special meeting of the state board of health on 16 December. Fearing that Cogswell would continue Tuttle's policies, Cooley did not initially inform him about the proposed board of entomology law. Linfield, however, actively lobbied Cogswell and succeeded in persuading him to testify in favor of the bill's passage.[50]

At the first meeting of the Montana State Board of Entomology, a defensive Cooley recommended that the U.S. Bureau of Entomology, which had recently received a fifteen-thousand-dollar appropriation for use in spotted fever tick eradication, be given exclusive rights to the tick eradication work, thus shutting the U.S. Public Health Service out of any involvement. The two other board members, Cogswell and the state veterinarian, W. J. Butler, however, consulted with Governor Stewart and formulated a plan by which more harmonious relations might be maintained between the state and the two federal agencies. Their proposal, carried over Cooley's objection, called for a conference with representatives of the two federal agencies to work out an acceptable compromise. At the meeting, held 11 April 1913, W. D. Hunter of the U.S. Bureau of Entomology and Lunsford D. Fricks of the U.S. Public Health Service agreed to divide tick control work in the Bitterroot Valley geographically. A line of division was set at Big Creek, southwest of Stevensville. Territory north of this line was declared the province of the U.S. Bureau of Entomology, with Cooley in charge of the work. The southern part of the valley would be under the jurisdiction of Fricks, representing the U.S. Public Health Service. On instructions from Service headquarters, however, Fricks was to report only to the secretary of the Montana State Board of Health.[51]

To residents of the Bitterroot, this division must have seemed peculiar, especially since each agency advocated different measures to rid the valley of its scourge. Initially the entomologists stood fast by their contention that within two or three years livestock dipping alone would reduce the spotted fever tick to levels such that the disease would no longer be a threat. Destruction of the small rodents that harbored the immature stages of the tick was described only as "an important secondary means of combating the tick." In contrast, Fricks, representing the medical position, held that a vigorously prosecuted, three-pronged program was necessary. Of equal importance to livestock dipping, Fricks argued, was an active campaign to destroy small rodents. In addition, he insisted that legislation should be passed restricting domestic stock from grazing on the infected west side of the river during tick season. In spite of these differences, the *Northwest Tribune* reported the conference as the beginning of a concerted war on the wood tick, never mentioning spotted fever.[52]

These different approaches led to a second conference on 18 July. Cooley argued that the division of responsibility was not proving effective. Fricks caused dissension, Cooley alleged, by claiming that "dipping would not get rid of the tick in thirty years." Cooley further asserted that Fricks did "not know any more about entomology" than Cooley did about medicine. Cooley's plan was to divide the work along professional specializations: the U.S. Bureau of Entomology should solely manage tick control operations; the U.S. Public Health Service, laboratory experiments; and the U.S. Bureau of Biological Survey, which Cooley hoped would reactivate its participation, ground squirrel eradication.[53]

Believing that it was "not fitting" for two federal agencies to "haggle with the state authorities" over the work, Fricks recommended to Surgeon General Blue that the U.S. Public Health Service withdraw from tick control work entirely. L. O. Howard, chief of the U.S. Bureau of Entomology, likewise suggested to Blue that the bureau's generous appropriation for tick eradication work would surely be renewed and would provide ample funds for the work. Howard argued that "perfect harmony" could be achieved if the Service did pathological work and left tick eradication to the entomologists.[54]

At U.S. Public Health Service headquarters, reaction to this new proposal was uniformly negative. Service leaders had battled since the 1870s for primacy in federal health matters, and they were not inclined to yield any of their hard-won authority. Blue notified Howard that the Service intended to continue its work and remarked that the surrender of functions was hardly cooperation, "at least in the best sense of the term." In a memo to his superior, Secretary of the Treasury William G. McAdoo, Blue reiterated the Service's longstanding position that spotted fever, in all its aspects, was essentially a public health problem. "It would be as logical," Blue wrote, "to turn over to the Bureau of Entomology the suppression of yellow fever epidemics, because the disease is spread by mosquitoes." If such a precedent were set, "it would also be necessary to turn over to the Bureau of Animal Industry the dipping of cattle because several domestic animals harbor the tick, [and] also a part of this work would have to be given to the Forestry Service because ticks are found in the Forest Reserves bordering the Bitter Root Valley."[55] Fricks, furthermore, was advised to revise his position, letting it be known that the Service would not withdraw "without a fight." Observing that Cooley would probably attempt to "slip the skids under you at the first opportunity," Blue cautioned Fricks, "Whatever you do, don't let any of them back you out of there."[56]

For five years, from 1913 through 1917, two federal agencies advocating two separate programs combated a tick known by two names. Since the dipping of livestock was the most visible aspect of both agencies' efforts—and the one most directly affecting the livelihood of valley residents—any problem with this undertaking jeopardized the future of the entire program. Unfortunately, the mild dipping solution available on the open market, which contained 0.169 percent of arsenious oxide, proved to be too weak to kill engorged female ticks. When the strength was increased to 0.228 percent—the concentration commonly used throughout the south to treat Texas cattle fever—the solution burned the hides of Montana cattle. As the search continued for an acceptable concentration, other quality control problems developed. On one occasion, for example, the kerosene and water in the dip separated when it was allowed to stand unused for several hours. When cattle were subsequently immersed, the solution burned the cows' udders.[57]

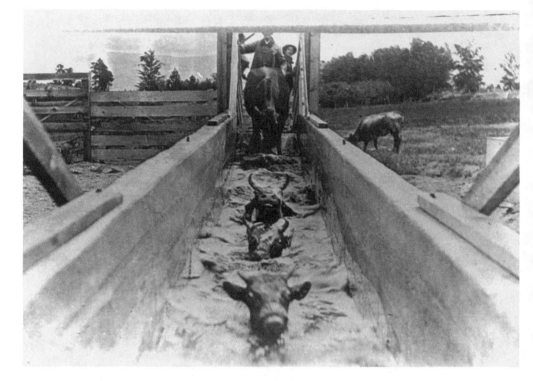

An arsenical solution killed ticks on the hides of livestock in the fifteen seconds it took to swim through the concrete dipping vat. Rocky Mountain wood ticks, however, preferred to attach themselves around the horns and ears of cattle. It was nearly impossible to submerge the heads of the cattle for longer than one second, which was insufficient time to do serious harm to engorged female ticks. (Courtesy of the National Archives and Records Administration.)

These difficulties, which might be expected in any new undertaking, generated significant ill-feeling in the owners of the afflicted stock. Local ranchers, who remained skeptical of the tick theory and who, during tick season, blamed the dip for any sickness or death among their stock, filed several lawsuits. The state attorney general exacerbated already strained relations when he ruled that the state was not liable for accidental death or damage to the ranchers' stock caused by the program.[58] By 1914 a less damaging arsenic dip was identified, but Bitterroot Valley ranchers who sustained real or imaginary losses from the dipping procedure were not inclined to be patient.[59]

In June 1913 the U.S. Public Health Service's vat at Hamilton was destroyed by vandalism, and later that month the U.S. Bureau of Entomology's vat at Florence was dynamited. No precipitating incident was traced to the Hamilton attack. In Florence, however, Carl and George Wemple, brothers aged nine and eleven who assisted at the vat on their family's property, had fallen ill with spotted fever. After George died, the vat was destroyed.[60] During his investigation of the incident, Cooley was advised that the people of Florence, whom he termed in exasperation "an ignorant, mean lot," felt no remorse over the dynamited vat. In fact, since many of them rejected the tick transmission theory outright, there existed "quite a hard feeling among them" about the dipping program. In response to the incidents, the Montana State Board of Entomology called for vigorous prosecution of anyone vandalizing the dipping vats. The board also increased its educational efforts among ranchers, utilizing circulars and demonstrations. Within a year the board reported that public attitude in the Stevensville and Florence districts had been so changed that it was no longer necessary to argue the question of tick transmission of spotted fever. Residents of the Lo Lo canyon area remained unconvinced and never installed a vat, but they refrained from taking violent action against other facilities in the program.[61]

To determine the relative extent of tick infestation in different sections of the Bitterroot and to serve as a check upon the efficacy of tick eradication measures, Willard V. King and Lunsford D. Fricks conducted tick surveys in their respective control districts. King examined livestock for tick infestation in the U.S. Bureau of Entomology's districts; Fricks undertook a more ambitious survey, gathering ticks from the riverbank, from the rolling benchlands, and even from the high reaches of the Bitterroot Mountains. He found practically no ticks on the cultivated lands, a zone of heavy infestation in the hills where horses and cattle were allowed to range, a zone of "moderate" infestation—up to 7,040 ticks per square mile—just above the range of domestic animals, and, finally, an extraordinarily heavy infestation, estimated at millions of ticks per square mile, in "goat country," the high mountainous area where large numbers of Rocky Mountain goats ranged. Because heavy infestations at the higher elevations constantly threatened the tick eradication efforts in the valley, Fricks concluded that ultimate success would depend upon "the creation of a tick-free zone extending as far as possible up into the Bitter Root Mountains."[62]

Both groups also took a census of livestock in the valley. Surprisingly, it revealed that relatively few animals ranged over the tick-infested areas. In the Victor district, for example, there were 1,865 animals, but only 350 cattle and 50 horses required regular dipping. The remaining 1,500 animals were either pastured on the tick-free bottomlands or classified as dairy cows or work horses, animals exempted from dipping if their owners agreed to remove ticks by hand.[63]

Since there were so few animals that actually needed to be dipped, Fricks strongly recommended that the grazing of livestock be restricted by law during the spring. "It would be cheaper," he noted, "to prohibit such grazing entirely than to construct and operate dipping vats." The Montana State Board of Entomology, however, consistently refused to adopt restrictions, arguing that they would generate hostility among the citizenry. After one meeting at which restrictions were considered and soundly defeated, Cooley wrote to King that "each member of the board, speaking for himself, said that he did not care to take the responsibility of voting such a regulation through."[64]

Fricks also maintained that the labor costs of ground squirrel eradication, viewed by Cooley as excessively expensive, could be controlled by inducing landowners themselves to do the work. To this end he procured twelve "squirrel destroyers," or carbon bisulphide pumps, like those used by the Service in the antiplague campaign on the Pacific coast. Farmers were offered free use of the pump for a specified period.[65]

In addition, Fricks suggested the novel idea that west side landowners substitute bands of sheep for their horses and cattle. Sheep had been grazed closely on the east side of the valley since about 1890, Fricks noted, and tick infestation there was practically nonexistent. He concluded that sheep grazing might be an economical method to rid the west side of ticks as well. It was known, moreover, that lanolin in sheep wool was repugnant to ticks and that the density of the wool made it difficult for male and female ticks to locate one another for mating. In an experiment Fricks conducted during 1913 with one small band of sheep, over 87 percent of 295 ticks placed in the wool of unshorn sheep were recovered dead. Moreover, most ticks recovered from sheep grazing naturally were found dead, and many engorged females appeared to be unfertilized.[66]

More importantly, sheep were known to eat the brush vegetation in which ticks dwelled. By herding them back toward the foothills as they grazed, Fricks argued, a habitat alien to the tick would be produced. Other large domestic and wild animals would be removed from sheep ranges, and some ticks would be destroyed simply by the grazing of sheep. Finally, Fricks observed that if further experiments with sheep proved successful, tick eradication could be placed on an industrial basis. This would significantly diminish the cost of spotted fever control work to the federal and Montana taxpayers.[67]

The chilly reception given to Fricks's theory by Cooley and King reflected the ongoing tension between the U.S. Public Health Service and the Montana State Board of Entomology. At Cooley's request, King repeated Fricks's experiment with a band of six sheep. His findings indicated that "the number of ticks which developed on the sheep were more than sufficient to maintain a normal supply." King did not explore whether sheep grazing might control the underbrush that harbored ticks. To Cooley, King wrote that "only in a special combination of circumstances can sheep be relied upon to effect reduction of the tick." He did not elaborate on what these circumstances were or whether they existed in the Bitterroot.[68]

Because Fricks's plan remained experimental and was never supported on a wide scale, moreover, it is difficult to assess its potential merits. Initially there was optimism among Bitterroot residents, and some ranchers added sheep to their stock.[69] Had the plan proved efficacious, of course, it would have merited praise for cost-effectiveness. Under the strained circumstances, no adequate trial was ever conducted.

By 1916 experience had demonstrated that rodent control and grazing restrictions would indeed be necessary if the Rocky Mountain wood tick was to be eliminated from the Bitterroot Valley. The "starvation" method used so successfully against the Texas cattle fever tick, *Margaropus annulatus*, simply did not work in Montana. That tick spent its entire life cycle on one animal, hence dipping killed all stages. The spotted fever tick, in contrast, fed on different animals in the larval, nymphal, and adult stages. The Texas cattle fever tick died after one year if unable to reach a host, but the hardier Rocky Mountain wood tick could remain unfed for three years or longer, after which it would feed and reproduce if placed on a host.[70]

Furthermore, Montana's climate interfered with dipping operations during the crucial early spring period. "One warm sunshiny day in March is sufficient to bring forth the adult ticks," Fricks wrote after one season in Montana, "and when this is followed by a week or more of freezing weather . . . during which it is impossible to use the dip, some females may be fertilized and drop off for egg laying before it is possible to destroy them." Complicating this situation further was the tick's predilection for attaching itself to cattle "around the horns, ears, and high up on the neck." The average time required by a cow to swim through the Victor vat was found to be fifteen seconds, and all ticks submerged that length of time were killed or incapacitated. The cattle, however, swam with their heads out of the solution. It was almost impossible to submerge them completely for longer than one second, a period insufficient to do serious harm to the engorged females in any strength that could be borne by the livestock.[71]

The entire spotted fever situation changed "materially" in the spring of 1915, when the disease was reported from eastern Montana. "To the surprise of us all," Cooley noted, two cases appeared in the northern part of Gallatin County, near Bozeman, and a few were reported near Billings. "Something like ten or a dozen" cases were reported from the flat, sagebrush country in eastern Montana near Miles City and others from Richland County, which bordered North Dakota.[72] Of thirty-five cases reported in 1915, only seven occurred in the Bitterroot Valley and Missoula areas, while twenty-three were reported from the newly discovered eastern areas of infection. The disease seemed to take the mild Idaho form in the eastern counties, for only two deaths were reported, compared with five among the Bitterroot Valley cases. W. F. Cogswell, secretary of the Montana State Board of Health, told the press that spotted fever had probably spread into eastern Montana from Wyoming. "The new cases are occurring along the Powder river, which has its source in Wyoming."[73]

Both the U.S. Public Health Service and the Montana State Board of Entomology launched investigations of this new appearance of spotted fever. The Service had detailed a young assistant surgeon, Roscoe Roy Spencer, to assist Fricks in 1915; Fricks sent Spencer to Miles City, Montana, to confirm the diagnosis of spotted fever by inoculating guinea pigs with the blood of patients.[74] The Montana State Board of Entomology focused on the ecology of eastern Montana spotted fever. Cooley assigned the project to Ralph Robinson Parker, a young assistant entomologist employed by the state board. Ten years later, these two "R.R.s," as they were often called, would collaborate on a vaccine against spotted fever, but at the end of the summer of 1915, Spencer returned to his rotating assignments as a new Service officer. Parker, on the other hand, continued to be intimately involved with spotted fever control work.

The twenty-seven-year-old son of a Massachusetts physician, Parker was a graduate student in entomology at Cooley's alma mater, the Massachusetts Agricultural College.[75] In 1914, Cooley had written to his mentor H. T. Fernald, seeking the name of a student who might be interested in studying flies and their relation to typhoid fever for the Montana State Board of Entomology. Fernald recommended Parker, and Cooley recruited him to work during that summer in the

Yellowstone valley. An extremely conscientious worker and meticulous record keeper, Parker surveyed the eastern Montana spotted fever situation in 1915 and returned in 1916 with his Ph.D. in hand to establish a field station at Powderville, Montana. With the assistance of his bride, Adah Nicolet Parker, the young entomologist investigated topography and vegetation in addition to the local species of ticks and their animal hosts. His most disturbing finding was that in this area, small animals, particularly rabbits, served as hosts to adult as well as immature stages of the tick. Dipping domestic stock would be futile if adult ticks matured on the widely distributed rabbits. The following year Parker gathered additional information in Musselshell, Montana, but he offered no concrete suggestions for tick control.[76]

As it became manifest that spotted fever would not be eradicated as simply and quickly as had Texas cattle fever, the Montana State Board of Entomology reluctantly adopted a regulation restricting, with some exceptions, the grazing of livestock in the Bitterroot Valley between 1 March and 15 July each year. Ground squirrel destruction also became a more important part of the U.S. Bureau of Entomology's control program. In the fall of 1916 a newspaper article reported on the expanded control program with no mention that the U.S. Public Health Service had advocated such methods since 1911. Fricks reacted to this article as Tuttle had before him: the entomologists, he believed, were claiming credit that rightly belonged to others. Fricks protested the perceived injustice, but the entomologists maintained that they had come to their conclusions independently.[77]

More substantive was an ongoing disagreement between Fricks and the Montana State Board of Entomology over grazing restrictions. The board's regulations authorized exemptions for persons who grazed their stock on state land under long-term leases. The state was loath to cancel these leases, even though many of the lessees were absentee owners, and the Montana State Board of Entomology argued for the exemptions on the grounds that some of the lessees had few other means of income. Fricks countered that this argument was wholly unacceptable. "By the same reasoning, many practices, such as piracy and highway robbery for instance, which are now under the ban of the law might easily be condoned."[78]

In December 1916, Fricks appealed to federal officials in Washington to put pressure on the state authorities. William P. Malburn, writing for the secretary of the treasury, accordingly reminded Governor Samuel V. Stewart of the "large sums of money which this Department has expended in the endeavor to control this disease in the State of Montana." He urged state authorities to adopt strict grazing restrictions immediately. The state board of health secretary, W. F. Cogswell, replied to this letter, explaining the exceptions, but Treasury Secretary William G. McAdoo was not appeased. Reiterating the federal financial investment, McAdoo warned that the state must enact and enforce more stringent grazing restrictions if the work of the U.S. Public Health Service was to be continued.[79]

Even as this exchange was occurring, the United States was being pulled relentlessly into World War I. President Woodrow Wilson had been reelected on the slogan "He Kept Us out of War," but a German declaration of unrestricted submarine warfare in January 1917, followed by the actual torpedoing of several ships, induced Wilson to change his position. By 6 April 1917 both houses of Congress had voted to declare war. The following day, at a meeting of the Montana State Board of Entomology, Fricks took the first step toward disengaging the U.S. Public Health Service from its commitment in Montana. He introduced a resolution declaring a portion of the territory on the west side of the Bitterroot tick free. In his report of this meeting to the surgeon general, Fricks noted that Willard V. King had admitted "for the first time, that the dipping of domestic animals had proven impracticable as a tick eradicative measure in the Bitter Root Valley." Furthermore, he continued, "the Board passed a resolution favoring the introduction of sheep for this purpose." Fricks recommended that the Service discontinue its work after 30 June 1917, since its position had been "vindicated." Surgeon General Blue concurred and informed Cogswell that the Service was withdrawing. Fricks, who had grown to love the Bitterroot Valley, was ordered to Memphis, Tennessee, to take charge of malaria control work for the duration of the war.[80]

After the withdrawal of the U.S. Public Health Service, the state board of entomology voted unanimously to ask the U.S. Bureau of Entomology to take over control work for the entire valley. Cooley wrote to Congresswoman Jeanette Rankin, whose father had died of spotted fever in 1904, for assistance in securing a larger appropriation for the work. The U.S. Bureau of Entomology, however, had changed its mind about participating. "The matter primarily is a question of public health," stated the secretary of agriculture in his reply to Rankin's inquiry. "It is believed that the question of eradication is one which should be dealt with by the State authorities and, if the assistance of the Federal Government is needed, the cooperation of the Health Service should be sought. While the Bureau of Entomology heretofore has done some work in connection with the eradication of the disease, it seems advisable hereafter for that Bureau to deal only with the entomological phases of the problem, such as the study of the life history and habits of the tick and similar matters."[81]

The absence of any federal assistance left Montana in a financially difficult position. The state board of entomology resolved to continue the work and in the spring of 1918 appointed Ralph R. Parker to take charge of control measures in the Bitterroot. During the previous fall, Parker had spent two months at Harvard University in productive research on the anatomy of ticks and was clearly the most knowledgeable entomologist available to Montana authorities. He worked with little money and few assistants, since many young men had volunteered for service in the military. The vats at Stevensville and Blodgett Creek leaked, the Victor vat needed repairs, and there was a problem getting water to the Florence vat. Local committees, however, supported Parker, advocating enforced dipping and expressing willingness to assume a larger share of the cost.[82]

After directing the control program for only a short time, Parker concluded that its priorities needed to be reordered. "I am seriously of the opinion," he wrote to Cooley, "that the work here will have to undergo a radical change . . . if we are to get real results. Frankly I am in favor of cutting out the dipping absolutely. I have no faith in it." He pointed out that Montana's cold spring made dipping impossible during late February and early March. "It seems to me that under the best of conditions . . . we cannot, by dipping get more than a scant 25% of the ticks that actually engorge on the animals." He concluded that ground squirrel control coupled with restrictions on grazing constituted a better approach.[83]

The entire program, moreover, was under some strain during this period. In spite of five years of tick control efforts, spotted fever had not been eradicated. There continued to be some opposition from some stock owners to grazing restrictions, and the game warden opposed the "indiscriminate" use of poisoned grain because of the hazard it posed to birds. In support of the program, Cooley argued that spotted fever cases had been reduced from eleven to three from 1913 to 1918. King published data indicating that the number of ticks had been reduced 80–90 percent, although he noted that the reduction varied from area to area. Given this unsettled situation, Cooley solicited testimonial letters from valley residents for the board's third biennial report, presumably to buttress the board's appropriation request.[84]

Although Montana lawmakers did increase the budget of the board for 1919 and 1920, they curtailed the appropriation in 1921.[85] Cooley and Parker had hoped to launch a broad-scale study of spotted fever in nature as a basis for developing more efficient and permanent methods to destroy the tick. In 1920, furthermore, Cooley recommended that tick control operations be extended into the mountainous regions, including possible extermination of the Rocky Mountain goat, which had been shown to serve as a major natural host for adult ticks. A few years later, this proposition became a minor cause célèbre as wildlife lovers came to the goat's defense. The author of a *Northwest Tribune* article entitled "The Mountain Goat or Taxpayers Goat" argued that the entire tick control program was a sink for money and had produced scant results. Unless it could be shown definitively that the program was effective, "a pause should be made before continuing to throw money into the bottomless well."[86]

The reduced appropriation in 1921 ironically coincided with a precipitous rise in the number of spotted fever cases in the Bitterroot — from four in 1920 to eleven in 1921. All eleven cases, moreover, proved fatal. Among the victims were two prominent Lo Lo residents, Montana State Senator Tyler Worden and his wife, who was president of the Montana Federation of Women's Clubs. All but two of the 1921 cases were acquired in the canyons running back into the Bitterroot Mountains, which indicated that although the tick control program had contributed to the safety of residents within the control districts, spotted fever remained a hazard in the valley. Worried state officials, fearing that the disease might be in a resurgence, petitioned the U.S. Public Health Service to return.[87]

A decade of tick control efforts had reduced the tick population but had not succeeded in ridding the Bitterroot of spotted fever. In assessing the work of this period, it is necessary to recall that in 1910, when the hope for a medical approach to spotted fever control seemed to die with Howard Taylor Ricketts, vector control offered the most promising method of combating the disease. Similar efforts against yellow fever and Texas cattle fever had produced stunning results, and doubtless Robert A. Cooley and his associates hoped to rid western Montana of its scourge with the same simple, effective measures. Cooley's personal clash with Thomas D. Tuttle, unfortunately, led the ambitious entomologist into a combatant posture with the U.S. Public Health Service that surely retarded adoption of control methods other than livestock dipping. The insistence of the Service that its officers deal only with the state health officer rather than with the Montana State Board of Entomology, moreover, exacerbated the situation. In retrospect, these quarrels may have cost Montana and federal taxpayers additional money, but at that time the control efforts themselves appeared to be the only recourse available by which virulent spotted fever in the Bitterroot could be attacked, and thus they provided a means for some type of active response against the deadly affliction.

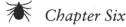 *Chapter Six*

A Wholly New Type of Microorganism

Nature makes so gradual a transition from the inanimate to the animate kingdom that the boundary lines which separate them are indistinct and doubtful.

Aristotle, *Historia Animalium*

From 1902, when Louis B. Wilson and William M. Chowning launched the first scientific investigation, until 1910, when Howard Taylor Ricketts died, bacteriological techniques had been the methods of choice among investigators of Rocky Mountain spotted fever. Using the microscope, blood smears, staining and fixing techniques, and animal inoculations, bacteriologists had demonstrated tick transmission and identified a suspected organism. Conclusive proof that this microorganism caused spotted fever eluded early researchers, however, because they could not cultivate the organism on artificial media, a requirement laid down by Robert Koch to demonstrate bacterial causation.[1] Serum therapy used successfully against some other diseases, furthermore, had failed to produce a dramatic cure for spotted fever, and, in any case, efforts to develop preventive or therapeutic medical strategies had died with Ricketts. With the armamentarium of bacteriology so depleted, investigators sought new approaches to identify spotted fever's mysterious etiological agent. During the second productive period of laboratory research on spotted fever, the methods of pathology supplanted those of bacteriology in unraveling this portion of the riddle.

The beginning of systematic study in disease pathology is usually traced to the work of Giovanni Battista Morgagni, an eighteenth-century professor of anatomy at the University of Padua. Morgagni noted particular lesions found at autopsy and suggested that they might explain clinical symptoms. His observations stimulated a systematized search to correlate pathological lesions with symptoms. By the mid nineteenth century, sufficient data had been gathered to distinguish among many diseases with similar characteristics. With improvements to the microscope after 1830, it became possible to study the fine structures of the body. In 1858, building on concurrent discoveries that plant and animal tissues were comprised of cells, Rudolf Virchow postulated the doctrine of cellular pathology—that disease occurred because of interaction between living cells and disease agents. After 1880, when the light microscope was perfected and the discovery of bacteria stimulated the development of staining methods and other techniques, careful studies of the cellular pathology—or histology, as it came to be called—of diseased tissue became possible.

Since the most pressing need during the early decades of histological study was information about such major infectious diseases as tuberculosis and typhoid fever, rare maladies such as Rocky Mountain spotted fever received little attention. Aside from Wilson and Chowning's autopsy notations on gross pathology, E. R. LeCount, an associate of Ricketts at Rush Medical College in Chicago, had by 1916 produced the sole histological study of spotted fever. LeCount's work was not exhaustive but rather constituted the initial findings of a larger study abruptly terminated by Ricketts's death. The microscopic changes caused by spotted fever infection, LeCount noted, were of two sorts. First, diffuse lesions, affecting entire groups of organs, were similar to the changes caused by other infectious diseases. Second and more important, he believed, were the "focal lesions" connected with the occlusion of blood vessels in sections of the skin, liver, kidney, spleen, and adrenal glands. Although LeCount also found capillaries and small veins in the lung and heart practically occluded with leukocytes, he concluded that "there were no serious consequences of these conditions with exception of minute hemorrhages beneath the endocardium." Likening the changes caused by excessive leukocytes and the focal lesions to those seen in typhoid fever, LeCount speculated that they were probably caused by the "action of the toxin of this disease." Some of the "so-called 'endothelial toxins' " he noted, were believed to be "liberated from the bodies of bacteria."[2]

In January 1916, Simeon Burt Wolbach, a pathologist at Harvard University School of Medicine, became interested in Rocky Mountain spotted fever. Trained under the distinguished pathologists William T. Councilman and Frank B. Mallory, Wolbach had in 1911 participated in studies of trypanosomiasis, parasitic protozoa, and tropical ulcers in Gambia, then a British colony, on the west coast of Africa.[3] The publications resulting from this work earned Wolbach promotions at Harvard, to associate professor of bacteriology in 1914 and to associate professor of pathology two years later. Wolbach began his work with strains of spotted fever obtained from Surgeon Lunsford D. Fricks of the U.S. Public Health Service, who was continuing his own bacteriological studies in addition to implementing tick control efforts.[4]

About the same time, Hideyo Noguchi, a bacteriologist at the Rockefeller Institute for Medical Research in New York also entered spotted fever investigations.[5] Having achieved prestigious status as a full member of the Rockefeller Institute in 1914, Noguchi was well known for his early work on snake venoms and his more recent work on spirochetes, especially on *Treponema pallidum*, the cause of syphilis. According to Noguchi's biographer, Isabel R. Plesset, Noguchi cast about during 1915 for an interesting new problem and selected Rocky Mountain spotted fever, which resembled his homeland's tsutsugamushi disease. In late 1915 or early 1916, Noguchi visited Fricks at the Hygienic Laboratory and obtained strains of spotted fever in guinea pigs. The entrance of this more senior, celebrated Rockefeller researcher into the spotted fever field prodded both Wolbach and Fricks to speed up their work.[6]

Fricks, who had already studied spotted fever for three years, hastened to publish the results of his microscopical research. In early 1916, at medical meetings in Missoula and Salt Lake City, Fricks announced that he had consistently found "extra corpuscular granules" in the blood of human and animal victims of spotted fever. These, he stated, occurred singly and in pairs and, when stained by the Giemsa method, appeared bright red and were highly refractile. He also found similar bodies "within or in close proximity to" the red blood cells. Those inside the red cell, he said, were "round or slightly elongated red chromatin bodies partially surrounded by or in close approximation to a somewhat larger deep-blue staining body." All of the chromatin bodies were one micron or less in diameter. Fricks concluded that the "morphological and tinctorial characteristics" of these bodies implied that they were of a protozoan nature.[7]

Wolbach, although just beginning his studies, had little regard for Fricks's presumed organism. Corresponding with the secretary of the Montana State Board of Health, W. F. Cogswell, Wolbach confided, "I am on an entirely different track and have great hopes of contributing something of importance." It would take time, he continued, to confirm his hypotheses, because he was using the "peculiarly difficult technique" of teasing apart tick tissues rather than crushing them. Initially, Wolbach had planned to supplement these laboratory studies of tick and guinea pig tissues by traveling to Montana to study human cases of the disease, and to this end he had requested that the Montana

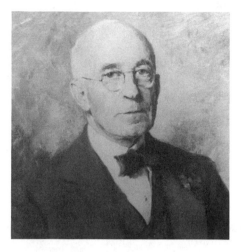

S. Burt Wolbach, a pathologist at Harvard University School of Medicine, described spotted fever as an infection of the circulatory system and identi-fied the causative organism in the tissues of infected ticks, experimental ani-mals, and human victims. Wolbach also recognized that the rickettsial organisms could not be cultured on lifeless media but required living cells in which to grow and replicate. (Courtesy of the National Library of Medicine.)

State Board of Entomology detail Ralph R. Parker to assist him. Robert A. Cooley, however, wanted Parker to spend the summer in Powderville studying Eastern Montana spotted fever, just recognized the previous year. All hope of studying human cases evaporated when Wolbach suffered an attack of appendicitis with complications that precluded any travel.[8]

Despite this setback, Wolbach determined to publish preliminary findings based solely on studies of tick and guinea pig tissues rather than risk losing priority to Noguchi.[9] His research had revealed, Wol-bach wrote to Cooley, that spotted fever affected "primarily the pe-ripheral blood vessels" and that the rash and necrosis were "secondary to the vascular lesions." These findings were "entirely consistent and confirmatory of clinical descriptions of the disease," he continued, and he expressed surprise that no one had previously paid attention to the tissues, which he regarded as essential.[10]

In mid 1916, Wolbach published two papers on these preliminary findings in the *Journal of Medical Research*. In the first he described a Gram-negative organism from 0.2 to 0.5 microns wide that occasionally occurred "in large numbers" and was concentrated in the "smooth muscle cells of affected arteries and veins." With Giemsa's stain the organisms stained "bluish," this being "in marked contrast to most bacteria, which take an intense reddish purple stain." Since this reddish purple coloration—usually achieved by using the Romanowsky stain—was regarded as the chromatin staining reaction, Wolbach noted that he was "somewhat at a loss to understand the description 'chromatin staining' by Ricketts as applied to this organism." This initial paper was followed a few months later by a second preliminary report on the organism in ticks. Although he had observed the organism throughout tick tissues, Wolbach concluded that there was no cellular reaction in the ticks to the presence of the parasites, "even when present in enormous numbers." This was indicative that the organism had evolved a symbiotic relationship with its tick host over centuries.[11]

Ironically, although it was Noguchi's perceived competition that stimulated the publication of Fricks's and Wolbach's papers, Noguchi himself did not make much progress during 1916 on spotted fever. His attention had turned instead to studies of the spirochete that caused Weil's disease, an organism that he identified as a new genus, *Leptospira*. Having read the papers published by both Fricks and Wolbach, Noguchi was inclined to support Fricks's protozoan theory. When he received a slide of Fricks's presumed organism, Noguchi replied that he, too, had "seen similar bodies several times" in his own work. It is not surprising that Noguchi, as a specialist in spirochetes, some of which were known to be arthropod-borne, was receptive to the possibility of a spotted fever organism with protozoan characteristics.[12]

Smarting under Noguchi's preference for Fricks's protozoan theory, Wolbach characterized Noguchi and his colleagues as "the skeptical autocrats at the Rockefeller Institute."[13] Such feelings of institutional rivalry also emerged at the Hygienic Laboratory. The director, George W. McCoy, wrote encouragingly to Fricks that no one at the laboratory was concerned about Wolbach's publication. They had concluded that Wolbach's organism was probably the same organism Fricks had seen. "Unless Noguchi has something a whole lot better than Wolbach," McCoy continued, "we should worry." He noted that the laboratory's histologist had thus far been unable to verify Wolbach's findings of the organism in tissues. Furthermore, Arthur M. Stimson, another researcher at the laboratory and later director of its Division of Scientific Research, was attempting to duplicate and verify Fricks's research. Unfortunately, McCoy informed Fricks, although Stimson had seen the "intracorpuscular bugs" once under the microscope, he had "not been able to find them since to show us." McCoy remained confident, however, that Fricks's work would soon be confirmed.[14]

It was, however, the pathological approach of Wolbach that would reveal definitively the etiology of spotted fever. As he continued his examination of guinea pig lesions and tick tissues, an entirely unanticipated phenomenon altered Wolbach's perception of the nature of the disease organism. By December 1916 he was certain that he had seen the organism multiplying "in the nuclei of the Malpighian tubules of ticks. This is the first instance known," he wrote to Cooley, "of a parasite multiplying inside of nuclei. As you see, I am getting away from the idea that the organism is a bacterium."[15]

In the spring of 1917, Wolbach was finally able come to Montana for several weeks, where he conducted two autopsies on spotted fever victims. To his surprise, the lesions of the disease in humans had an "exact similarity" to those in animals. Commenting on this "remarkable feature," of spotted fever, Wolbach asserted, "There is probably no other disease of man which is so accurately duplicated in animals."[16]

In 1918, Wolbach published a third preliminary report, this one on spotted fever in humans. In this paper, and in his report to the chairmen of the Montana state boards of health and entomology, Wolbach stated emphatically, "It is possible now to define Rocky Mountain Spotted Fever as a disease of the peripheral blood vessels, a specific endangiitis caused by the minute parasite described in my first report."[17] Moreover, Wolbach had decided that the spotted fever organism was indeed unique. "My opinion regarding the organism," he wrote Cooley, "is that it represents a wholly new type of micro-organism and that it probably stands intermediate between the bacteria and protozoa as does spirochaeta."[18]

Because of this intellectually exciting discovery, Wolbach hoped to launch a large-scale research project on spotted fever at Harvard. He invited Ralph R. Parker, who had investigated tick anatomy at Harvard for a brief period in 1917, to assist with entomological studies for "one or two years" under a special grant from the university—an offer that appeared hard to turn down in Parker's mind. World War I and the 1918 influenza pandemic, however, thwarted these plans. Wolbach dropped spotted fever work for a time in order to study influenza. He wrote to Cooley: "Some day and as soon as possible we shall see an adequately organized research on Spotted Fever; but that can not be until the war is over. We are stripped to the last man here and the calls for men are so urgent that it will be impossible to put through my intention now."[19]

During that tumultuous summer, a tragedy in Noguchi's laboratory at the Rockefeller Institute helped to confirm that Wolbach's organism was indeed the cause of spotted fever. Noguchi had been hospitalized in May 1917 with typhoid fever and had suffered relapses that prevented his return to the laboratory for nearly a year. During his absence, all of Noguchi's cultures were maintained by his laboratory assistant, twenty-three-year-old Stephen Molinscek. Shortly after Noguchi's return to the laboratory in March 1918, Molinscek fell ill. Noguchi later contended that Molinscek had scratched his hand or arm with a needle, but Molinscek told his attending physician that he could not remember any laboratory accident. On 18 March, Molinscek was hospitalized after developing symptoms that were provisionally diagnosed as Brill's disease, spotted fever, or possibly typhoid.[20]

Noguchi himself cultured Molinscek's blood to rule out a laboratory spirochetal infection. Typhoid was also eliminated after several Widal tests gave negative results. When Molinscek died a week later, however, the diagnosis was still uncertain. Samples of Molinscek's tissues were sent to Wolbach at Harvard for examination, and he confirmed typical spotted fever organisms in the vascular lesions. Guinea pigs inoculated with Molinscek's blood showed characteristic spotted fever signs, hence the attending physician concluded that spotted fever had been the cause.[21]

By accepting Wolbach's diagnosis of Molinscek's terminal illness, the Rockefeller Institute in effect confirmed Wolbach's research. Following this incident, the Harvard pathologist prepared a definitive paper on Rocky Mountain spotted fever that occupied the entire 197 pages of the November 1919 issue of the *Journal of Medical Research*. In addition to presenting an exhaustive review of the literature, clinical observations, epidemiological evidence, an analysis of the life cycle of the tick vector, and a detailed description of his histological method, Wolbach expanded his discussion of the differences he had observed between the spotted fever organism and bacteria. He particularly emphasized the fact that the organism invaded the nuclei of tick cells, often "completely filling and even distending the nucleus." Noting his early reluctance to accept the intranuclear bodies as forms of the spotted fever organism, Wolbach emphasized that he now regarded them "as the most characteristic form in infected ticks." He reiterated, moreover, that this phenomenon was the impetus for concluding that the agent of spotted fever indeed represented "a new form of microorganism." He proposed that it be called *Dermacentroxenus rickettsi*, taking the genus name from the tick known to carry the disease and choosing the species name "in honor of Ricketts who first saw it in the blood."[22]

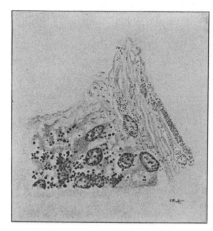

S. Burt Wolbach's drawing of the spotted fever organism in the tissues of infected animals. Wolbach's name for the organism, *Dermacentroxenus rickettsi,* was later supplanted by the currently accepted designation, *Rickettsia rickettsii.* (Reproduced from S. Burt Wolbach, "Studies on Rocky Mountain Spotted Fever," *Journal of Medical Research* 41 [1919]: 1–197.)

Wolbach did not accept Ricketts's description of nonpathogenic organisms in the eggs of uninfected ticks. Robert A. Cooley prepared slides of noninfective tick eggs for Wolbach and identified short rods as identical with those that Ricketts had described. These short rods, Wolbach maintained, were not the spotted fever organism, which in tick eggs exhibited a lanceolate form. Ricketts had been misled, Wolbach concluded, by having the "misfortune" to work with ticks contaminated with the rod-shaped bacteria as well as with the spotted fever organism.[23] Later researchers, however, confirmed Ricketts's finding of nonpathogenic rickettsiae in many noninfective ticks.

Between 1916, when Wolbach wrote his first preliminary report, and 1919, when he published the comprehensive study, he apparently resolved his questions about the different coloration Ricketts had observed and described. Control of acidity in laboratory studies was not well understood before 1920, and, as Edmund V. Cowdry at the Rockefeller Institute noted, by varying the composition of Giemsa's stain, either the red or the blue coloration could be enhanced. "The frequently noted tendency to be colored less intensely than ordinary bacteria with Giemsa's stain," Cowdry observed, was also difficult to estimate quantitatively and varied "within wide limits."[24] Because of this, it is impossible to ascertain whether the organism described by Lunsford D. Fricks—despite his repeated protestations to the contrary—was identical to Wolbach's. After 1917, when Fricks was assigned to malaria control operations in Tennessee, he made no more effort to defend the organism he had identified.[25]

In addition to the difficulty of identifying the spotted fever organism under the microscope, the riddle of its relationship to typhus—the disease it most closely resembled—likewise remained unsolved. Although the louse-borne nature of typhus had already been firmly established, its microbial etiology remained shrouded in mystery. In 1914, Harry Plotz and his colleagues in the Department of Pathology, Mount Sinai Hospital, New York, identified a Gram-positive bacillus associated with the blood of typhus fever victims and typhus-infected lice. They argued that this bacillus might play an important causative role in the disease. Two years later, a Brazilian researcher, Henrique da Rocha Lima, described red staining, "bluntly elliptical, olive-shaped" organisms "somewhat smaller than the smallest bacteria," which had the ability to penetrate the digestive tract cells of lice and there to multiply rapidly. Like spotted fever, these presumed typhus organisms resisted all efforts at cultivation. Even so, da Rocha Lima maintained that they were the etiological agents of typhus, and he named them *Rickettsia prowazeki* in honor of Ricketts and of the Polish investigator Stanislaus von Prowazek, both martyrs in typhus research.[26]

Wolbach, however, declined to classify the spotted fever organism with that of typhus. In arguing for two different genus names, he noted that Ricketts's descriptions of the typhus and spotted fever organisms had been "markedly different."[27] Wolbach's name, *Dermacentroxenus rickettsi*, was to stand as the designation for the spotted fever organism for more than two decades as he and other researchers investigated a variety of so-called Rickettsia-bodies and their connection to what came to be called the typhus-like diseases. Between 1910 and 1930 reports began to be published from nearly every continent about diseases exhibiting a high fever and rash, usually occurring after a tick, mite, or insect bite. Although the geographical isolation of most of these diseases precluded intensive laboratory study, they added anecdotal evidence that these were indeed a distinct class of diseases.

In 1910, Alfred Conor of the Pasteur Institute in Tunis reported with a colleague on a peculiar eruptive fever in Tunisia. Clearly different from known Mediterranean fevers, this malady caused a rash that was "difficult to classify in the nosological framework of skin diseases." Although the lesions, which appeared "first on the abdomen, then on the whole surface of the body, including the face," were not "spots or stains or pimples," Conor believed that the best description for them was "pimply lesions." This designation, he admitted, might "lack precision," but for want of a more explicit term, it appeared most useful. Many patients ill with the disease were observed to have bites, but these were attributed to "small mosquitoes," and tick bites were never mentioned.[28]

The same year, an American physician, Nathan E. Brill, described an unknown disease he had studied in 221 patients for more than a decade. In 1898, Brill had reported on apparent typhoid cases that produced no Widal reaction and displayed symptoms of typhus fever. Having pursued this mysterious fever for so many years, Brill convincingly demonstrated that it was a distinct, previously undescribed disease. No arthropods of any type were connected with this illness, but because of the thoroughness with which Brill presented his case, "Brill's disease" immediately attracted the attention of the research community and became a catch all for unknown, typhus-like symptoms.[29]

European researchers at colonial stations in Africa also enriched the literature by describing a typhus-like disease in southern Africa. In 1911, José F. Sant'Anna reported in *Parasitology* that he had seen six patients in Lourenço Marques, in Portuguese East Africa, who suffered headache, joint pains, lymph gland inflammation, and a slight papular eruption on the fourth or fifth day. These symptoms occurred after the victims were exposed to the bites of larval ticks, which were so numerous in the grass of Lourenço Marques "as to constitute a veritable scourge." Identified primarily as *Amblyomma hebraeum* larvae, the ticks were especially prevalent in July and August. Because cases occurred infrequently and victims recovered spontaneously, few hospitals had experience with the disease.[30]

Sant'Anna's report stimulated G. H. F. Nuttall, the editor of *Parasitology*, to report his own correspondence about tick-borne fevers in southern Africa. A Johannesburg physician, G. E. Turner, Nuttall stated, had identified similar cases resulting from the bite of *Amblyomma hebraeum* ticks. Turner described at the site of the tick bite "a kind of bleb over the bite," from which some "watery material" could be squeezed out, after which a small sore formed. Later, this lesion would be known as the *tâche noire*, or eschar, of the disease. Victims, Turner observed, were usually new arrivals to the area, for local inhabitants seemingly had immunity. C. W. Howard, an entomologist in Lourenço Marques, also reported additional cases. Howard recounted his own bout with the fever, which had occurred "some years ago," just after his arrival and following a tick bite. He also noted that the well-known researchers Edward Hindle and Frederick Breinl had contracted a similar fever at Runcorn Research Laboratories, near Liverpool, while they were studying *Amblyomma he-*

braeum larvae sent from Capetown. Because all of these cases were presumably connected to the bite of a tick, Nuttall proposed that the African diseases be called tick-bite fever in order to distinguish them from the more general name, tick fever, which, he maintained, was closely identified with Rocky Mountain spotted fever and with relapsing fever.[31]

J. G. McNaught, a member of the Royal Army Medical Corps in South Africa, held a different position about this unknown African fever. In a paper delivered to the South African Medical Congress in 1911, McNaught sought to distinguish it from paratyphoid fever, with which it had been confused. Although clinical symptoms in cases seen by McNaught were virtually identical to Nuttall's tick-bite fever, McNaught had observed tick bites in only a few cases and had been unable to find any "blood parasites" in blood smears. Having just read Nathan Brill's paper, moreover, McNaught argued that the unknown diseases in South Africa must be the same disease because of their clinical similarity.[32]

In 1917, J. W. D. Megaw of the Indian Medical Service added a new disease to the growing list by describing his own encounter with a fever contracted after a tick bite near Lucknow in the Kumaon Hills of the Himalayas. Quoting from the 1913 unpublished report of a colleague about a disease identified as typhus in the same vicinity, Megaw determined that his illness was identical. He maintained, however, that this disease was not typhus but rather a disease similar to Brill's disease. He argued, in fact, that all the typhus-like diseases with the exception of typhus itself should provisionally be classified as Brill's disease. The etiological agent, he speculated, was "probably an invisible virus," which was likely to have been "conveyed from man to man or from another animal to man by a biting insect or tick."[33]

In the Far East, typhus-like fevers were reported from the Federated Malay States, Australia, and Japan.[34] Although knowledge about those in Australia and the Malay States was limited to clinical descriptions, the disease known for centuries in Asia and called tsutsugamushi in Japan was subjected to closer scientific scrutiny.[35] In 1810, Hakuju Hashimoto described a *tsutsuga*, meaning "disease," along the tributaries of the Shinano River. A similar disease, thought to be carried by mites, or *mushi* in Japanese, had been known at least since the sixteenth century in southern China. Laboratory investigations of tsutsugamushi began in Japan in the early 1890s when it captured the attention of Shiramiro Kitasato, who returned from his work with Robert Koch in Germany to found the Institute for Infectious Diseases in Tokyo. Maintaining that the bite of a red mite transmitted the disease, Kitasato believed that he had seen a protozoan body in the red blood cells of patients. This theory gained support from the distinguished Tokyo physician Masaki Ogata, himself a specialist in protozoa. Many of Kitasato's colleagues at the Institute for Infectious Diseases, however, favored a theory of bacterial causation. A third theory held that tsutsugamushi was the result of a toxin contained in the body of the red mite. In 1908, U.S. Army surgeons Percy M. Ashburn and Charles F. Craig, who had confirmed Charles Wardell Stiles's findings that a protozoan organism was not the etiological agent of Rocky Mountain spotted fever, conducted a comparative study of spotted fever and tsutsugamushi. Although they noted these different theories, they concluded only that tsutsugamushi and spotted fever were distinct disease entities.[36]

Completing the group of typhus-like diseases known during the first two decades of the twentieth century was yet another, newly discovered during World War I. Known by various names, including Wolhynian fever, quintan fever, Polish fever, Meuse fever, and Russian intermittent fever, the descriptive appellation given to the disease by the British armies in northern France seemed most appropriate: trench fever. This disease never killed, but it caused much misery and loss of manpower in all the warring armies. Studies by several commissions, including one sponsored by the American Red Cross, showed that trench fever was a member of the typhus family, clinically characterized by headache, joint and muscle pains, a high fever, and a rash. Half the cases suffered relapses after the first bout.[37]

The Great War of 1914–18 in Europe provided the stimulus for further intensive research on epidemic typhus itself. Although typhus did not harass the armies of western European nations, it did ravage those of Russia, Serbia, and Poland. After the war ended, it settled with vengeance on Polish civilians. During the 1915 Serbian epidemic, it was reported that every fifth man in the army was ill, and 135,000 died. The Soviet revolution, which ended the war in Russia, did not bring relief from this malady. Between 1919 and 1922, more than 10 million cases of typhus were reported.[38] Known to be a disease of cold climates and the winter months, typhus spread rapidly via its louse vector in the fur-lined clothing common in northeastern Europe.

In 1919, S. Burt Wolbach was invited by Richard P. Strong, medical director of the League of Red Cross Societies, to head a commission to study typhus in Poland.[39] Since Ralph R. Parker's 1917 work on the anatomy of the tick had proven useful, Wolbach invited Parker to accompany the group for entomological studies on lice. After some discussion, the Montana State Board of Entomology approved Parker's participation. Unfortunately, after Parker had traveled to Massachusetts to join the group, he was stricken with a respiratory illness complicated by heart problems and was unable to make the journey.[40] An entomologist from the Lister Institute, Arthur W. Bacot, replaced Parker, but shortly after arriving in Poland, Bacot became ill with trench fever and had to return to England. "We seemed to be doomed to disappointment with entomologists," Wolbach wrote in frustration.[41]

The work of the commission, therefore, focused primarily on "a minute histo-pathological study" of typhus lesions in humans and in lice. This was necessary, Wolbach maintained, in order to understand typhus as a disease, and particularly "for appraising relationships between lesions found and presumptive etiological agents which might be encountered." Bacteriological methods, he noted, were deliberately given second importance, "pending the development of indications during the research."[42] In his 1919 paper on Rocky Mountain spotted fever, Wolbach had noted the arguments surrounding da Rocha Lima's claim that *Rickettsia prowazeki* was the cause of typhus. The Brazilian had not demonstrated the organism in vascular lesions of typhus patients, and such a demonstration, Wolbach believed, "would do much to settle the question." And indeed, the Red Cross typhus commission seemed to produce an irrefutable confirmation of da Rocha Lima's findings. "We conclude," Wolbach wrote in the commission's report, "that *Rickettsia prowazeki* is the cause of typhus." They had found not only "the virus of typhus and *Rickettsia prowazeki*" inseparable in infective lice, but also "bodies indistinguishable from *Rickettsia prowazeki*, demonstrable with great regularity, in the lesions of typhus in man."[43]

Wolbach also incorporated into the commission's report a summary of knowledge about Rickettsia-bodies. Although he observed that "a satisfactory definition of rickettsia is not possible at present," it was possible to note the properties that the organisms held in common. They all had a bacterium like morphology but were smaller than bacteria. The difficulty of staining them with solutions used for bacteria was "a striking feature," as was "the failure to retain the stain by Gram's method." There were no motile forms. None of the rickettsiae pathogenic for humans had been successfully cultured. All had arthropod hosts, were highly specific for that host, and, except for typhus, were transmitted through the eggs of the female arthropod.[44]

No general acquiescence to the view that Rickettsia-bodies represented a new form of microorganism, however, was forthcoming from the worldwide scientific community. Julius Schwalbe, Berlin corre-

spondent for the *Journal of the American Medical Association*, remarked in June 1921 that, despite numerous investigations on the
etiology of typhus, there was still no common agreement. Because
Rickettsia-bodies had not been cultured on artificial media, many researchers continued to reject them as the etiological agents of the
typhus-like diseases and to support instead bacterial, protozoan, or
viral etiologies. In 1920, for instance, a Brazilian researcher claimed
that typhus was caused by a protozoan organism of the *Herpetomanas*
genus, a group that he regarded as "piroplasms in a farther advanced
stage of evolution."[45] The *Piroplasma* genus to which he referred, of
course, was the one in which Wilson and Chowning had placed their
presumed spotted fever organism. Two years later, another Brazilian
claimed to have cultured a different typhus organism, which he described as a bacterium, on ascitic agar, a lifeless medium.[46] H. M.
Woodcock, a fellow at University College, London, preferred to dis-
pense entirely with the concept of disease-causing Rickettsia-bodies.
He argued that they were merely the end process of cell lysis and hence
the cause of the typhus-like diseases was "an abnormal haemetabolic
enzyme." In 1921, Harry Plotz's colleagues in New York compared
Plotz's bacillus with Rickettsia-bodies and determined only that they
were different. They withheld judgment on the precise relationship
between typhus and either organism. Not even discussing Wolbach's
claim that Rickettsia-bodies were unique organisms, they focused only
on the bacterial or protozoan nature of the organisms, concluding that
the evidence remained insufficient to classify them as either.[47]

One red herring that complicated the picture further emerged from
the 1916 discovery of Viennese physician Edmund Weil and his English
associate Arthur Felix that a strain of *Bacillus proteus* was agglutinated
by the sera of typhus patients.[48] Weil and Felix subsequently identified
other strains of *B. proteus* and numbered them sequentially as X-1,
X-2, etcetera. They also introduced terms to designate the motility of
the organisms: *O* organisms were nonmotile while *H* organisms were
motile. Their work showed that the *O* or nonmotile *B. proteus* organisms agglutinated more specifically than did the *H* organisms. Of
all the strains they isolated, OX-19 gave the best results.[49]

What Weil and Felix had developed was the first serological test for
typhus, which quickly became known as the Weil-Felix reaction. In
1922, W. J. Wilson confirmed in the *Lancet* that "although the nature
of the specific etiologic agent in typhus is still uncertain, and although
no simple laboratory test apart from animal experimentation is yet
available for its recognition," the Weil-Felix test using OX-19 provided
a specific laboratory diagnostic tool for confirming clinical diagnosis.

In 1921, moreover, a new strain of B. *proteus* was identified by A. N. Kingsbury, an Englishman. It appeared to be a modification of OX-19 with distinct antigenic differences. Called the OX-K strain after Kingsbury, it agglutinated sera of tsutsugamushi patients in low dilution and that of victims of the typhus-like disease of Malaya—later shown to be an antigenic variant of tsutsugamushi—in high dilution.[50]

Although subsequent studies revealed that the Weil-Felix reaction was caused by a chance antigenic "fit" between the B. *proteus* and the typhus organism, a few bacteriologists declared that this bacillus was the "exciting organism" of typhus. It was soon demonstrated, however, that B. *proteus* alone would not induce typhus. Other investigators, including Felix himself, argued that B. *proteus* and the typhus virus were simply variants of the same organism. Another champion of this theory was Max H. Kuczynski of Berlin, whose assistant, Elisabeth Brandt, died of a laboratory-acquired Rocky Mountain spotted fever infection. Kuczynski claimed to have cultured a spotted fever variant of the B. *proteus* organism, but his experiments were never replicated in other laboratories.[51]

Finally, a few researchers, including the respected Europeans Frederick Breinl and Rudolf Weigl, maintained that filterable viruses were the actual agents of the typhus-like diseases. In this theory, Rickettsia-bodies were considered either coincidental or a variant form of the viral agent. The agents of spotted fever and typhus had been demonstrated to be unfilterable, but that of trench fever had been filtered by the American Trench Fever Commission.[52] "Filterability," it should be noted, was one of two links among a variety of unidentified submicroscopic agents of disease and was not an entirely precise term, since experimental conditions such as the type of filter and the pressures exerted could vary. The other link between these agents, of course, was their inability to be cultured on lifeless media.

Several investigators, including S. Burt Wolbach and Rockefeller Institute researcher Peter J. Olitsky, attempted to convince their scientific associates that Rickettsia-bodies, like the filterable viruses, were obligate intracellular parasites—that is, they multiplied only within living cells. Such pathogens, they argued, would have to be grown using the emerging method of tissue culture, and they experimented with various tissue and media combinations. Unfortunately, the crude tissue culture techniques then available did not support luxurious multiplication of rickettsial organisms. The limitations of technique impeded a clear demonstration that Rickettsia-bodies required the presence of living cells to multiply.[53]

Although definitive proof eluded him, Wolbach continued to argue

that the unique characteristics of Rickettsia-bodies demanded modification of Koch's postulates. Dismayed that many researchers adhered
uncritically to the criteria established for bacterial diseases no matter
what laboratory investigations revealed, Wolbach spoke out forcefully
in a 1925 speech to the New York State Association of Public Health
Laboratories.

> I wish to emphasize and to insist on the importance of methods which may
> be employed in the face of failure to cultivate insect-borne microorganisms in
> artificial mediums. Properly conducted experiments in which the insect vector
> serves as culture tube, after natural or artificial introduction of the "virus,"
> have yielded evidence fully as reliable and in my opinion less open to mis-
> construction than in vitro cultivation. I feel it to be a duty to challenge skep-
> ticism based on rigid adherence to Koch's postulates when dealing with insect-
> borne diseases. . . . I do not know what to say to those who, in the face of
> the evidence I have assembled, may still insist that *Rickettsia prowazeki* is not
> the cause of typhus, but simply invariably accompanies the virus of typhus,
> particularly to those who assume, like Breinl and Weigl, that the virus of
> typhus in man may be in ultramicroscopic form. The same line of reasoning
> may be applied to all infectious agents, whether or not cultivated in test tubes.[54]

The controversy over the relationship of Rickettsia-bodies to disease
was finally settled only as a consequence of developments in research
on the filterable viruses. Wolbach himself had remarked as early as
1912 that "when our knowledge of filterable viruses is more complete,
our conception of living matter will change considerably, and . . . we
shall cease to attempt to classify the filterable viruses as animal or
plant."[55] His views were supported by many of the leaders of virus
research, notably Thomas Rivers at the Rockefeller Institute and
W. G. MacCullum of Johns Hopkins University School of Medicine.
At the 1925 meeting of the American Association for the Advancement
of Science, for example, MacCullum observed that progress in viral
research had been slow because "we still use blindly the methods of
investigation worked out for bacteriology." He suggested that "totally
different mediums" might be necessary for the cultivation of viruses
in addition to a conception of their nature different from existing
views.[56]

The concept of microbial pathogens as minute plants or animals,
however, was slow to change. In a 1930 editorial, the *Journal of the
American Medical Association* observed that viruses might merely be
"unusually small or unusually flaccid bacteria or protozoa," a concept
that "would not introduce any new factors into current pathologic
theory." There were, however, bacteriologists who proposed a "non-
microbic 'liquid life' " theory and botanists who entertained the hypothesis that viruses were "self-propagating toxins, enzymes, or 'mor-

bidic bions.' " Should either theory be correct, the *Journal* noted, "such transmissible biochemical perversion would necessitate radical revisions of present methods of research and clinical attack."[57]

In 1935 the need for such a radical revision in concept was proven when Wendell M. Stanley, a biochemist at the Rockefeller Institute, crystallized the tobacco mosaic virus. Stanley, who later won a Nobel prize for his work, viewed the virus as an "autocatalytic protein, which, for the present, may be assumed to require the presence of living cells for multiplication."[58] Before this revolutionary discovery, viral research had focused primarily on study of the infectious diseases caused by the submicroscopic agents. Subsequently, the techniques of the relatively new discipline of biochemistry were employed in an intense period of study that revealed the nucleic acid and protein composition of viruses—findings that rekindled discussion about the definition of life itself.[59]

By the late 1930s viruses were accepted as different entities from bacteria or protozoa, as was their property of multiplying only inside living cells. With this change in concept, the rigid adherence to Koch's postulates decried by Wolbach finally ceased to be a major barrier to proving etiology in viral and rickettsial diseases. Because of their common characteristic of intracellular multiplication, moreover, the viral and rickettsial diseases came to be thought of as one group. In 1939 the papers from a symposium at the Harvard School of Public Health were published as the first in a long line of studies entitled *Virus and Rickettsial Diseases*.[60]

By the time this conference was held, the diseases caused by the pathogenic *Rickettsiae* were termed *rickettsial* diseases more often than *typhus-like* diseases, although the etiology of many geographically isolated maladies in this group remained unclear. Wide usage of the lower-case *r* implied a general acceptance of the concept that these organisms were the etiological agents of a separate class of diseases. New laboratory techniques introduced in 1939—which will be discussed in chapter 9—had also proved useful for the immunological typing of rickettsial diseases. With these methods human rickettsial diseases were classified into three groups: the typhus group, the Rocky Mountain spotted fever group, and the tsutsugamushi group.[61]

Because these organisms were so small and so difficult to study, their taxonomic classification remained fluid for some time. Da Rocha Lima's designation *Rickettsia prowazeki* was honored as the type species for the typhus organism, but in 1927 Emile Brumpt, a French parasitologist, challenged Wolbach's genus designation of the spotted fever organism, *Dermacentroxenus*. Brumpt contended that it should be classed in the genus *Rickettsia* with the *rickettsi* species designation being preserved. In 1936, Henry Pinkerton of the Department of Pathology at Harvard University School of Medicine observed that Brumpt had not considered the intranuclear location of the spotted fever organism nor "the important morphological differences between it and *Rickettsia prowazeki*." Thus Pinkerton supported the separate genus proposed by his mentor, Wolbach. In 1940, Cornelius B. Philip, an entomologist who had worked with Rocky Mountain spotted fever investigations in Montana and who was, at that time, on the staff of the Army Medical School in Washington, D.C., attempted to bring some order into rickettsial taxonomy. In a Mayo Foundation lecture, Philip proposed that *Rickettsia* be adopted as the genus name for all the pathogenic rickettsiae, with *Dermacentroxenus* retained as a subgenus designation for the spotted fever organism. By the 1957 publication of the seventh edition of *Bergey's Manual of Determinative Bacteriology*, the definitive reference work on bacteriology, Philip's taxonomic criteria had been accepted, as evidenced in his authorship of the section on rickettsiae. The editors of the *Manual*, moreover, had adopted an international convention of doubling the final *i* of most species names. In this way the Rocky Mountain spotted fever organism received the name by which it is now called, *Rickettsia rickettsii*.[62]

Although in 1921 such standardization had not been achieved, international research on the typhus-like diseases had provided investigators with clues that would prove fruitful during the ensuing decade. Wolbach's emphasis on pathological study of the tissues in rickettsial diseases, for example, provided strong, if not universally accepted, evidence that a new type of microbe caused spotted fever and epidemic typhus. In the United States most investigators accepted Wolbach's findings and used his techniques to confirm clinical diagnoses of rickettsial diseases at post-mortem. When the U.S. Public Health Service returned to the Bitterroot Valley in 1922 to cooperate with Montana state authorities in seeking a medical solution to the problem of Rocky Mountain spotted fever, Wolbach's research provided the theoretical basis on which the renewed investigations were conducted.

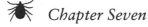

Chapter Seven

The Spencer-Parker Vaccine

We must also keep in mind that discoveries are usually not made by one man alone, but that many brains and many hands are needed before a discovery is made for which one man receives the credit.

Henry E. Sigerist, *A History of Medicine*

By the early 1920s the etiological agent of Rocky Mountain spotted fever had been identified and tick control efforts had been implemented for ten years, yet the disease continued to claim many victims and affect living conditions in Montana's Bitterroot Valley. In 1921 case incidence climbed precipitously to eleven cases and eleven deaths—a 100 percent mortality rate. In some areas of the valley, land prices had dropped from $125 to $15 per acre. Potential income from tourism was likewise threatened by the presence of the disease in the valley.[1] Disturbed by these problems and unsatisfied with the results of earlier control measures, local citizens clamored for additional federal assistance in attacking the problem. "A crisis has been reached in the Spotted Fever situation," wrote the manager of the Missoula Chamber of Commerce to W. F. Cogswell, secretary of the Montana State Board of Health. "A greater number of deaths from this dreaded disease has occurred this year than in the past, despite the fact that the people generally are aware of the malady and take precautions against it. The people are aroused to a very emphatic desire that the United States Public Health Service take an active hand in the fight to overcome this disease."[2]

Exacerbating the situation was the laboratory-acquired spotted fever death of Arthur H. McCray, Montana's first full-time state bacteriologist. McCray had assumed the post in October 1917 and had taken up spotted fever research during his spare time, hoping "to derive a curative serum for the treatment of the disease." In early June 1919, however, while working in the laboratory, he was infected. McCray died on 14 June 1919.[3]

As secretary of the state board of health and president of the state board of entomology, Cogswell wired the newly appointed surgeon general, Hugh S. Cumming, and appealed to the Montana delegation in Congress for assistance in persuading the U.S. Public Health Service to reenter the work. The surgeon general sent Thomas Parran, a rising Service administrator and later surgeon general himself, to evaluate the situation. Parran's visit was widely hailed in the Montana press as the beginning of renewed federal support for spotted fever research.[4] Parran was unsure if future cooperative measures would be productive, because of past tensions between state and federal authorities over jurisdiction in tick control efforts. A meeting with local civic groups, however, convinced him that the general public in the valley seemed "to be awakened to the menace of this disease" and was "very anxious" for the Service to assist in its eradication.[5]

To emphasize the state's cooperative intentions, Cogswell obtained pledges of twenty-eight hundred dollars from Missoula civic clubs to defray initial expenses of the work, and he secured an abandoned school building near Hamilton to serve as a laboratory. The "substantial, two story brick school building" that came to be known as the "schoolhouse lab" was located on the infected west side of the river about two miles from Hamilton.[6] Its West Valley Road site in the river bottom area, however, was considered free from infected ticks. A consolidation of schools in Hamilton had left it empty. Lunsford D. Fricks, who inspected the facility at the request of the surgeon general, enthusiastically wrote:

This new laboratory is a much more elaborate affair than any field laboratory which has been previously used in conducting spotted fever investigations. It is excellently lighted—kept well heated and has two sheds on the same school lot which can be used for storing automobiles and supplies. Dr. [Ralph R.] Parker has installed the necessary shelving, animal cages, and other equipment including laboratory animals. . . . In addition to Dr. Parker there are at present five employees in the laboratory—three at $150 each per month and two, a clerk and janitor, at $90 each. These men have been employed in equipping the laboratory, making maps, caring for animals and the building, and will be ready to begin field investigations at any time the season permits.[7]

Such concrete efforts by Montana authorities proved convincing, hence on 4 March 1922, Cumming detailed to Montana Roscoe Roy Spencer, the young Passed Assistant Surgeon who in 1915 had assisted Fricks in spotted fever work. The thirty-four-year-old Spencer was born in 1888 in West Point, Virginia, the last of five children of Branch Worsham Spencer and Emma Roy Burke Spencer. He took his A.B. degree in 1909 at Richmond University, and in 1913 he received the

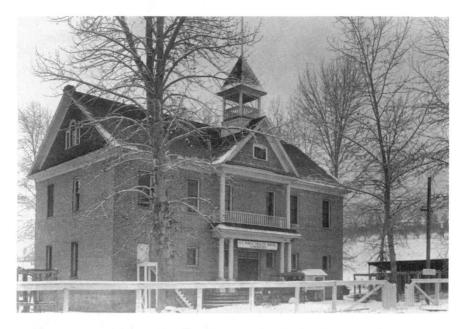

The sign over the door identifies this abandoned schoolhouse on the west side of the Bitterroot River as a U.S. Public Health Service Laboratory. Widely known in the 1920s as the "schoolhouse lab," this was the site where Roscoe R. Spencer and Ralph R. Parker ground up ticks to make a vaccine against spotted fever. (Courtesy of the Rocky Mountain Laboratories, NIAID.)

M.D. degree from Johns Hopkins University School of Medicine. Believing that he could "never assume a radiant bedside manner," Spencer joined the U.S. Public Health Service in 1914 as an assistant in the Hygienic Laboratory and was commissioned an Assistant Surgeon later that year by President Woodrow Wilson. During his 1915 work on spotted fever, Spencer had not been impressed by Fricks's research. After being recalled to Washington in the fall, Spencer assumed he would have no further involvement with the disease. For the next seven years, he completed the usual tour of duty stations, including plague control in Pensacola, Florida.[8]

Although Ralph R. Parker had been in charge of the board of entomology's work since 1918, the Service insisted that Spencer be placed in charge of spotted fever investigations in 1922, "simply because," as Fricks explained to Cogswell, who had complained, "from a Service standpoint Dr. Spencer out-ranks Dr. Parker. This is a fixed rule in the Service, as you perhaps know, from which it would be impossible to deviate." Spencer, of course, was a physician, and Parker, an entomologist. The arrangement threatened to rekindle the old antagonism between the two groups, because Parker saw no reason to relinquish his position of authority. Cogswell, however, "had a talk" with Parker about the delicacy of the situation, soothing his injured ego with the assurance that Spencer "could come in no other capacity." Parker decided to accept the situation without further protest. When Spencer arrived, the two men amicably agreed that all publications about spotted fever would be joint.[9]

Initially, Spencer and Parker planned an ambitious program of field investigations that would be supplemented with laboratory studies as time permitted. Parker planned a broad study on the relationship that ecological factors — the distribution of vegetation, rodents, and ticks — might have to human disease and to one another. Believing that there was a natural cycle regulating spotted fever in nature, Parker especially wanted to continue his work on the links among rabbits, their ticks, and spotted fever.[10] The field studies needed to implement such a program, however, were costly, time-consuming, and of questionable value to an improved tick control program. Fricks, who reviewed the plan for the Service, believed that sufficient investigational work had already been done to assure practical control through grazing restrictions and rodent destruction. Spencer, too, soon lost his enthusiasm for Parker's wide-ranging entomological studies. For the moment, however, Spencer let matters ride and concentrated on laboratory studies, hoping that a medical solution to the spotted fever problem might be found.[11]

Laboratory methods for identifying natural spotted fever infection in ticks had not changed significantly since Howard Taylor Ricketts identified the guinea pig as an experimental animal. Groups of suspect ticks were secured by a wire mesh collar on guinea pigs and allowed to engorge for several days, after which the animals were watched for symptoms of the disease. In Spencer's work with plague in Pensacola, however, fleas had been ground up and injected into the peritoneal cavities of guinea pigs, a method that shortened the waiting period by several days. Spencer suggested to Parker that they try the same method with ticks to test for spotted fever infection. Initially they allowed ticks to feed on infected animals for a time, after which they were ground up and injected into guinea pigs. This experiment worked well — five of the six pigs developed spotted fever. Continuing on this course, they separated 1,500 ticks into 102 lots, and, without allowing them to feed first, ground them up and inoculated them into guinea pigs. Sur-

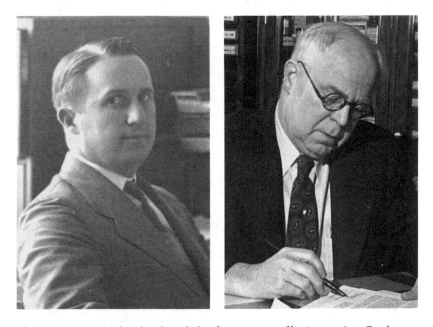

The two "R.R.s" who developed the first vaccine effective against Rocky Mountain spotted fever: Roscoe R. Spencer, a physician in the U.S. Public Health Service (left) and Ralph R. Parker, a Montana entomologist appointed as a Special Expert to the Service. When the vaccine had been demonstrated effective, Spencer returned to other Service assignments in Washington, D.C. Parker continued as director of the Rocky Mountain Laboratory until his death in 1949. (Courtesy of the National Library of Medicine and the Rocky Mountain Laboratories, NIAID.)

prisingly, none of the animals developed spotted fever. Many proved immune to subsequent direct inoculations of known lethal doses.[12]

These results appeared to indicate that Spencer's new method was a failure. As Louis Pasteur observed, however, chance favors the prepared mind. No conclusion was drawn about the results of the experiments until Henry Cowan, a field assistant, killed a mountain goat and brought it into the laboratory because it carried many engorged ticks. These ticks, too, were emulsified and injected, and they unquestionably produced spotted fever in guinea pigs. Spencer and Parker simultaneously realized the significance of their findings. The only difference between the ticks that produced immunity and those that caused spotted fever was that the latter had already had a blood meal on an animal. A jubilant but cautious Spencer wrote of this insight and its potential implications to Surgeon General Hugh S. Cumming.

One might be justified in inferring from these results that the virus in the tick . . . requires fresh animal blood to stimulate its growth and multiplication. There is good reason to believe that the inoculated ticks which conferred immunity would have produced fever if fed. In other words the virus needs to be primed with fresh animal blood before it can become infective. . . . Up to the present time all attempts to attenuate the virus in vitro have met with failure but there appears now a possibility of attenuating it in the body of the tick over a long period of time.[13]

Before Spencer suggested the short cut of emulsifying and injecting ticks, no change in virulence of the spotted fever organism had been suspected. By altering the method, Spencer unintentionally introduced a new way of viewing the process. The resulting insight also explained two observations by earlier investigators. First, as Spencer noted: "this view fits in with the fact that a tick must be attached for some hours before it becomes infective. The very earliest time of infectivity as determined by Ricketts was 1¼ hours of feeding and 8 to 10 hours as an average." Second, it illuminated the origin of cases of spotted fever that had no history of tick bite. Spencer had already demonstrated that the internal organs of infected animals would communicate the disease when rubbed on shaved or scarified skin.[14] Since engorged ticks contained highly virulent organisms, a person who had crushed such a tick might transfer the disease on the hands to any abrasion or cut in the skin.

Once again, a fresh approach yielded results where previous investigations had stalled. With his new insight, Spencer reviewed the earlier work of Ricketts and Fricks, in which each had produced immunity in guinea pigs by inoculating them with the eggs of infected ticks, and found it suggested promising avenues for research. Enthusiastically he wrote to Fricks, "These experiments of yours and Rickett's [sic] appear to me now highly significant." Observing that they had apparently attenuated the organism in tick eggs over time, Spencer predicted, "If I am correct in this assumption, it appears to me that in this direction lies the road to successful vaccination of people."[15]

Before more conclusive experiments could be undertaken, however, Spencer's observation about the potentially infectious nature of engorged ticks on abraded skin was confirmed in a tragic manner. William Edwin Gettinger, an undergraduate student at Montana State Agricultural College in Bozeman, had been hired at his "earnest request" as a student assistant for the summer. Born 16 July 1899 in Melrose, Iowa, Gettinger had studied entomology with Robert A. Cooley and was saving money to attend medical school. After the serendipitous discovery in April, Gettinger assisted Spencer in dissecting ticks and making stain smears of their organs in order to test them for the presence of rickettsiae. Although never bitten by a tick, Gettinger apparently rubbed at a pimple on his neck repeatedly while working in the laboratory. In late June he fell ill with typical spotted fever symptoms. It was a fulminating case, and the young man was soon delirious. Until he died on 30 June 1922, a few weeks before his twenty-third birthday, Gettinger "imagined himself in the laboratory and talked of it constantly." Gettinger's death brought to three the number of laboratory-acquired spotted fever cases in Montana and gave re-newed impetus to development of a successful vaccine.[16]

At the end of the summer, Spencer left the schoolhouse laboratory in Parker's care and returned to the Hygienic Laboratory in Wash-ington, D.C., to continue his experiments. Methodically he explored various properties of the spotted fever organism in light of the previous spring's discovery. Spencer demonstrated that spotted fever rickettsiae would remain infective in animal tissues if kept in 100 percent glycerine at a temperature constantly below $-10°$ C and that rickettsiae could readily be demonstrated in ticks after incubation or after feeding the ticks.[17]

Confident that laboratory work would soon provide medical inter-vention for the disease, Spencer apparently decided that his doubts about the cost and benefits of Parker's broad-ranging ecological studies were well founded. He therefore recommended that the control work be abolished or cut back severely. Spencer's memo, however, ran into trouble with Hygienic Laboratory director George McCoy and Surgeon General Hugh Cumming, both of whom rejected the recommendation. Although they gave no reason for their decision, it is likely that earlier battles between Service physicians and Montana entomologists con-vinced them that tolerance was preferable to confrontation.[18]

At about this same time, Hideyo Noguchi at the Rockefeller Institute again became interested in the spotted fever problem. Proceeding along the older path of research investigated by Ricketts, Noguchi announced in November 1922 that he had developed an immune serum for treating a person infected with spotted fever. Instead of using horses, as Ricketts had, Noguchi produced his serum in rabbits, declaring that it was superior, "both in potency and quantity." In guinea pigs, Noguchi wrote, 1 cc of the serum suppressed a spotted fever infection if given within twenty-four hours of the tick bite. Noguchi argued that guinea pig and human susceptibility to the disease were comparable and recommended an immediate injection of about 16 cc for adults "in every instance when the bite of a tick gives reason to suspect a possible infection with spotted fever."[19]

In Montana the news of Noguchi's serum was greeted with some skepticism. Remembering the abortive efforts of Ricketts and his colleagues in a similar attempt, Cooley remarked, "I do not see that there is anything particularly new in . . . [the serum] excepting, perhaps, that he has figured out the minimum dosage for a guinea pig and computed the dosage for man." Nonetheless, state board of health secretary W. F. Cogswell wrote to Noguchi, requesting that he make his serum available for prophylactic purposes in Montana. It was doubtful that the serum could function as a vaccine, Noguchi replied, because, being a foreign protein, it would be quickly eliminated from the body. He suggested that instead it would be useful to give the serum to anyone bitten by an infected tick.[20]

During the next few months, Noguchi went one step farther and developed a prophylactic vaccine by adding infected guinea pig blood to the immune rabbit serum. This serovaccine gave full protection to guinea pigs. Because of the danger of using live virus, Noguchi studied the immunizing power of a heated vaccine. He concluded that heating the mixture to 56–60° C for twenty minutes did not destroy the immunizing property, although it did "markedly" reduce it.[21] A decade before, Ricketts had pursued similar studies and abandoned them.

Tick season in 1923 offered the first opportunity for Noguchi's serovaccine to be tested in humans. Since Noguchi planned to come to Montana for the tests, the Montana State Board of Health capitalized on his visit to further its longstanding goal of educating the public that spotted fever was a regional problem, not limited to Montana. In March 1923 the board issued a call to the state and local health officers of the Rocky Mountain region to meet on 5 and 6 April in Missoula to discuss the current status of Rocky Mountain spotted fever in their states. Noguchi would, of course, be present to discuss his new vaccine. S. Burt Wolbach was likewise invited, as were representatives of the U.S. Public Health Service.[22]

Papers were presented on a wide variety of subjects relating to spotted fever, but Noguchi's presence and announcement of a vaccine overshadowed all other concerns. Because of Noguchi's Japanese origins and connection with the prestigious Rockefeller Institute, the Montana press devoted nearly as much space to descriptions of the famous investigator as to information about the conference. "Intensely alive, intensely, Orientally polite—and, most intensely, devoted to science and humanity. That is Doctor Noguchi," exclaimed one Missoula reporter. Under the banner headline "Spotted Fever Heroes," another article noted that nine Japanese residents of Missoula had volunteered to take the first human injections of their countryman's vaccine.[23]

Although the method of preparing the vaccine given to the Japanese volunteers was not described, Noguchi apparently was willing to risk administering the live virus mixture in order to achieve protection. This certainly seems to have been his plan when he offered the vaccine to members of the schoolhouse laboratory in Hamilton. In an oral history memoir, Spencer recalled insisting that the vaccine be heated to 45° C in order to kill the rickettsiae. Noguchi reportedly opposed this move, but he eventually complied and vaccinated five members of the laboratory staff. Later, other Bitterroot Valley residents volunteered, bringing to 152 the total number of people who took Noguchi's serovaccine. A number of them became ill with serum sickness, possibly because the vaccine contained two types of foreign proteins — those in the rabbit serum and those in guinea pig blood.[24]

The real measure of the vaccine, of course, was whether it would prevent the disease or lessen its severity if contracted. Initially there was an indication that it was efficacious. In July after he was vaccinated in April, Ralph R. Parker sustained a laboratory accident in which he knocked a syringe full of infected blood off a table. It stuck in his leg as it fell. "I didn't think anything of it for a few seconds," he wrote to Cooley, "and then it dawned on me what I had done." Parker immediately treated the wound with iodine and "burned it out" with nitric acid. "I am not worrying much. . . . I think the vaccine is all right. . . . I feel that there is no danger, but of course will feel uneasy for a few days."[25] Parker did not become ill, but whether the vaccine or luck protected him was unclear.

A second case produced a different outcome. It occurred in George Michky, Jr., son of the laboratory's janitor.[26] The child had been vaccinated with Noguchi's vaccine, and although he recovered, he suffered a long illness. Widely publicized, the case cast doubt on the value of the vaccine. Noguchi maintained that one case proved very little but noted that he was attempting to develop a safe way to administer the more potent unheated vaccine to humans. Spencer and Parker's immediate response to the Michky case was to make a large, painted sign, visible to all approaching the schoolhouse laboratory, warning them of the danger and advising them that they entered at their own risk.[27]

Noguchi discontinued his spotted fever research in November 1923, when he departed New York for Brazil and turned his attention to yellow fever. Upon his return in 1925 he resumed the work, searching for a way to produce a safe, potent, unheated serovaccine. Both Wolbach and Parker viewed this work as promising, but Noguchi was unable to protect monkeys with the preparation, a step he believed essential before testing the vaccine on humans. Increasingly, he became preoccupied with identifying the causative organism of yellow fever. After asserting that a spirochete was the guilty organism, Noguchi found his work attacked by other researchers. In 1928 he traveled to Africa with hopes of vindicating his research, but instead he contracted yellow fever and died.[28]

Because of the inconclusive results obtained with Noguchi's serovaccine, Roscoe R. Spencer pressed on with his own work after returning to the Hygienic Laboratory. During the fall and winter of 1923–24, he continued to seek a means to attenuate the organism and produce a vaccine. By injecting guinea pigs with various dilutions of an emulsion made from the engorged ticks, he determined that 1/5,000 of a tick would cause infection in a guinea pig. He refined his previous experiments on the virulence of the spotted fever organism in hibernating, warmed, and engorged ticks. He determined that the organism in tick tissues was unfilterable, a point not examined by Ricketts and Wolbach before him. Curiously, Spencer found that rickettsiae could not be demonstrated in some infective ticks. Subsequent studies threw no additional light on this problem.[29]

Even with much new information, Spencer could identify no method for translating it into a usable vaccine. The key that unlocked the puzzle came from a Czechoslovakian researcher working in Austria on a vaccine for typhus, spotted fever's closest rickettsial relative. Worldwide work on the typhus-like diseases was abstracted in several journals, including the *Journal of the American Medical Association*, and through these summaries Spencer kept abreast of each new development. In February 1924 he spotted the *Journal's* abstract of an article originally published by Frederick Breinl in the *Journal of Infectious Diseases*. Instead of attempting to make a typhus vaccine using the standard tactic of mixing typhus organisms in blood with immune serum, Breinl demonstrated that rabbits were actively immunized "by injecting emulsified louse intestines, to which phenol has been added." Protection was achieved, he speculated, because of the immunizing properties of quantities of dead typhus organisms present before the phenol was added.[30]

Spencer seized upon Breinl's method, even though he concluded that Breinl's explanation of how immunity was produced was not applicable to spotted fever. As soon as he returned to Montana in late February 1924, Spencer prepared a vaccine from infected ticks. From his experiments on changes in spotted fever virulence in fasting and engorged ticks, Spencer knew he needed to use fully engorged ticks to obtain a vaccine that would maximize protective value. Using a mortar and pestle, he ground up the ticks in a salt solution to which 0.5 percent phenol had been added to kill the rickettsiae. Each 1 cc dose contained the equivalent of one tick, and since he had determined the minimum infectious dose to be 1/5,000 of a tick, each guinea pig received 5,000 infectious doses of killed vaccine in the injection. In every guinea pig so inoculated, the vaccine prevented illness when the animal was injected with infectious spotted fever blood fourteen days later.[31]

By May, Spencer had sufficient confidence in the vaccine to inoculate himself with it. Although it caused no adverse reaction, Parker and the rest of the staff remained wary of taking the vaccine until further tests had been conducted.[32] There was certainly reason for caution. Preparing a human vaccine from an arthropod vector had never before been attempted. Breinl had protected animals from typhus, but his louse intestine vaccine had not been used on humans. Rabies vaccine, of course, was made from the dried spinal cords of infected rabbits and smallpox vaccine from the pus in cowpox scabs, hence the concept of utilizing animal tissues was not new. Noguchi's vaccine, containing two foreign proteins, however, had caused adverse reactions. Doubtless this memory dampened the staff's enthusiasm for an unproven vaccine containing tick proteins.

Testing of the vaccine was delayed during the spring and summer of 1924 because of a newly identified illness among laboratory workers. Shortly after Spencer arrived in Montana, Parker queried him about peculiar lesions observed in the laboratory's rabbits. Spencer believed the lesions were caused by tularemia, a disease with symptoms similar to bubonic plague. Tularemia had first been described in 1911 by the Hygienic Laboratory's director, George W. McCoy, as a plague-like disease of rodents, which he had found while doing research on plague in Tulare County, California. He named the disease after this location. Another Hygienic Laboratory researcher, Edward Francis, had become an expert on tularemia, demonstrating that humans could be infected through handling infected rabbits or through the bites of infected ticks, deer flies, and other arthropods. Spencer thus wrote to Francis about his suspicions, and the senior man confirmed the diagnosis. The discovery of tularemia in laboratory animals stimulated the staff of the Hamilton laboratory to expand their studies into a second tick-borne disease. More important to the spotted fever work, however, was the highly contagious nature of tularemia. In July, Spencer and Sam Maclay, an assistant bacteriologist, came down with the disease. Both recovered, but Spencer was quite ill for several weeks. After Spencer returned east, Parker himself contracted the disease and was ill for seven weeks.[33]

During Parker's bout with tularemia, George Henry Cowan contracted spotted fever. The son of Bitterroot Valley pioneers, Cowan had the longest continuous record in the state in spotted fever research. He had begun working for the U.S. Bureau of Entomology in 1913, and his exemplary record had earned him a promotion in 1917 to chief deputy in tick control work under the Montana State Board of Entomology. When the U.S. Public Health Service took over the work in 1921, Cowan had been made a field assistant. His duties included making rough maps in the field, trapping experimental animals, and collecting ticks from animals and special localities.[34]

Because Cowan had escaped spotted fever despite a decade of dangerous work, one Montana newspaper speculated that, "as many other natives have done, he perhaps came to regard himself as immune" to the disease. He apparently contracted spotted fever in the laboratory through handling infected material, for there was no evidence of a tick bite. As the thirty-eight-year-old man became sicker, his physician administered some of Spencer's vaccine in hope that it might have a therapeutic effect. This effort was in vain: Cowan died on 29 October 1924. Parker wired Spencer about Cowan's death and in the same telegram requested enough vaccine to inoculate the laboratory staff.[35]

During the winter of 1924–25, Spencer tested his vaccine on monkeys as well as on guinea pigs. Monkeys provided an animal model so much closer to humans that Hideyo Noguchi had written to Spencer, "If you can protect *Macacus rhesus* with your vaccine, I shall be convinced that it will protect man." Spencer inoculated eight monkeys with his vaccine, leaving five others unvaccinated as controls. An immunity test two weeks later produced frank spotted fever in the controls, but all of the vaccinated monkeys remained healthy. He also tested for evidence of human antibodies to the vaccine by injecting guinea pigs with combinations of serum from vaccinated persons and infective blood serum. These results indicated that the vaccine did indeed produce antibodies to spotted fever.[36]

When Spencer returned to Montana in the spring of 1925, enough vaccine was prepared to vaccinate thirty-four people in the Bitterroot Valley—primarily laboratory and field staff and other residents whose occupations exposed them to spotted fever infection. Since human dosage had not been worked out precisely, the vaccine was administered in two to four doses of 1 or 2 cc at five-day intervals. No severe reactions were encountered, but most people reported local redness,

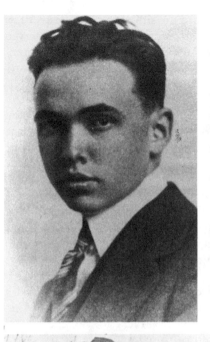

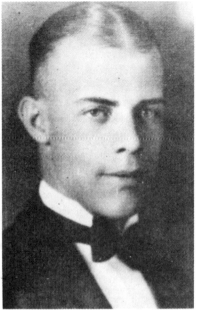

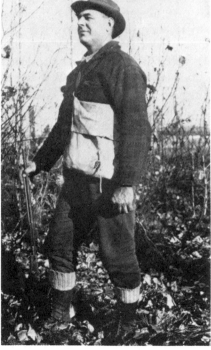

During the effort to develop a vaccine against spotted fever, three workers at the schoolhouse laboratory became martyrs to laboratory-acquired infections. William Edwin Gettinger (top left), a student assistant with the U.S. Public Health Service, died in 1922; George Henry Cowan (bottom), a field assistant with the Montana State Board of Entomology and the U.S. Public Health Service, in 1924; and Albert LeRoy Kerlee (top right), also a student assistant to the Service, in 1928. (Courtesy of the Rocky Mountain Laboratories, NIAID.)

swelling, and heat for two days around the site of the injection. A few also suffered headaches and muscular pains. One recipient observed that his "hand became swollen and the arm was somewhat uncomfortable for a while," but that he was able to continue his regularly scheduled activities. "I imagine that it looked worse than it felt," he commented.[37]

The first test of the vaccine's effectiveness came unexpectedly in April, when E. O. Everson, a forty-three-year-old employee of the Montana State Board of Entomology, contracted spotted fever. He had actively sought vaccination because he dipped tick-infected cattle and often picked engorged ticks off by hand. The course of his illness was mild, and although convalescence was prolonged, he recovered. Spencer noted that it was impossible to state without reservation "that the vaccine modified the course and severity of the infection." Four unvaccinated victims of spotted fever that spring, however, died within ten days, and since the disease in persons over forty was nearly always fatal, Everson's recovery augured well.[38]

The apparent success of the vaccine on a small scale produced a large demand for it the following year, even though it remained an experimental product. Spencer underwent surgery for appendicitis in March 1926 and was unable to return to Montana, but Parker and his staff produced enough vaccine to inoculate over four hundred persons, ranging in age from four to seventy, in the Bitterroot Valley and in Idaho. In the southern valley town of Darby, school was dismissed in order to allow people to be vaccinated. Each person received 2 cc of vaccine in each of two injections one week apart. Few severe reactions to the injections occurred; none was fatal.[39]

Ralph R. Parker and L. B. Byington, whom the U.S. Public Health Service had detailed to Montana in Spencer's place, were equally interested in analyzing the vaccine's effectiveness against the mild Idaho form of spotted fever. A large concentration of Basque sheepherders, whose occupation rendered them particularly vulnerable to spotted fever, provided an ideal population for a trial of the vaccine in Idaho. Since infection often took place on the range far from medical assistance, the incapacitation of a sheepherder often meant loss of many sheep to the owners. Idaho stock owners thus urged their sheepherders to take the vaccine. Because some resisted and, in any case, there was insufficient vaccine to inoculate all of them, those not vaccinated served as controls in studying the new product's effectiveness. None of the 94 sheepherders vaccinated in 1926 developed spotted fever, while thirteen cases occurred among 180 who had not been vaccinated. When this test was repeated in 1927, one case occurred among 99 vaccinated men as opposed to nine cases among 184 controls.[40]

Three cases of spotted fever at the laboratory further increased confidence in the vaccine's value. Two young vaccinated laboratory attendants, Martin Nolan and Frank P. Merritt, suffered only mild bouts with the disease. When the sixty-two-year-old janitor, Alex Chaffin, fell ill, the vaccine's protective power was demonstrated most impressively. Parker observed that Chaffin's recovery was a first "for a man of his years" in the Bitterroot. "It is believed," Parker continued, "that these . . . cases place the value of the vaccine outside any realm of doubt."[41]

A four-year retrospective study of spotted fever in the Bitterroot later confirmed these empirical observations of the vaccine's efficacy. Spencer and Parker excluded the high-risk laboratory workers and examined the records of 1,208 residents of a known infected zone on the west side of the valley. Of these, 496 chose to be vaccinated, while 712 refused and thereby served as controls in the study. Over the four-year period, only three cases of spotted fever occurred in vaccinated persons, and none was fatal. In contrast, nine cases occurred in the control group, seven—or 77.7 percent—of which were fatal.[42]

For the next fifteen years, Parker continued to gather extensive records from which he published data confirming the efficacy of the vaccine. Overall, vaccinated adults experienced a 74.24 percent lower fatality rate than did the unvaccinated. In Idaho, where the disease had never been virulent, the number of cases decreased markedly as the number of vaccinated persons increased. Scientific objectivity rejected the obvious conclusion that the vaccine fully protected people, for, as Parker acknowledged, other factors such as ecological shifts that were not well understood could be responsible. Nonetheless, the partial correlation convinced most people of the vaccine's protective power and increased demand throughout the west.[43]

Developing the best method to mass produce the vaccine involved a trial-and-error process. Parker worked with his chief technician, Earl W. Malone—who alone among all employees involved with the vaccine-making process escaped spotted fever infection—to find a technique that would yield a consistent level of protection in all lots. Initially they made the vaccine in the fall before its distribution in the spring. Eventually, Parker and Malone learned not only that the vaccine remained potent after a year's storage but also that a more potent vaccine resulted if ticks were stored in the cold room for a year before being used. Preservatives posed another problem. Carbolic acid, or phenol, was originally used, but it was found insufficient to kill all contaminating organisms. Parker switched to formalin for a period, but it

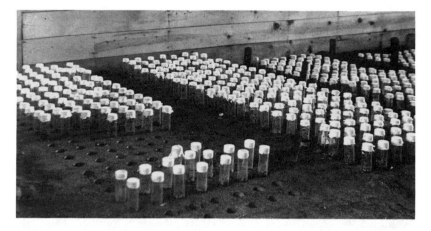

Tubes containing ticks were stoppered with cotton to permit oxygen to enter. Their open bottoms were buried in the damp earth. (Courtesy of the Rocky Mountain Laboratories, NIAID.)

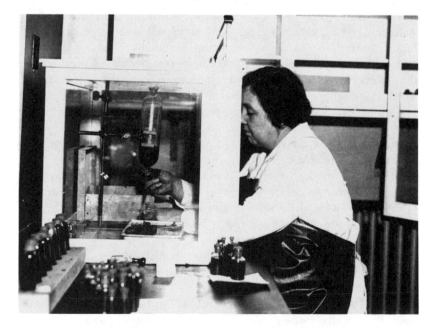

A laboratory technician decants Spencer-Parker vaccine into bottles for shipment, 1931. (Courtesy of the Rocky Mountain Laboratories, NIAID.)

caused the vaccine to appear cloudy. Finally he adopted a combination of the two preservatives. Although the formalin caused a slight stinging for about five minutes after a patient was injected, it ensured a sterile product and generated no other side effects.[44]

The standard method finally adopted was expensive, time-consuming, and dangerous. It required four to six thousand rabbits and twenty to thirty thousand guinea pigs for feeding the ticks in all stages of their development, for maintaining passage strains of spotted fever, and for potency testing of the vaccine. Initially, field workers collected thirty to forty thousand adult ticks, which were placed on rabbits to feed and mate. After mating, the male ticks died. The females were collected and placed on a wire cloth over moist sand on a tray in an incubator, where they produced some hundred million eggs and then died themselves.

Approximately 80 percent of the eggs hatched into larvae after a five- to six-week incubation period. At this point, adult female rabbits were infected with spotted fever. On the first day the rabbits ran a high fever, they were placed in "infesting bags," to which the larvae of four female ticks were added. This number was the maximum that could feed without exsanguinating the rabbits. Left alone for twenty-four hours, the larvae attached to the rabbits and the bags could be removed. Rabbits and ticks were placed in wire cages and covered with white cage bags to prevent the ticks from escaping. After four or five days, about one-fourth of the larvae succeeded in engorging and dropped from the rabbits to be caught in the cage bags.

The next step involved emptying the cage bags into a "tick picker" containing a series of screens designed to separate out waste food and rabbit feces from the larval ticks. The recovered larvae were put back into the incubator to molt into nymphs, a process that took about a month. The feeding process was then repeated on a new series of infected female rabbits, although fewer nymphs—about four hundred—were placed on each rabbit. After the engorged nymphs were separated by the tick picker, they were washed and separated from further debris in a converted cream separator and dried with a hair drier. Next they were placed in pillboxes, two hundred nymphs to a box, and returned to a low humidity incubator at 22° C for several weeks until they molted into adults. About one million of the one hundred million original eggs survived to adulthood. They were stored for six months to a year in a refrigeration room that simulated a normal Montana mountain winter temperature.

When ready to be used for vaccine production, the ticks were taken from storage and placed into a "tick separator," an ingenious device in which live ticks were separated from dead ticks and any cast skin from the last molt. The separator consisted of a cylindrical sheet metal container, into which the stored ticks were placed, and an attached glass tube. In a lighted cabinet, the ticks migrated toward the light—that is, into the glass tube—leaving the dead ticks and refuse behind. These ticks were warmed in the incubator and fed on guinea pigs for three days to reactivate the virus. They were then soaked for twenty-four hours in a Merthiolate solution to sterilize the surface of their bodies, after which they were divided into lots by weight. Covered with a salt solution containing a 2 percent mixture of phenol and formalin, each lot was emulsified in a Waring blender for two minutes. To the deep orange liquid produced was added additional phenol-formalin-saline diluent to bring the volume to 200 cc. This crude vaccine was stored for a week at room temperature to kill the rickettsiae and any contaminating organisms.

Finally, the vaccine was diluted with another 600 cc of saline without additional preservatives, bringing the volume to nearly a quart and reducing the concentration of the phenol-formalin preservatives to 0.5 percent. The vaccine thus produced contained one "tick equivalent" in each cc. After a few additional weeks of storage in a cold room, the vaccine was centrifuged in order to remove the tick tissue. Guinea pigs were inoculated with each lot of vaccine to test potency, and sterility tests were performed by the biologics control section of the Hygienic Laboratory in Washington, D.C. The lots that passed these tests were bottled, labeled, and shipped.[45]

The enthusiastic reception given the tick vaccine across the northwestern states was welcome, but some of the attendant publicity was not so well received. Bitterroot Valley residents, acutely sensitive to spotted fever's effect on property values, were outraged in 1927 when Paul de Kruif chronicled the saga of vaccine development for the magazine *Country Gentleman*.[46] A former bacteriologist who had abandoned his career at the Rockefeller Institute to become a popular science writer, de Kruif was renowned for his hyperbolic style. Although a generation of scientists was inspired by de Kruif's book *Microbe Hunters*, residents of the Bitterroot found little to praise in his description of their valley crouching in fear of spotted fever. "When the snow begins to melt on the hills the terror of the spotted fever begins to stalk in the Bitter Root Valley," de Kruif wrote. "In that sad territory the doors of the empty ranch houses creaked and whined on the hinges, singing a lonesome song for fathers who had died and brothers and sisters and mothers who had gone away." De Kruif's style riveted readers and sold magazines, but Bitterroot businessmen were convinced that the article would discourage prospective home-owners and businesses from purchasing land in the valley.[47]

Shortly after the article was published, the *Northwest Tribune* ran an article under the banner headline "Bitter Root Valley Is Up in Arms." Missoula and other Montana cities were also reported to be "ablaze with a wave of indignation." Commercial clubs in Victor, Stevensville, and Darby joined with the Hamilton Chamber of Commerce to send a protesting telegram to the editors of *Country Gentleman.* Another article called de Kruif's story an "absurd fairy tale." Believing that de Kruif must have obtained material for his story from employees of the schoolhouse laboratory, George L. Knight, secretary of the Hamilton Chamber of Commerce, wrote Montana Congressman Scott Leavitt, requesting that laboratory employees be restricted in what they could say to reporters. "We have no objection whatever to the facts being printed," Knight asserted. "The statements that we do object to are the ones which have in the past been dressed up by information exaggerated and over-drawn." Surgeon General Cumming responded, but his instructions were couched as "merely a caution" that employees should be careful what they said to the press, so information would not be abused.[48]

It was not only articles in the popular press that elicited hostility from the guardians of the valley's public image. In 1926, W. F. Cogswell, secretary of the Montana State Board of Health, found himself at the center of unintended controversy. A man from Dillon, Montana, whose daughter's geology class at Vassar College was scheduled to make a field trip to the west side of the Bitterroot, inquired of Cogswell whether the outing would be safe. Cogswell replied that, as state health officer, he would do all in his power to prevent such a field trip in the spring. This letter stimulated an "indignation" meeting of the Hamilton Chamber of Commerce, whose secretary threatened "dire and sundry things" against Cogswell, including trying to get him fired. In the view of the Chamber of Commerce, Cogswell had gone out of his way "to give the Bitter Root Valley a black eye." When pressed, however, secretary Otto Bolen admitted that he would not want his own daughter going into the Bitterroot mountains during active tick season, and he agreed to discuss with Cogswell how future inquiries should be handled.[49]

Although the danger of living in the Bitterroot Valley was periodically overstated or minimized, the peril in which the staff of the schoolhouse laboratory worked was never questioned. In August 1926, Ralph R. Parker suffered an especially bad moment. His wife Adah found a tick attached to herself that, when tested, produced spotted fever in laboratory guinea pigs. Fortunately, Mrs. Parker had been vaccinated in May, and the tick was discovered before it had become well engorged. She showed preliminary symptoms of spotted fever but never came down with a full case. A relieved Parker noted: "The facts appear to be good circumstantial evidence of the value of the vaccine, but it is far from a pleasant thing to accumulate evidence from one's own wife. The curse of this work is not the danger to one's self but the continual fear of bringing infection home."[50]

With the discovery of tularemia in the laboratory's rabbits, moreover, another hazard was added to the burden under which researchers and their staff labored. In May 1925, Earl W. Malone, the chief vaccine maker, contracted tularemia. His incapacitation brought to six the number of spotted fever or tularemia infections among the laboratory staff in just one year. Infected ticks from the vaccine-making process often were found attached to laboratory personnel, and the schoolhouse design of the laboratory even allowed dogs to wander in occasionally. As the dangers compounded, the staff came to believe that the only way to make the work safer was to build a new laboratory.[51]

Beginning in early 1925, the Montana State Board of Entomology explored possible sources of funding for a new facility, the total cost of which was estimated to be fifty thousand dollars. Robert A. Cooley wrote to the Anaconda Copper Mining Company, the Rockefeller Foundation, and the U.S. Public Health Service, but all hesitated to commit the necessary monies. Since spotted fever was known only in the northwestern states, the Service preferred that these states pool their funds to support vaccine production. Although some interest was expressed by a former state health officer in Wyoming, none of the northwestern state governments appropriated funds for the venture.[52]

In early 1926 the quest for a new laboratory took on additional urgency when the original owners of the schoolhouse laboratory petitioned to recover their property. A stipulation in the deed provided that the property would revert to the Waddell family if the building ceased to be used as a school. Since the Waddells had "mentioned a price at which they would sell," Cooley presumed that their aim was "to get a sum of money from somebody for the property."[53] The school board opposed the petition, claiming that a population increase might eventually require that the building be reclaimed as a school. In 1927 a court hearing the case decided in favor of the Waddells.

The Montana State Board of Entomology seized upon this ruling to press the state legislature for a new building. Old friends of the spotted fever researchers came to their aid in this effort. S. Burt Wolbach, who stopped at the laboratory during a western trip, felt compelled to write

Hygienic Laboratory director George W. McCoy that he considered the schoolhouse "the most dangerous place" he visited. Describing laboratory conditions as disgraceful, Wolbach asked McCoy's help in moving federal or state authorities to secure a new facility. W. F. Cogswell, secretary of the state board of health, also appealed to the surgeon general for documentation that would impress the state legislature. Surgeon General Cumming complied, intimating that a new laboratory was necessary to "make continued studies by Service personnel possible."[54]

When the state legislature convened in January 1927, it appropriated sixty thousand dollars to build a new laboratory and twenty-five thousand dollars per year for operating expenses during the next biennium. Once the question of funding had been resolved, another prickly issue arose: where should the new laboratory be located? Spencer argued for Missoula, a larger town than Hamilton and home of the University of Montana. Faculty members favored such a move, and Spencer asserted that the infected ticks posed no threat to the campus. "I carry yearly thousands of infected ticks with me to Washington, and ship hundreds more to New York and abroad." The state board of entomology, however, preferred that the new laboratory be located in Hamilton. Because of additional research planned by the board, Cooley stated, "we need to be nearer to the field than we would be in Missoula. For the vaccine work I think we could have gotten along very nicely as far away as Missoula but, all things considered, the Board was of the opinion it would be better at Hamilton." The board's position prevailed when the Hamilton Chamber of Commerce purchased and donated to the state a tract of land on which the laboratory would be built.[55]

Many Bitterroot Valley residents vehemently opposed the location just outside the business district in Hamilton, in an area known as Pine Grove. Of primary importance was that, for the first time ever, a spotted fever laboratory was to be built on the uninfected east side of the river. Since no one knew why spotted fever was restricted to the west side, it is not surprising that there was opposition to a facility that would be rearing millions of infected ticks in a previously safe area. For two decades, furthermore, the economic fortunes of the Bitterroot Valley had fluctuated with the success or failure of schemes to irrigate the dry benchlands. In 1920, after the collapse of one of these efforts, a bankruptcy court had ordered residents to form an irrigation district to raise needed water revenues. The president and Board of Commissioners of this new Bitter Root Irrigation District viewed a laboratory in Hamilton as a threat. Siting it there, they protested, would "cause a general feeling that the entire valley was so infected, causing unjust damage to the East Side farming lands."[56] To protect their interests, they filed suit against the state boards of health and entomology and against the state board of examiners.

Most of those complaining were residents of Pine Grove who felt that their own property values were threatened. E. R. Hammond, an employee of the local Light and Water Company, described as the "principal agitator," was joined by other prominent Hamilton residents, including a physician, a dentist, a pharmacist, a judge, and an engineer for the Bitter Root Irrigation Company. When the first stirrings of opposition appeared, proponents of the new laboratory dismissed it as "Cigar Store, Drug Store, Bridge Club and street corner discussion." Although the case remained on the court's calendar, a number of the plaintiffs soon dropped out, realizing that they would be responsible for court costs if the ruling went against them.[57]

Cooley welcomed this fight. He believed that erecting the laboratory in Hamilton would do much to clear away superstition that had surrounded spotted fever for decades. He thus rebuffed an alternative proposal from Victor officials, who hoped to entice the laboratory to their city. Setting out his opinions in a letter to Cogswell, Cooley stated:

The psychological influence of bringing this laboratory into town will be considerable. One great difficulty in the past has been that people have looked upon spotted fever as a mystery about which the less said the better. There has been too much *unreasonable* fear of it. To bring the laboratory into town will help, gradually, to allay unreasonable fear, and will help to educate everyone. Some day residents in that vicinity will say to visitors who come to the valley that "We used to be afraid to go across the river. Now we have the laboratory right in town." This will do much to reassure people who think of settling and making business investments.[58]

On 27 July 1927 the case was heard by Judge George B. Winston of the Fourth Montana Judicial District. The plaintiffs' testimony focused on the dangers already documented at the schoolhouse laboratory. Field assistants were described as coming back with ticks "on their horses and clothing, and their beds, and they will ride up to the institution." Since field workers were seeking "the most malignant and wild—the most virulent and dangerous ticks," there was fear that they would carry them home if the laboratory was in Hamilton. It was noted that ticks had escaped in the yard of the laboratory and alleged that the janitor had been "the sole protector of the community." Countering suggestions that children playing near the proposed site would be at risk, Cogswell testified that there would be no chance for the experimentally infected ticks to escape from the laboratory. The vivid

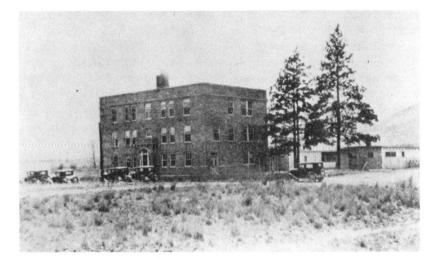

Built by the state of Montana in 1928 for spotted fever vaccine production, this laboratory was located in Hamilton, Montana, on the uninfected east side of the Bitterroot River. To prevent infected ticks from escaping, it incorporated many special features, such as rounded seams where walls met floors and a moat around its perimeter, across which ticks reportedly could not swim. (Courtesy of the Rocky Mountain Laboratories, NIAID.)

testimony caught the attention of the *Journal of the American Medical Association*, which reported that "the question of how fast these ticks travel is said to have enlivened the court proceedings." Judge Winston ultimately sided with the researchers and ruled that construction of the laboratory, begun in mid June, should continue.[59]

With the court case behind them, the sponsors of the new laboratory concentrated on tick proofing the facility, which was occupied in May 1928. The laboratory was built of reinforced concrete, brick faced. Around the perimeter of the building was a moat containing water, across which ticks supposedly could not swim. Outside it was a "tick yard," used, in part, for storing hibernating ticks. An animal house was attached to the main building, and the whole complex was surrounded by a fence to keep out "rodents, domestic animals, and boys." In addition to several laboratory rooms, refrigeration rooms, and general offices, there were specially designed tick-rearing and vaccine-producing rooms. The joints between floor and walls were all rounded to prevent ticks from hiding. A chamber through which workers passed on entering or leaving the tick-rearing room contained mirrors for examining their bodies. Eventually a device was also installed to heat their stored clothing to 150° F for six minutes in order to kill any ticks hiding in the fabric seams.[60]

These extraordinary precautions, solicitous public relations, and evidence that no children playing near the laboratory became infected soothed the tensions raised by construction of the facility. Within a few years, in fact, the problem reversed itself: townspeople visited the laboratory so often as to make themselves a nuisance. It had become, Cooley noted, "a rather popular place for visitors to go. People in town like to take their guests out there and show them through the building." Fearing that an accidental infection might take place, Parker ordered all employees to get permission before taking visitors through the building.[61]

Parker had some cause for concern, because even with the best advice on constructing the building, unanticipated dangers were eventually discovered. Infected ticks were found hiding around the windows and screens, in a pile of sacks that had lain undisturbed for some time in the corner of a room, and in the nickel caps around pipes going through the floor. Ticks also escaped via the cage sacks used in the tick-rearing process. After each use, these sacks were sent down a chute into a creosote solution that was supposed to kill any remaining ticks before the sacks were washed. The solution was discovered to be ineffective when ticks were found in the laboratory's backyard where the sacks were dried. Subsequently the bags were soaked in kerosene and boiled in soap before washing.[62]

Ironically, none of these precautions would have prevented a laboratory-acquired spotted fever infection that occurred at the schoolhouse laboratory just three months before the new facility was completed. No infected tick was found attached to LeRoy Kerlee, a Bitterroot Valley native and student volunteer at the laboratory, who became ill on 4 February 1928. W. F. Cogswell speculated that Kerlee might have contracted the disease through a skin abrasion or by rubbing his eye with a contaminated finger. Because Kerlee had received injections of the Spencer-Parker vaccine, his illness provoked suspicions among some local doctors that the vaccine itself had caused the disease. Roscoe R. Spencer and Ralph R. Parker launched an immediate investigation of the case, which revealed that the young man had not received the full vaccine regimen. On 1 and 6 September 1927, Kerlee had received 1 and 2 cc, respectively, of vaccine—whereas two injections of 2 cc each were the norm. Spencer's research had shown that the vaccine's protective power lasted only a few months, so Kerlee's immunity had probably not been carried over into 1928. On 30 January

1928, Kerlee had taken 1 cc of vaccine, only one-fourth of the complete series. Records on the lot of vaccine showed that it had protected all six guinea pigs on which it was tested. Parker speculated that Kerlee had been infected either before receiving the 1928 injection or almost immediately thereafter.[63]

There was some indication that these minimal doses of vaccine affected the course of Kerlee's illness. Four days after the onset of symptoms, he seemed to rebound. He got out of bed and shaved but soon felt exhausted. This short period of remission, Parker believed, indicated that the virus and the antibodies produced by the vaccine were "fighting" and that the vaccine almost won on that morning.[64] When Kerlee's temperature shot up to 104° F that same afternoon, he was taken to the hospital. His condition deteriorated rapidly, and a week later, on 15 February, he died. In death the promising young scientist was honored almost like a military hero. His brother, refusing to be intimidated by the deadly disease, applied before the funeral for a position at the laboratory.

Kerlee's death unsettled Bitterroot citizens and threatened the vaccine program at the laboratory. In an effort to allay fears, Cogswell published a newspaper article trying to explain to Bitterroot Valley residents that this singular case did not invalidate the effectiveness of the Spencer-Parker vaccine. He noted that occasionally vaccines failed in individuals even though they were effective on a broad scale. Furthermore, he argued, the spotted fever strains maintained at the laboratory were the "most virulent form of the poison, much more virulent than that found in nature." At the laboratory itself, a morose Spencer wrote Surgeon General Cumming that the situation had "caused a gloom to be cast over our personnel." Not only had they lost a friend, Spencer noted, but fear generated by the death had prompted Lawrence McNeal, who was in charge of the infected-tick-rearing room, to resign effective 20 February. "This position in the tick room is the most dangerous in our laboratory," Spencer observed, and informed the surgeon general that it was impossible to replace McNeal with another immune individual.[65]

Spencer's depression hastened his decision to leave Montana. In contrast to his U.S. Public Health Service colleague Lunsford D. Fricks, Spencer had never come to love living in the Bitterroot Valley. Both he and his wife preferred the sophistication of Washington, D.C., to the isolation of Hamilton, and neither enjoyed the Bitterroot's cool climate. Uneasy with the dangers of spotted fever research, Mrs. Spencer was "very anxious" that her husband finish his work and move on into something new. Spencer himself admitted that the intellectual challenge of the work lay in vaccine development—the mechanics of vaccine production did not interest him. He therefore asked for and was granted orders relieving him of duty in Montana at the end of the summer of 1928.[66]

Over the next two years, as credit for their achievement began to be accorded to Spencer and Parker, the old physician-entomologist rivalry surfaced momentarily. In August 1928, Parker presented a paper on the spotted fever work to the Section on Medical and Veterinary Entomology of the Fourth International Entomological Congress at Ithaca, New York. Spencer learned from a friend that Parker never mentioned Spencer's name.[67] This news arrived while Spencer was preparing an exhibit for the American Medical Association. Reacting in an admittedly vindictive manner, he left Parker's name off the exhibit, which was awarded the 1930 Billings Medal by the association.[68] Except for this unfortunate display by both men, the two regarded each other highly. After Spencer left Montana, he held a variety of positions within the U.S. Public Health Service. From 1943 to 1947 he served as the second director of the National Cancer Institute. After retiring from the Service in 1952, Spencer lived thirty more years in retirement. He died 10 January 1982 in Virginia. He published several popular articles on spotted fever, hoping to educate the public about the disease and about the methods of medical research.[69]

With Spencer's departure from Montana in 1928, Parker was designated a special expert by the Service and placed in charge of the new laboratory, despite some concern that his lack of an M.D. degree would strain the laboratory's relations with physicians. Fricks, who made yearly inspection tours in the northwest states for the Service, thought the state health officers would find it "more agreeable" if "a medical officer were again placed in charge of these activities," but Service administrators supported Parker's appointment. The surgeon general commented that "Dr. Parker's excellent work should break down any opposition to him on the part of doctors in the Northwest." Indeed, although Parker did not acquire another professional staff member until October 1930, he managed to supervise vaccine production while continuing his studies on the natural history of spotted fever. Parker's appetite for work, his maintenance of detailed records, and his careful attention to correspondence won him the respect and admiration of Service officers and state health officials alike.[70]

A thornier problem concerned long-term funding for vaccine production. The Montana state legislature constructed the laboratory building, and the State Board of Entomology conducted field investigations on entomological problems, but neither wanted to support

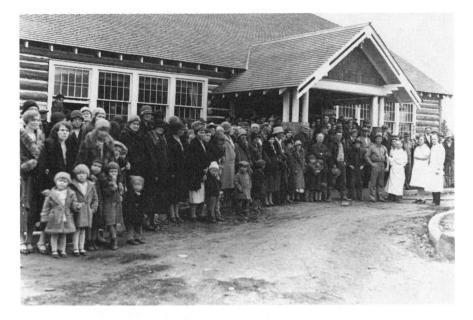

In 1931 people lined up outside this school in Darby, Montana, to be vaccinated against spotted fever at a free clinic sponsored by the U.S. Public Health Service. R. R. Hayward, M.D., a local physician, administered the vaccine. (Courtesy of the Rocky Mountain Laboratories, NIAID.)

the costly vaccine program. The U.S. Public Health Service had agreed to fund vaccine development, assuming that a successful product would be produced commercially or by state health departments. Producing a vaccine from ground-up ticks, however, limited the location of any production facility and imposed costs and dangers that made it an intimidating venture. George W. McCoy, director of the Hygienic Laboratory, summed up the dilemma when he toured the northwest states in April 1928 to assess the impact of the Spencer-Parker vaccine.

The question as to the means of supplying the vaccine ultimately, if the early promising results of its use are fulfilled, is a difficult one. No commercial firm is likely to be interested in its manufacture and sale. It seems to be an unprofitable field for the Service once the research features are disposed of and for each state to manufacture its own supply would be most wasteful by reason of the necessity for the duplication of plant and personnel. Perhaps a pooling of the interests of the several states concerned would be the logical procedure.[71]

Although the future of vaccine production remained uncertain, most people in the Bitterroot Valley and in other western areas welcomed the vaccine, accepting its theoretical underpinnings about microorganisms, antibodies, and tick transmission without the skepticism that had characterized their forebears. Parker's statistics and their own experience validated the vaccine's effectiveness. Scientifically the Spencer-Parker vaccine was a tour de force, the first human vaccine prepared from the bodies of arthropod vectors and the first effective medical intervention against spotted fever. Spencer and Parker owed much to the earlier investigators who had struggled with Rocky Mountain spotted fever for more than two decades as well as to international research on typhus and its related maladies. Their own ingenuity and persistence, however, especially in culturing rickettsiae in their tick hosts and in devising the complex process for making the vaccine, had produced the long-sought preventive, and for that achievement they won the respect and gratitude of people throughout the Rocky Mountain states.

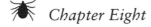

Chapter Eight

Spotted Fever outside the Rockies

*Disease is very old and nothing about it has changed. It is we who change
as we learn to recognize what was formerly imperceptible.*

John Martin Charcot, *De l'expectation en médecine*

In 1926, a young girl in Terre Haute, Indiana, was playing in a pile
of gravel when she discovered a "brown and black bug the size of a
'butter bean' " attached to her scalp behind her right ear. Although
she had not been out of the immediate vicinity, she later developed a
high fever and headache, which were accompanied by a rash and a
"pronounced sleepy condition" from which it was difficult to rouse
her even for food, liquids, and medication. Her physician diagnosed
Rocky Mountain spotted fever.[1] Similar isolated cases of spotted fever
outside the Rocky Mountain region had been reported, but their numbers seemed too small to be significant.

East of the Mississippi River, physicians usually diagnosed cases
displaying the symptom complex of high fever, headache, stupor, and
a rash as typhus fever or Brill's disease. These two diseases had been
viewed as identical since 1912, when John F. Anderson and Joseph
Goldberger demonstrated that Brill's disease and epidemic typhus fever
produced cross-immunity in guinea pigs. Brill's disease, with its milder
clinical course and lower mortality, often became the default diagnosis
when physicians encountered typhus-like symptoms with no reports
of lice or of contagiousness.[2] In 1926, however, U.S. Public Health
Service investigator Kenneth F. Maxcy demonstrated in a brilliant
epidemiological study that an "endemic" form of typhus existed in
the southeastern states. Although clinically indistinguishable from epidemic typhus, endemic typhus produced a lower mortality rate, consistently under 5 percent. Classic, epidemic typhus was clearly contagious, while endemic typhus occurred sporadically. No lice were
associated with endemic typhus cases, but some sort of vector seemed
to play a role in the disease. Maxcy suggested that a parasite of the

147

rat might be one potential vector. Since no arthropod vector had been associated with Brill's disease, it appeared that endemic typhus represented a third distinct manifestation of typhus.[3]

Maxcy's work did not explain the odd cases of typhus-like symptoms in the east that varied from all three patterns. In 1930, for instance, a Virginia physician, R. D. Glasser, reported a case of typhus-like fever following the bite of an *Amblyomma americanum* tick. This tick, though known as an occasional parasite of man, had never before been implicated in the transmission of disease. Glasser also thought the case noteworthy because animals injected with the victim's blood did not show typical typhus signs. Moreover, the Weil-Felix test for typhus produced consistently negative results.[4]

Glasser's report might have remained yet another medical curiosity had not the National Capital Area itself suffered an increase in what were presumed to be endemic typhus cases in 1930. In late June the *Washington Post* noted several cases from Alexandria and Fort Humphreys, Virginia, northward through rural Maryland. Additional cases were soon reported, one in the city of Baltimore. By mid July, when nineteen cases with five deaths had been reported, federal and state health officials from Virginia, Maryland, Delaware, and Pennsylvania held a conference in Baltimore and agreed to cooperate in a broad epidemiological and laboratory study of the typhus problem.[5]

Representing the federal government at this meeting was U.S. Public Health Service officer Rolla Eugene Dyer, who had taken up Kenneth F. Maxcy's work on typhus in 1929, when Maxcy resigned from the Service to accept an appointment at the University of Virginia. Born in Ohio and reared in Kentucky, Dyer had studied medicine at the University of Texas Medical Branch.[6] He entered the Service in 1916 and rose rapidly through the ranks, rotating through the usual duty stations until 1921, when he joined the Hygienic Laboratory staff. Within a year, he had been named assistant director of the laboratory. In 1925 he published an authoritative paper on scarlet fever antitoxin, and in 1929 the laboratory director, George W. McCoy, asked him to set up a typhus unit, assigning two Service officers, Lucius F. Badger and Adolph S. Rumreich, to assist him.

Dyer, Badger, and Rumreich operated out of laboratory buildings at Twenty-fifth and E Streets, N.W., in Washington, D.C. These red brick buildings had housed the Hygienic Laboratory since 1904, and, after the laboratory was renamed the National Institute of Health (NIH) in May 1930, they remained the principal locus of service research until 1938, when operations were transferred to a much larger campus in Bethesda, Maryland.[7] In their laboratory the NIH typhus

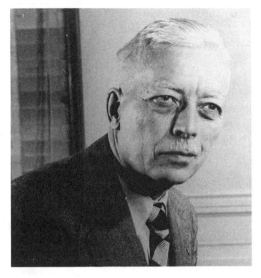

Rolla E. Dyer, who headed
the National Institute of
Health (NIH) typhus unit
and later served as director
of the NIH, demonstrated in
1931 that Rocky Mountain
spotted fever was also present on the east coast of the
United States. (Courtesy of
the National Library of
Medicine.)

team injected blood from a Virginia case into guinea pigs, hoping to
establish a strain of typhus in the experimental animal. Before conclusive observations could be made, Dyer was called to Garfield Hospital in Washington to see a case diagnosed as typhus fever. He asked
Roscoe R. Spencer to go with him and provide an additional opinion.
"We saw the patient and decided that the doctor was right, that the
patient had typhus fever," Dyer recalled in an oral history memoir,
"but as we walked down the hill, Spencer remarked, 'If I had seen
that case in Montana, I would have called it spotted fever.' " Spencer's
uncertainty triggered a new line of thinking in Dyer's mind. Upon
returning to the NIH, he sent to Montana for a strain of spotted fever,
which he established in guinea pigs. When he tested it against those
strains isolated from rural Virginia patients, he had a clear answer:
the rural cases were not typhus at all. They were Rocky Mountain
spotted fever.[8]

Armed with this critical information, Dyer, Badger, and Rumreich
launched a full-scale study of the two diseases along the eastern seaboard. "Most of the cases living in rural districts," they reported, as
well as "urban dwellers vacationing in the country, suffered from a
very severe disease, which did not correspond to the clinical picture
of endemic typhus, and which resembled spotted fever of the Rocky
Mountains more closely than it did any other disease. A quite high
proportion of these cases gave a history of tick bite within a short
time preceding onset." They analyzed the geographic distribution, gen-

eral symptoms, nervous and mental symptoms, and complications of 100 selected cases that included both Rocky Mountain spotted fever and typhus. Disturbances of the central nervous system were more severe in the patients with spotted fever. Convalescence was more prolonged and was often accompanied by deafness, visual disturbances, slurred speech, and mental confusion that persisted for weeks. No deaths occurred among the endemic typhus cases, while among "93 cases of the Rocky Mountain spotted fever type . . . 21 died—a case fatality rate of 22.6 percent." The *Journal of the American Medical Association* found this work of great interest. It would "help to clear up another obscure type of disease," the *Journal* opined, "and will place the public in the eastern part of the United States on guard against being bitten by ticks."[9]

One key question, however, remained unanswered. How did the victims of typhus and Rocky Mountain spotted fever contract their illnesses? Almost half of the spotted fever cases reported a definite history of tick bite within three weeks before the onset of symptoms. A few victims remembered crushing engorged ticks removed from dogs. All the cases, moreover, occurred under conditions in which tick bite was possible. In contrast, the relation between victims of endemic typhus and any arthropod was less clear. The epidemiological evidence confirmed Maxcy's suggestion that rodents were somehow involved: 78 percent of the typhus cases had occurred in close association with rats. Only 16 percent of typhus victims, however, reported actual contact with rats and only 8 percent recalled having received flea bites. To answer these questions, the NIH typhus unit launched another study. Experimentally, they soon demonstrated that spotted fever could be preserved in the body of the American dog tick, *Dermacentor variabilis*. The key to demonstrating tick transmission, however, was locating infected ticks in nature. By 1932, Badger accomplished this, collecting naturally infected *D. variabilis* from a farm in Virginia on which a human case had occurred.[10]

Even before the spotted fever vector was confirmed, the typhus unit recovered typhus rickettsiae from fleas on rats caught at typhus foci in Baltimore, Maryland, and in Savannah, Georgia. Dyer announced this exciting finding in a paper presented at the 1931 annual meeting of the American Medical Association. The news precipitated animated discussion among other rickettsial researchers present. Hans Zinsser of Harvard University Medical School, who, with his Mexican collaborator M. Ruiz Castaneda and a Swiss pathologist, Herman Mooser, had recently demonstrated that rats were one reservoir of endemic typhus fever in Mexico, was not convinced that fleas were

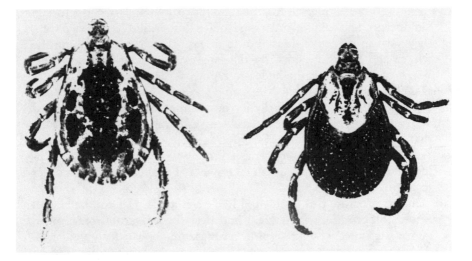

The common dog tick, *Dermacentor variabilis*, is the principal vector of spotted fever in the eastern United States. (Courtesy of the Rocky Mountain Laboratories, NIAID.)

the sole vector. Zinsser favored the bedbug because of his personal experience in Vera Cruz, Mexico, a town teeming with rats and fleas but free from typhus. Kenneth F. Maxcy argued that epidemiologic evidence clearly ruled out bedbugs, and Rolla E. Dyer buttressed Maxcy's position by noting that Zinsser himself admitted the possibility of mild or subclinical cases of unrecognized typhus in Vera Cruz.[11]

This debate reflected the vigor of rickettsial research in the early 1930s. Zinsser optimistically predicted that both typhus and spotted fever investigations in the United States were reaching a "coordinating phase" because of "a gradual encirclement" by epidemiologic and experimental methods.[12] His positivism was doubtless influenced by the expansion of knowledge about typhus in Mexico to which Zinsser and his associates had recently contributed. Their discoveries had helped to establish additional criteria by which typhus-like diseases across the globe, including Rocky Mountain spotted fever, could be studied.

The disease called tabardillo, or Mexican typhus fever, for example, changed scientific identities during the studies of Zinsser, Castaneda, and Mooser. The Mexican people had used the descriptive term, meaning "red cloak" to describe fevers that exhibited a particular symptomatic rash, whether they occurred in summer or winter and whether the mortality was high or low. When Howard Taylor Ricketts, Joseph Goldberger, and John F. Anderson studied "tabardillo" in Mexico City, they saw an epidemic, louse-borne disease that occurred during the winter and spring months. By the late 1920s, however, researchers began to realize that the endemic typhus fever described by Maxcy was also widespread in the Mexican highlands. Also called tabardillo, this disease occurred primarily in the summer and fall and exhibited a low mortality. During the intensive investigation of this new disease that followed, the name *tabardillo*, as well as the phrase *Mexican typhus fever*, soon became identified solely with endemic typhus. Epidemic typhus in Mexico became known as European typhus in order to distinguish it.[13]

In 1917, before this distinction had been made, U.S. Public Health Service officer Mather H. Neill had described a scrotal reaction in guinea pigs infected with "typhus fever" from the Mexican highlands. Although Neill noted that it was milder than the reaction induced by spotted fever, it had not been observed in guinea pigs inoculated with European strains of typhus or with Brill's disease. Neill's paper was nearly forgotten until 1928, when Mooser cited it to support his own similar findings. He also described cells packed with rickettsiae in the tunica vaginalis, the lining over the testes. These cells came to be called Mooser cells, and the tunic reaction in guinea pigs, which served as a test to distinguish between endemic and epidemic typhus, became known as the Neill-Mooser phenomenon.[14] This form of typhus fever was generally transmitted by the rat flea, but if introduced into a louse-infested population, it could become epidemic like its better-known relative. Mooser thus pointed out that the name *endemic typhus* was not truly descriptive. In 1932 he proposed the name *murine typhus* to indicate that the disease was a natural infection of the rat.[15]

Although such new information helped to distinguish epidemic and murine typhus, Brill's disease remained a puzzling phenomenon. In the laboratory it appeared to be identical with epidemic typhus, yet its milder symptoms resembled the murine disease. In 1934, Zinsser conducted an epidemiological study as rigorous as Maxcy's work on murine typhus that identified victims of Brill's disease as European immigrants who had come from regions where epidemic typhus was prevalent. He concluded that Brill's disease—later called Brill-Zinsser disease—was really a recrudescence of an earlier attack of epidemic typhus. This indicated, Zinsser argued, that typhus rickettsiae could remain dormant in the human body, making typhus a disease in which humans, rather than rodents or arthropods, served as the natural reservoir. If a patient with Brill's disease was fed on by lice, the insects could become infected and transmit the disease to others. By this means, apparently spontaneous epidemics of typhus might be started. Laboratory studies in the early 1950s confirmed Zinsser's epidemiological reasoning.[16]

Across the Atlantic Ocean, Sir William Hames declared at a 1930 meeting of the Royal Society of Medicine in London that "typhus in the tropics" was "coming to judgment like a Daniel," with research "throwing much new light upon dark corners of the epidemiological world." The paper that elicited Hames's enthusiastic comment was given by William Fletcher, a British physician working in Kuala Lumpur, capital of the Federated Malay States. In a review of the typhus-like diseases, Fletcher had observed that they were widely distributed across the warmer parts of the globe, from New York and Marseilles in the northern hemisphere to Adelaide in the southern. They comprised, Fletcher argued, a list of names rather than a list of diseases: shop typhus, scrub typhus, tropical typhus, sporadic typhus, twelve-day fever, and many others. Plainly, some rational criterion for grouping these maladies was needed.[17]

During the 1920s, J. W. D. Megaw of the Indian Medical Service had proposed classification according to arthropod vectors: (1) louse typhus; (2) tick typhus; (3) mite typhus; (4) typhus-like fevers transmitted by unknown vectors.[18] Fletcher advocated a simpler scheme based on geographic location. "The typhus-like fevers fall into two distinct groups: a rural group and an urban group." Rural types included Indian tick typhus; tropical scrub typhus of Malaya, Mossman fever of Australia, Rhodesian fever, and possibly *fièvre exanthématique* of Marseilles. The urban group was comprised of endemic typhus, shop typhus of Malaya, Sumatra, and Java, and *typhus endémique bénin* of Toulon.[19]

Fletcher made a strong case for separating epidemic typhus itself from all the others. In contrast to the well-known contagiousness of classic typhus, he argued, the other diseases were all noncontagious. "A case of typhus is a matter of public concern," he noted, pointing out that no public health authority in any country quarantined cases of Brill's disease or murine typhus. Other investigators, especially Charles Nicolle, who had originally identified the louse vector of epidemic typhus, believed that the classic disease belonged to the same family as murine typhus. Nicolle proposed a "unity" theory of typhus, arguing that the endemic form of the disease, because of its association with rodents, must be an older form. Epidemic typhus he regarded as an "evolved" form of the endemic organism.[20]

The lack of agreement about the classification and nature of these diseases underscored both the vigor of the field and the limitations of existing laboratory technique. Inability to grow concentrated quantities of rickettsial organisms in anything other than their arthropod vectors inhibited more direct study of the immunological relationships among the rickettsiae. The tiny size of rickettsial organisms obscured the details of their morphology. Rickettsial disease research, in which work on Rocky Mountain spotted fever was grounded, thus continued to be oriented toward the various typhus-like diseases, rather than toward the causative organisms themselves.

Most interesting to Rocky Mountain spotted fever investigators were foreign reports of new tick-borne rickettsial diseases. During 1927 and 1928 in Marseilles, France, an unusual typhus-like fever was reported. Unlike typhus, the rash of this fever extended to victims' faces, and a persistent "black spot" was identified as a possible point of infection. In 1930, French parasitologist Emile Brumpt, professor at the Faculté de Médicine in Paris, diagnosed the Marseilles epidemic as north African *fièvre boutonneuse*—the disease Alfred Conor had described in 1910 in Tunis. In his laboratory, Brumpt transmitted this "Marseilles exanthematic fever" to man through adult ticks reared from nymphs obtained on dogs in Marseilles. Since ships traveled regularly between Marseilles and north African ports, Brumpt suggested that the disease had been transported across the Mediterranean in the bodies of stowaway ticks, and he proposed that the causative rickettsia be named *R. conori* after Conor.[21]

Confirmation of *fièvre boutonneuse* as a new tick-borne rickettsiosis stimulated comparative research with Rocky Mountain spotted fever on both sides of the Atlantic. In July 1932, Brumpt visited the Spotted Fever Laboratory in Hamilton, Montana, and collected infected ticks, which he took back to Paris. He received one injection of the Spencer-Parker vaccine, but he had such a severe reaction that he did not take the prescribed second dose. In February 1933, after returning to France and initiating his research, Brumpt fell ill. It was finally determined that he suffered from Rocky Mountain spotted fever, but diagnosis was difficult because he was in delirium and no previous case of spotted fever had been observed in France. Brumpt was transferred to the Hôpital Pasteur and eventually recovered.[22]

At the university in Paris, Brumpt's illness produced a "considerable stir." Although he was probably infected through a wound in his hand during a necropsy on an infected guinea pig, rumors circulated that a "vial containing the ticks had been carelessly broken by a laboratory assistant, that the ticks had been scattered over the laboratory, and that Professor Brumpt had been bitten." Students refused to return to the building until all tick vials were destroyed and infected guinea pigs were killed. The press announced to the public that Rocky Mountain spotted fever could not spread in France "by reason of the climatic conditions," and although this argument may have had little value, it calmed the public mind. As soon as he recovered, Brumpt requested sufficient spotted fever vaccine to inoculate ten members of his laboratory staff.[23]

On the western side of the Atlantic, NIH investigator Lucius F. Badger also studied the immunological relationship between Rocky Mountain spotted fever and *fièvre boutonneuse*, which Americans came to call boutonneuse fever. Badger concluded that the diseases were immunologically identical, but shortly afterward, Gordon E. Davis and Ralph R. Parker at the Spotted Fever Laboratory in Montana reported that spotted fever vaccine did not protect against boutonneuse fever. They speculated that the European disease was less closely related to spotted fever than was another new tick-borne disease in Brazil.[24]

Identified in 1929 as São Paulo "typhus," this disease struck sixty-eight people between October 1929 and December 1931. Like the Bitterroot Valley strain of Rocky Mountain spotted fever, it exacted a high mortality: 80 percent of the victims died. Ecologically, São Paulo in the 1920s was similar to the Bitterroot Valley at the turn of the century. During the 1880s, Brazilian coffee planters, having watched the decline of slavery in South America, encouraged the importation of thousands of European immigrants, principally from Italy. This mass immigration had rapidly changed São Paulo from a small city to a thriving metropolis that strained its public health resources. By the 1920s many previously rural areas were becoming suburbs of the city. Human invasion of the habitat of several local ticks, most notably *Amblyomma cajennense*, accounted for the apparently sudden appearance of the disease. In 1933, São Paulo typhus was identified in the nearby Brazilian state Minas Gerais, which had also experienced a recent population spurt.[25]

Early research on São Paulo typhus was conducted by José Lemos Monteiro of São Paulo's Butantan Institute, a facility famous for research on snake venoms.[26] Lemos Monteiro showed the close relationship between Rocky Mountain spotted fever rickettsiae and the rickettsial organism that caused the affliction in São Paulo. He asserted that São Paulo typhus was "a native disease" with its own individuality, and he proposed calling its causative organism *Rickettsia brasiliensis*. Emmanuel Dias and Amilcar Vianna Martins at the Oswald Cruz Institute in Rio de Janeiro and at the Ezequiel Dias Institute in Bello Horizonte supported Lemos Monteiro, proposing that the disease be called *febre maculosa brasileira* in Portuguese, or Brazilian spotted fever in English.[27]

In 1933, however, a series of papers in *Public Health Reports* refuted the concept of a new disease. Parker and Davis at the Spotted Fever Laboratory found that convalescent serum from patients with São Paulo typhus was protective against Rocky Mountain spotted fever, which indicated a close relationship between the organisms. A week later, Rolla E. Dyer stated that the two diseases were identical. Over the next few months, Parker and Davis published two additional papers concluding that the "essential identity of these typhus-like diseases appears to be well established."[28]

More importantly, these studies directly affected residents of the stricken Brazilian towns, for they indicated that the Spencer-Parker vaccine should offer protection against São Paulo typhus. And, indeed, once the identity of the diseases had been confirmed, Brazilian scientists persuaded their government to attempt large-scale production of the vaccine at the Butantan Institute. José Lemos Monteiro and his assistant, Edison de Andrade Dias, traveled to Montana in the fall of 1933 to study production methods and to appeal for a supply of vaccine until Brazil could produce its own. Although supplies were short in Montana, 1.5 liters of the vaccine were sent to São Paulo.[29]

While visiting the Spotted Fever Laboratory, Lemos Monteiro and de Andrade Dias had been routinely inoculated with spotted fever vaccine, Lemos Monteiro taking two doses and de Andrade Dias a single dose. In November 1935, however, when they began grinding ticks in São Paulo to manufacture the vaccine, both became infected with spotted fever. The Spencer-Parker vaccine they had received a year and a half earlier may have lengthened the incubation period of the disease, which was observed to have been long. Tragically, it did not save them: Lemos Monteiro died seven days after becoming ill, and de Andrade Dias survived for only five days. At the Spotted Fever Laboratory, Ralph R. Parker recorded these fatalities, noting that, ironically, the lot of vaccine on which they had been working displayed a high immunizing value. After this tragedy, Emmanuel Dias and Amilcar Vianna Martins took over the Brazilian vaccine program. Tick eradication methods for São Paulo were also investigated, but they proved disappointing, hence vaccination was adopted as the primary prophylactic measure.[30]

In 1937 another virulent epidemic was reported from Tobia, Colombia, a narrow, rural, river valley community located near Bogotá in the eastern range of the Andean highlands. Symptoms of victims and guinea pig reactions to inoculations with blood all pointed toward an infection of the Rocky Mountain spotted fever type, and rickettsiae were identified in guinea pig tissues. Furthermore, the arthropod vectors of all the major typhus-like diseases, including the tick that transmitted São Paulo typhus, were present in the valley. From July 1934 to August 1936, sixty-five people had contracted the disease, and only three had survived—a mortality rate of 95 percent.[31]

By the early 1940s, Tobia petechial fever, as it was called, had been unmasked as another focus of Rocky Mountain spotted fever in the western hemisphere. Luis Patiño-Camargo, director of Instituto Federico Lleras in Bogotá, treated patients, amassed epidemiological data, and compared strains of the infectious agent against rickettsial strains in ticks obtained from Parker in Montana. In the course of this work, one of Patiño-Camargo's countrymen, Héctor Calderón Cuervo, became yet another martyr to laboratory-acquired spotted fever.[32] In 1941, Colombian authorities requested a half-liter of the Spencer-Parker vaccine for the afflicted area. One health official wrote that when the first vaccinations were performed, "the local civil authorities were present and the Reverend Father José Antonio Rodriguez, who blessed the vaccine and gave a speech regarding the great benefits of this prophylactic medium and the interest which the National Government has taken toward freeing the region of this deadly disease."[33]

Even as Rocky Mountain spotted fever was being unveiled in these South American countries, certain aspects of the disease in the United States seemed to become more baffling. In 1931, when spotted fever was identified in the eastern part of the nation, the NIH typhus unit noted that it killed about 25 percent of infected guinea pigs. In contrast, death was "the rule" for those infected with the Bitterroot Valley strain. Guinea pigs showed a scrotal reaction with the western strain, but it had been noted only once in those inoculated with the eastern strain. "With these differences in mind," Dyer, Badger, and Rumreich designated the disease in the east "as the *eastern* type of Rocky Mountain spotted fever in contrast to the *western* type of the disease."[34]

Almost at once, Ralph R. Parker took issue with the suggestion that the disease occurred in two different forms. The problem, he believed, lay in the limited experience of most investigators with spotted fever's variations.

Most textbook articles on Rocky Mountain spotted fever and a very considerable proportion of the papers by those who have studied spotted fever in and out of the laboratory are too highly colored by the fact that *all* have done most or all of their work with strains from the Bitter Root Valley. Not only is this true, but it is also true that the Bitter Root Valley strains with which they have worked have been particularly selected for virulence and scrotal-lesion-producing power. As a result, all of us, I believe, have become too much inclined to look upon high fever and scrotal lesions as being part of the typical symptomatology of Rocky Mountain spotted fever in guinea pigs. . . . I have, however, had extensive opportunity to observe guinea pig reactions to strains of lesser virulence, not only from other western points, but also many times from the Bitter Root Valley. . . . I know, therefore, that there is a marked difference in guinea pig reactions to different strains and even to the same strain at different times, and for that reason the differences which Drs. Dyer, Badger and Rumreich have noted do not to me seem to have the possible differentiating significance which they apparently do to them.[35]

Parker also cited documented differences in the clinical manifestations of the disease in humans throughout the western states. Because the eastern and western strains produced full cross-immunity, Parker argued that, barring other differences of which he was unaware, they were no more different than were those in Montana and in Idaho. "My personal opinion," he concluded, "is that we will find Rocky Mountain spotted fever very widely distributed *in nature* in the United States, and that possibly human cases are occurring over a much larger territory than that from which they have thus far been recognized."[36]

Although Parker's arguments were logical and grounded in personal experience, his superiors in Washington, D.C., believed that further investigations were required, especially by pathologists. At the NIH, Ralph D. Lillie took up the question. The thirty-five-year-old Lillie had taken both his undergraduate training and his M.D. at Stanford University, earning the latter in 1920. At Stanford he was influenced by William Ophüls, a noted pathologist and student of Johannes Orth, who in turn had studied under the pioneer cellular pathologist Rudolf Virchow. Highly respected, Lillie had collaborated with other NIH researchers on problems ranging from pellagra to chemical and pharmacological toxicology to infectious diseases.[37]

In 1931, Lillie conducted autopsies on four victims of eastern spotted fever and studied histological material on a fifth. His comparisons to the western type of the disease were made not on direct observations but on published findings of the twenty autopsies done since 1897. From this limited number of cases, Lillie observed that certain differences could be noted between eastern and western spotted fever. Bronchopneumonia, he found, was more frequent in the eastern type and perhaps suggested a relationship to typhus, in which "pneumonias have often been seen." He also noted fatty changes in the liver, enlargement of the spleen, and scrotal gangrene as more frequent in the western type. Focal brain lesions, which Lillie found "constantly present" in the eastern cases, were never mentioned in the autopsy reports of western cases. These and other differences, most notably the more prominent cutaneous hemorrhages in western spotted fever, associated with "its more acutely fatal course," led him to conclude tentatively that the diseases were indeed different.[38]

During the next eight years, only two pathological studies of eastern spotted fever cases were published, and none appeared on western cases. Lillie himself studied the disease in guinea pigs and in chick embryos.[39] As epidemiological experience with the disease in the east accumulated, however, it became clear that geography had little relevance to spotted fever's severity. In 1935, F. R. Maillard and E. L. Hazen of the New York State Department of Health noted a 30 percent mortality rate among ten cases that had occurred in upstate New York between 1926 and 1934. By 1941 the NIH typhus unit and other U.S. Public Health Service investigators had isolated virulent strains of the disease in ticks on the east coast and strains of low virulence in the west. When mortality rates were compared over large areas in each region, moreover, there was virtually no difference.[40]

Two 1940 clinical studies of larger groups of patients also challenged the designations *eastern* and *western* types of spotted fever. Investigators working at Walter Reed General Hospital reported on seven cases that occurred between 1931 and 1939. Eugene P. Campbell and his collaborator Walter H. Ketchum concluded that they found "little, if any, clinical basis for differentiating" the two spotted fevers. The second study, conducted by Alfred L. Florman and Joseph Hafkenschiel of the Johns Hopkins Hospital, was based on six adult and fifteen pediatric patients. They reported a 23.8 percent mortality, close to the 28.1 percent mortality for the western states compiled by the NIH typhus unit. Florman and Hafkenschiel also challenged Lillie's distinction that cases of eastern spotted fever often had bronchopneumonia whereas the western type did not. Only one of their twenty-one patients had bronchopneumonia. Scrotal necrosis was absent in Lillie's cases, but Florman and Hafkenschiel published a picture of this phenomenon in one of their cases. "It would seem," they concluded, "that severity of infection, rather than geography or vector, is of importance in determining the pathological picture."[41]

By 1940, Lillie himself had accumulated detailed pathological information on fourteen new cases of spotted fever. "This additional material," he wrote in a definitive 1941 study on the pathology of the disease, "tends to amplify the picture of the disease process and clarify some of the apparent disagreements between the 1931 report and the earlier reports based on cases occurring in the Rocky Mountain area." The differences noted in his 1931 paper—bronchopneumonia and brain lesions in the eastern cases and scrotal necrosis and enlarged

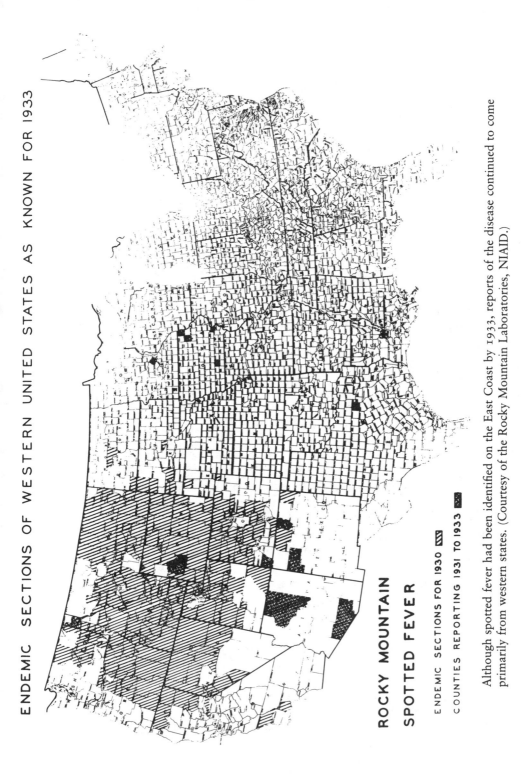

ENDEMIC SECTIONS OF WESTERN UNITED STATES AS KNOWN FOR 1933

ROCKY MOUNTAIN
SPOTTED FEVER

ENDEMIC SECTIONS FOR 1930

COUNTIES REPORTING 1931 TO 1933

Although spotted fever had been identified on the East Coast by 1933, reports of the disease continued to come primarily from western states. (Courtesy of the Rocky Mountain Laboratories, NIAID.)

spleen in the western cases—were more closely related to the length of illness than to inherent differences. Patients dying within ten days—a more common occurrence in the Bitterroot Valley but documented also in the east—demonstrated scrotal gangrene, enlarged spleens, and the severely darkened rash that had evoked some of the earliest descriptions of the disease, "black measles" and "blue disease." In contrast, all patients in whom the disease lasted more than twelve days exhibited brain lesions, more pronounced involvement of the heart and large vessels, and a tendency toward complications such as bronchopneumonia. Reiterating a point from S. Burt Wolbach's 1919 paper, Lillie emphasized that the fundamental lesion in spotted fever was found in the circulatory system, where *Rickettsia rickettsii* caused the endothelial cells to swell and even burst, resulting in occlusion of the small vessels or promoting the formation of blood clots. Tersely summing up a decade of pathological research, Lillie ended the debate over the differences in the disease east and west: "It may be concluded that there is no essential difference in the lesions of Rocky Mountain spotted fever whether in the Rocky Mountain area or on the eastern seaboard of the United States."[42]

Coincidently with these laboratory studies, entomologists were exploring a new tactic to control tick populations. In 1930, when Emile Brumpt identified boutonneuse fever in Marseilles, he had recommended two procedures to help control the disease. The first was not unusual: dogs should be bathed in an arsenical solution to kill ticks. Brumpt's second suggestion, however, was aimed at achieving biological control of ticks by exploiting natural host-parasite relationships. For some years he had studied a small insect, *Ixodiphagus caucurtei*, which burrowed into ticks and destroyed them from the inside. He now proposed that they be introduced into Marseilles to kill ticks by parasitizing their bodies.[43]

Brumpt's idea was not new—in the 1880s a famous and successful experiment in biological control had been carried out in California against a scale insect of citrus trees. In that instance, a small beetle imported from Australia had successfully parasitized the scale insect and effected complete control within two years. Based on this precedent, efforts to parasitize ticks had already been tried in the United States with mixed success. In 1926, Wolbach had acquired tick parasites from Brumpt to experiment with biological control of the large dog tick population that plagued summer residents of islands off the Massachusetts coast. Released on the islands of Naushon and Martha's Vineyard, the tick parasites survived for three years, but their numbers annually diminished, and they failed to become established. The difficulty with utilizing such natural tick control methods lay in the fact that these insects were native to tropical and subtropical areas and did not thrive in colder climates. For some time, however, there was hope that some species of tick parasites might be adapted to the northern United States. One candidate was *Hunterellus hookeri*, prevalent in Texas and commonly called the chalcid fly.[44]

In Montana, Robert A. Cooley took up the question of whether either the French or Texas tick parasite could be used to reduce the spotted fever tick population. In July 1926 he obtained a supply of the French insects from Wolbach and later received *Hunterellus hookeri* through the U.S. Bureau of Entomology. By 1928, Cooley's assistant at the Hamilton laboratory, Glen Kohls, had reared over three hundred thousand of the French parasites. They were liberated in the Bitterroot Mountains to see if they would parasitize the spotted fever tick under natural conditions.[45]

As this project got underway, Cooley laid plans to travel to Africa, the original home of tick parasites. Believing that other parasites might yet be undiscovered, Cooley planned to search for new ones and to learn more about their natural habits. In 1927 he applied to the Rockefeller Foundation for funding to make such a trip, but the foundation rejected the proposal as falling outside the narrow medical criteria for which they gave grants. Cooley raised the needed funds from the Montana State Board of Entomology, commercial firms, and a wealthy brother in New York, and in April 1928 he sailed for Africa.[46]

Although Cooley found tick parasites in the province of Transvaal, South Africa, they did not adapt to the cold Montana climate any better than the French species, which had not survived the winter of 1928–29 while he was gone. In 1931, when Cooley retired from university teaching and joined the Spotted Fever Laboratory in Hamilton as a staff entomologist, he began experimenting with a new method known as latent parasitism. Previously the insects had been released at the proper time to attack feeding nymphal ticks, but latent parasitism called for releasing the insects at a time when they would attack larval ticks. Theoretically, the parasites remained in the larvae as they molted into nymphs and there overwintered in a latent condition. Parasite development proceeded the next spring when nymphs found a new host. During the summer of 1932, Cooley tried this method, releasing *Hunterellus hookeri* parasites in Montana, Idaho, Oregon, and Colorado.[47]

As the United States sank deeper into the Great Depression, Cooley waited anxiously for the spring of 1933, when he could check the results of his work. Curtailment of funds prompted by the Depression, however, made it impossible to determine the results of these releases, except in western Montana. These restricted studies revealed that at least some of the parasites had survived the winter. It was also clear, however, that in contrast to the situation in tropical climes, only one generation of parasites each year was likely in the Rocky Mountain area.[48]

By 1934 the constraints of the Depression forced an end to the tick parasite experiments. Cooley had showed that *Hunterellus hookeri* could survive under western conditions for two years if allowed to overwinter as latent parasites in unfed nymphal ticks. The work had not, obviously, produced the hoped-for effective and low-cost means to reduce the tick population that carried Rocky Mountain spotted fever. Like Lunsford D. Fricks's abortive sheep-grazing theory, however, such a biological control system would have been a triumph had it proved workable. In 1934, Cooley transferred his attention to another long-term interest, building the Spotted Fever Laboratory's tick reference collection. In 1935 that collection contained eighty-three identified species and twenty-two unidentified species of ticks from all continents.[49]

The end of the tick parasite experiments also marked the beginning of the end of all government-sponsored tick eradication efforts in the Bitterroot Valley. State and county appropriations for the work had already been drastically reduced during the Depression. In 1935, A. L. Strand, who had succeeded Cooley in 1931 as secretary of the Montana State Board of Entomology, called a meeting with the U.S. Public Health Service, the U.S. Bureau of Biological Survey, the U.S. Forest Service, and "other interested parties" to discuss any practical way to reduce ticks over wide areas in Montana. Ralph R. Parker and others with experience in tick control measures offered very little hope that anything would work. During the Depression, men in the Civilian Conservation Corps camps in the Bitterroot Valley had been employed to collect ticks and assist in various tick control efforts. Parker argued that their efforts would have been better used in reforestation of marginal land on the western edge of the Bitterroot Valley next to the mountains. After this meeting, organized tick eradication efforts in western Montana were suspended. The next few years brought additional checks on tick parasites and occasional bits of promising information about the ability of the insects to survive in cold climates. Ground squirrel eradication and some stock dipping were continued by individual initiative, but no further attempt was made to eradicate ticks from mountainous or marginal lands.[50]

From the time its efficacy was first demonstrated, the Spencer-Parker vaccine was embraced throughout the west as the principal defense against Rocky Mountain spotted fever. Because of the peculiar nature of this tick tissue vaccine, however, long-term funding for vaccine production had never been resolved. The U.S. Public Health Service, which had funded vaccine development, hoped that other afflicted western states might pool resources with Montana to produce it, but all such requests had routinely been ignored.[51] As demand for the vaccine grew outside Montana, the state thus sought to shift the fiscal burden for future vaccine production to the federal government.

Momentum for shifting responsibility from state to federal shoulders increased in June 1930, when all three members of the Montana State Board of Entomology attended the Salt Lake City meeting of the western branch of the American Public Health Association. They were successful in having a study committee appointed, chaired by W. F. Cogswell, secretary of the Montana State Board of Health and president of the state board of entomology. Comprised of the state health officers of Wyoming, Idaho, Arizona, California, and Oregon, the committee met in Hamilton on 24 September 1930 and passed a resolution that the U.S. Public Health Service, through a congressional act, should take over the work of the Spotted Fever Laboratory, including the tick parasite research.[52]

The following month, Cogswell presented the resolution to the national meeting of the association in Fort Worth, Texas. The president, A. J. Chesley, made particular mention of the spotted fever problem in his presidential address, and Surgeon General Hugh S. Cumming of the U.S. Public Health Service called a luncheon meeting of all those interested in the disease. Since one case of spotted fever had been reported in Texas and two in Nebraska, Cumming went on record in support of Cogswell by stating that spotted fever was a national problem. After this, to no one's surprise, the annual meeting adopted the committee's resolution. Cogswell followed up with a well-organized lobbying campaign. He sent out a circular letter to all state health officers seeking support for the legislation and for an adequate appropriation. Thirty-nine representatives of state health departments pledged to work actively in the effort.[53]

On Friday, 30 January 1931, Senator T. J. Walsh of Montana introduced S. 5959, *A Bill Authorizing the Purchase of the State Laboratory at Hamilton, Montana, Constructed for the Prevention, Eradication, and Cure of Spotted Fever*, into the third session of the seventy-first Congress. In a speech accompanying the introduction of the bill, Walsh emphasized the danger of vaccine production and noted the increased demand from other western states. New York Senator Royal

Copeland, a homeopathic physician with a strong record of supporting public health measures, backed Walsh, citing as a precedent the transfer of the quarantine station at the port of New York to the federal government.[54]

The proposal also found support from Senator Hiram Bingham of Connecticut, who had initiated an inquiry about vaccine production at the urging of his state health commissioner, Stanley H. Osborn, a member of Cogswell's army of public health lobbyists. Bingham queried Treasury Secretary Andrew Mellon, in whose department the U.S. Public Health Service was then located, about support for the Service's plans to take action against spotted fever. The senator pointed out to Mellon that cases known outside the Rocky Mountain region had been traced to the common dog tick, *Dermacentor variabilis*, which was plentiful east of the Mississippi River and thus a potential vector through which the disease might spread. Secretary Mellon replied that he had already approved a $35,620 increase in funds for spotted fever work in fiscal year 1932, a decision that augured well for the favorable consideration of Senator Walsh's bill.[55]

As was customary for health-related legislation, Walsh's bill was referred to the Senate Commerce Committee, and its proponents stepped up their lobbying efforts. Prominent members of the General Federation of Women's Clubs contacted committee members and other key administration officials. Surgeon General Cumming kept a tally of letters received from members of Congress about the purchase of the laboratory. In addition to the expected letters of support from western states, members of the congressional delegations from Alabama, Ohio, Connecticut, and Maryland all wrote to praise the bill. Osborn next spurred Bingham into soliciting support from President Herbert Hoover, who the previous year had demonstrated an interest in public health matters by assisting the passage of a U.S. Public Health Service reform act and the Ransdell Act renaming the Hygienic Laboratory the National Institute of Health. Hoover was receptive, and his support provided the leverage needed for timely and favorable recommendations from the Budget Bureau and the Treasury Department, essential requirements for the passage of any bill.[56]

So effective was the work of the organized proponents and so popular was the work of the laboratory that only one incident blemished the bill's forward march to passage in the Congress. A provision for Robert A. Cooley's tick parasite work prompted one congressman to write to the secretary of agriculture, asking if that work was not more appropriately done under the auspices of the U.S. Bureau of Entomology. Echoing the decades-old question of the relation between professional

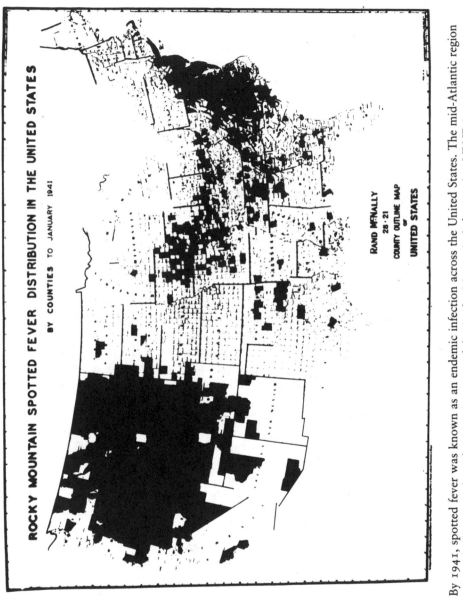

By 1941, spotted fever was known as an endemic infection across the United States. The mid-Atlantic region reported a large number of cases. (Courtesy of the Rocky Mountain Laboratories, NIAID.)

entomologists and medical researchers, this issue arose just before the bill was to come before Congress. Perhaps lulled by the generally favorable response to the bill, Cooley and Ralph R. Parker were jarred by the news that the tick parasite research might be cut. Parker telegraphed the surgeon general that the Montana state legislature had not appropriated additional monies for entomological work, assuming that the U.S. Public Health Service would take it over. Assistant Surgeon General Lewis R. Thompson replied that although the Service had not intended to take up the work, the surgeon general would allow it to be funded out of the spotted fever appropriation rather than see it discontinued. In addition, Thompson intervened with the secretary of agriculture, assuring him that if the bill passed, there would be no dispute along these lines. The secretary, settling the matter, wrote the inquiring congressman that he was in favor of the passage of the bill.[57]

On 17 February, two weeks after its introduction, the bill was reported favorably out of committee without hearings and with only two minor changes in its language.[58] Although it was not on the approved calendar of the Senate, on 20 February, Senator Walsh asked unanimous consent for immediate consideration of the bill. Unanimous consent was required for any bill not already scheduled, and since the Senate was in the closing days of its session, the bill would have been delayed for some time had any senator objected. Walsh described it as "a matter of very great importance and particular urgency," noting that its consideration should not lead to a time-consuming debate because there was no opposition. Doubtless, the publication that very week of the NIH finding that spotted fever existed in Virginia and along the eastern seaboard enhanced the Senate's willingness to grant unanimous consent. The bill was read, the amendments accepted, the bill read a third time and passed without a recorded vote. On 27 February the House of Representatives approved the bill, and President Hoover signed it on 2 March as Public Law No. 744. Two days later, Hoover also signed an implementing appropriations act that authorized $150,000 for spotted fever work during fiscal years 1931 and 1932.[59]

Unfortunately, this legislation was enacted just as the Great Depression tightened its grip on the United States. Within a year, the effects of economic calamity became everywhere evident in federal programs. "Sad news is coming from Capitol Hill, daily," Roscoe R. Spencer wrote to Parker in March 1932. "It seems our salaries will be cut inevitably and I don't know what is going to happen to appropriations."[60] Spencer's worst fears were confirmed in early 1933, as Franklin D. Roosevelt prepared to assume the presidency. The budget Roosevelt inherited from Herbert Hoover proposed a reduction of 25 percent for the U.S. Public Health Service. Rural sanitation work was to be virtually eliminated, cut from $150,000 per year to only $4,500, and the Division of Mental Hygiene's budget was to be cut by nearly 50 percent. Research programs were also hard hit. Although the maintenance appropriation of the NIH was slated to drop only about 25 percent, from $54,775 to $42,300, "field investigations" were to be slashed from $353,564 to only $54,000. This broad category covered a variety of research programs from cancer studies in cooperation with Harvard University to research on scarlet fever, infantile paralysis, and silicosis. The proposed budget also eliminated the appropriation for spotted fever work and stipulated that the Hamilton laboratory be shut down and the vaccine work discontinued.[61]

Surgeon General Cumming countered the Treasury Department's proposal with one that preserved as many professional positions as possible and maintained research programs, if on a reduced scale. Of the work at the Spotted Fever Laboratory he wrote to Undersecretary of the Treasury Arthur A. Ballantine:

If the government should discontinue this activity in the light of our present knowledge, the persons responsible for such action would in my opinion be morally responsible for the deaths which will occur as a result of the lack of this material. . . . I may add that only a few days ago a request was received from the Army for a large quantity of this material to be used for the protection of its forces in the field. The Service has been unable to persuade any other agency, official or non-official, to undertake the preparation of this material because of its danger.[62]

Cumming prevailed, and under Roosevelt's New Deal program, there was no further threat to the laboratory's existence.[63]

During this economically constrained period, Ralph R. Parker sought to keep his small group of researchers in the mainstream of scientific research by adopting practices already in place at the National Institute of Health. He initiated monthly staff meetings at which the work of each scientist was discussed. Recent journal literature was reviewed at meetings like the NIH's long-established Journal Club.[64] Under Parker's guidance, the laboratory expanded its work into other arthropod-borne diseases. Growth in the laboratory's tick reference collection and expertise of staff entomologists contributed to the facility's fame as a center for diseases of nature. In the 1933 outbreak of encephalitis in Saint Louis, Missouri, and the 1935 discovery of bubonic plague in rodents near Dillon, Montana, entomological experts from the laboratory cooperated with U.S. Public Health Service physicians in identifying the arthropod vectors and devising means to control the diseases.[65]

Tularemia, which had first been recognized as a problem in the laboratory animals used to test spotted fever vaccine, became another disease of nature in which laboratory staff developed expertise. Research in the early 1930s indicated that, in contrast to what had been believed, mild strains of tularemia could be demonstrated in nature. The laboratory experimentally secured mechanical transmission of the disease with the deer fly and black fly and demonstrated that the feces of some arthropods were infective. In 1934, two entomologists, Cornelius B. Philip and William L. Jellison, investigated an epizootic of tularemia among sheep near Ringling, Montana. Curiously, none of the ranch employees became infected, even though they hand-picked ticks from sheep and skinned those that died.[66]

Two other newly discovered tick-borne diseases were also investigated at the laboratory. Tick paralysis, a mysterious disease that paralyzed a victim's motor nerves, was found to be caused only by the bite of the female wood tick, *Dermacentor andersoni*. Believed to be caused by a toxin, the paralysis began in the legs and slowly ascended. If the tick was not removed before the paralysis reached the respiratory muscles, the patient died. Once the tick had been removed, however, the patient recovered rapidly. In 1926 a report received from Colorado launched a study of a disease that came to be called Colorado tick fever. By the early 1930s this tick-borne infection could be characterized only as "a probable disease entity," but continuing reports confirmed it as a viral malady having symptoms similar to those of spotted fever with a shorter, milder course and no rash. Usually there were two distinct periods of fever separated by a symptomless day or two.[67]

In addition to these investigations, researchers at the Spotted Fever Laboratory discovered an entirely new rickettsial disease. During the summer of 1935, Gordon E. Davis, a bacteriologist, isolated a filter-passing agent from *Dermacentor andersoni* ticks brought in by a laboratory attendant, Lawrence Humble, in connection with the tick-collecting work of the Civilian Conservation Corps (CCC) camp near Nine Mile, Montana. The following year a similar agent was also found in *D. occidentalis* ticks from southwest Oregon, California, and British Columbia. Initial investigation suggested that it caused a disease of wild animals, but in March 1936, Parker wrote the surgeon general that he and Davis were practically certain that the organism was the agent of a disease in man. This new malady, which caused headache, high fever, body aches and pains — in short, all the symptoms of known rickettsial diseases except for a widespread rash — was soon designated Nine Mile fever, and Herald R. Cox, a newly arrived bacteriologist whose work will be discussed more thoroughly in the chapter 9, took up the study of the causative agent. By 1938, Davis and Cox had published a description of their work on this mysterious agent, and Cox went on to characterize it as a rickettsia, for which he suggested the name *Rickettsia diaporica.*[68] This new organism, it was discovered, was present in many lots of the Spencer-Parker vaccine, hence vaccine recipients were unwittingly inoculated against Nine Mile fever as well. Since the laboratory believed its vaccine to be free from contaminating organisms, however, this discovery caused great concern.[69]

The year before Davis and Cox published their description of the organism, in a twist of scientific fate, an Australian physician, Edward Holbrook Derrick, published an account of a mysterious disease with similar symptoms occurring among abattoir workers in Queensland. Derrick designated it Q fever, the *Q* for "query," since little was then known about the illness. His countryman and a distinguished virologist, Frank Macfarlane Burnet, swiftly identified the agent as a rickettsia. By the end of the decade, investigators on both sides of the Pacific had confirmed that the two diseases were identical. The priority of the Australian name *Q fever* supplanted the designation *Nine Mile fever* for this disease, which later was found to exist around the globe. When the Q fever organism was classed as a separate genus from other rickettsia, it was named *Coxiella burnetii* after Cox and Burnet who had initially described it.[70]

Such productive research at the Spotted Fever Laboratory during the Depression years was clearly secondary to and protected by the demonstratively useful production of Rocky Mountain spotted fever vaccine.[71] During the early 1930s, the greatest demand for the vaccine came from the Bitterroot Valley and from Harney County, Oregon. In 1933 requests for the vaccine increased considerably from the eastern states, and the laboratory forwarded approximately 10,500 cc to the NIH for distribution on the east coast. In addition, vaccine was needed by the CCC camps in western national forests. Because demand for the vaccine always outstripped supply, the U.S. Public Health Service ruled that the civilian population was entitled to first consideration. Only the Bitterroot Valley CCC camps were certain to receive the vaccine. To mitigate this problem, the corps allocated special funds in December 1933, and CCC personnel in the Bitterroot flagged ticks for the extra batch of vaccine. Since adult ticks alone were used, the yield was low: only 40.8 liters out of 123 produced met potency standards. Even so, this amount was adequate to protect personnel in all highly infected areas of the west.[72]

In December 1934 this tenuous situation was strained when newspapers reported that the president might double the number of men

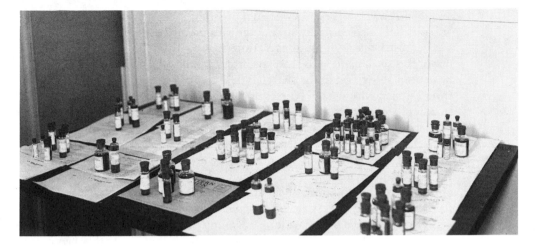

Demand for the Spencer-Parker vaccine always outstripped supply. Here bottles of vaccine await shipment, resting on orders in letters and telegrams from across the United States. (Courtesy of the Rocky Mountain Laboratories, NIAID.)

in the CCC camps. By April 1935 the rumor had become fact. Nearly two hundred new camps were scheduled, including two in the Bitter-root and a number of others near the northern Rocky Mountain spotted fever region where the need for vaccine was most urgent. Parker feared that the vaccine supply would be severely strained by these developments, especially since the laboratory's budget never seemed secure. For fiscal year 1934, for example, the appropriation had initially been cut from $86,649 to $49,000. Eventually, an additional $17,000 was released, and the CCC had contributed $20,000 toward the special lot of vaccine for the camps. In fact, the growing demand from the corps probably helped to stabilize the laboratory's budget. For fiscal 1935, $71,000 was allocated, with an additional $20,000 expected from the CCC.[73]

Many western citizens also complained directly to their congressmen about inadequate appropriations for vaccine work, often prodded by newspaper reporters, who were always prepared to question the priorities of government.[74] This rising demand for the Spencer-Parker vaccine was carefully documented by Ralph R. Parker, who attached copies of many of the letters to his monthly reports to the surgeon general. A physician in Prineville, Oregon, Parker noted, penned the following plea: "Can you let me have any amount of serum? Ticks awful bad and people panicky. Send if possible." Many isolated farmers and ranchers also earnestly sought the vaccine. "We are 50 miles from the nearest Doctor . . . and each time we ask there, they are always out of this serum and in the rare instances when some of our neighbors have been able to get it, the charge is $2.00 each," wrote R. S. Mefford from Decker, Montana.[75] Nurses and druggists also requested vaccine to administer to persons far distant from physicians. Their pleas were in vain, because laboratory policy restricted vaccine distribution to physicians and state or local health authorities.

In part, this policy was adopted to assure that vaccine recipients would be supervised by a physician in the event of untoward side effects, with the additional benefit that statistics on the vaccine's effectiveness would be easy to collect.[76] U.S. Public Health Service policy was also influenced by the widely prevailing philosophy of the medical profession in the United States. Championed by the AMA, this view held that physicians alone should administer all such vaccines and collect a fee for the service from all who were able to pay.[77] The vaccine itself was supplied by the laboratory at no charge.

Bitterroot Valley residents especially resented this policy in 1935, when they were asked to pay for the vaccine after ten years of receiving it free while the Service tested its efficacy. A. C. Baker of Hamilton complained to Montana Senator B. K. Wheeler that "the poor people of this valley" should continue to be vaccinated at no cost. "You take a poor family that has from six to 10 children, to pay $1.00 per child would be a serious hardship. The consequences will be, that they will not take the vaccine and then you will see the death list grow this year from the spotted fever." Responding to the senator's inquiry about the matter, Parker noted that the Service had actually planned to discontinue free vaccinations in 1933 but "because of the general existing financial situation," free vaccinations had been continued for two additional years. He also pointed out that valley residents could travel to Missoula and receive the vaccine free from the county health officer and that local physicians in Ravalli County were scaling their fees and vaccinating without charge "the families of those who are on relief." Other Montana counties offered free health department clinics, also, and during the 1940s, the Ravalli County health department instituted such a program.[78]

Other groups willing to pay a fee if only they could obtain the vaccine included physicians and hospital associations representing construction companies with large crews of men working in the field. Because of the limited amount of vaccine, Parker resisted sending lots to these people, believing that it was being used "to decrease compensation costs for construction companies employing common labor."[79] Parker finally asked the Service for guidelines on how the limited supply of vaccine should be allocated. Taking a somewhat more liberal view, Assistant Surgeon General Lewis R. Thompson, chief of the Scientific Research Division, summarized the Service's rationale:

I believe the first principle that should concern us is to get the vaccine into the more dangerous areas first. Requests from such areas should be filled to a greater extent than in the less dangerous areas. Second, I believe that the people who deserve the first consideration are those whose work takes them into dangerous areas. I do not believe the city man has the same call upon us as the country man, even if he has a now and then exposure. Third, I do not think that we should favor Federal employees, although I can see that here and there you may find individuals or groups which have as much right, by reason of the nature of their work, as civilians. Fourth, I believe that the question of decreasing compensation hazards for construction companies should not be taken into consideration but that such cases should be weighed in the same manner as all others.[80]

Fortunately for Parker, who remained the principal person besieged with pleas for more vaccine, empirical experience with vaccine production over the years had led to many improvements that increased

TABLE 3. *Production of Spencer-Parker Vaccine, 1928–1940*

Year	Liters (gross)	Liters (net)
1928	12.8	*
1929	25.2	*
1930	55.0	*
1931	117.2	*
1932	153.2	*
1933	205.1	*
1934	212	171
1935	315.6	248.4
1936	506.8 (360)**	274
1937	591.2 (309.6)**	462.4
1938	592.4	362.9
1939	756	495
1940	559	515

SOURCE: RML, *Annual Reports*, 1928–40.
NOTES: The widest use of the vaccine was during this period. After 1940, both tick tissue and yolk sac vaccine were produced. Tick tissue vaccine was temporarily discontinued during World War II and never returned to prewar levels. In 1948, when Lederle Laboratories began producing yolk sac vaccine commercially, production of tick tissue vaccine ceased.
*Information not given
**In 1936 the laboratory began storing a portion of vaccine for use in future years. The figures given in parentheses represent the number of liters used during the year that were also manufactured during that year.

the volume available for distribution. These advances, which were noted in chapter 7, enabled the laboratory to produce 205.1 liters of vaccine by 1933, an increase of 3,600 percent over the tiny amount produced in 1926, the first year in which vaccine production had been attempted (see Table 3 for a summary of liters produced, 1928–40).[81] Another major step forward was the 1935 discovery that vaccine could be stored without loss of potency, thus allowing some reserve stock to be maintained. Even with such improvements, the process remained expensive. Each liter of the vaccine cost about $375 to produce.[82]

Although the Spencer-Parker vaccine was embraced by thousands of people as the only hope against Rocky Mountain spotted fever, Ralph R. Parker and the NIH typhus unit continued to search for a simpler, less dangerous, and cheaper method of vaccine preparation. The discovery that spotted fever existed in the eastern United States and in South America underscored the national and international significance of this quest. After the U.S. Public Health Service assumed full responsibility for producing spotted fever vaccine, the burden of developing any new method rested on its investigators. Although the Great Depression hindered an all-out attack on the problem, research at last proved fruitful. The discovery of this improved method and its broad applications to rickettsial disease research are the subjects to which we now turn.

Chapter Nine

Dr. Cox's Versatile Egg

An active field of science is like an immense anthill; the individual almost vanishes into the mass of minds tumbling over each other, carrying information from place to place, passing it around at the speed of light.

Lewis Thomas, *The Lives of a Cell*

Rearing millions of ticks each year and converting them into Rocky Mountain spotted fever vaccine was a service for which residents of infected areas were profoundly grateful. Numerous people who grew up in Montana during the 1920s and 1930s recall with wry affection the sore, red arms they dutifully endured each year in order to be protected from the dread disease.[1] The danger, expense, and sheer awkwardness of making vaccine out of ground-up ticks, however, weighed heavily on laboratory staff members. Toward the end of the 1930s, a new method for preparing spotted fever vaccine was developed that also proved applicable to other rickettsial diseases. It also permitted the development of a more discriminatory diagnostic test and opened the way to fundamental studies on rickettsial organisms. The discovery of this technique was informed by productive research on the filterable viruses, and its subsequent applications were hastened by the medical problems of World War II.

It was clear that the key to a better vaccine was finding some medium other than ticks in which rickettsiae would thrive. The relatively new method of tissue culture held great promise for solving the problem. In this technique, small fragments of tissue, such as minced chick embryo, were placed in plasma, serum, or some other "natural" medium enhanced with nutrients. Strict asepsis was needed to prevent contamination, but, if properly maintained, the tissue culture would grow and could be inoculated with microorganisms known to multiply in the cultured cells. Because the nourishing media and the tissues often varied in composition, however, quantitative control was extremely difficult to maintain.[2] In 1923, S. Burt Wolbach and M. J. Schlesinger at Harvard University experimented with tissue plasma cultures and were able to keep rickettsiae alive for four generations.[3] Unfortunately,

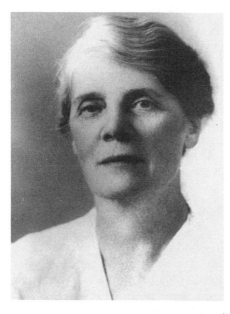

Ida A. Bengtson, the first woman on the professional staff at the Hygienic Laboratory of the U.S. Public Health Service, investigated alternative methods for producing spotted fever vaccine. In 1937 she reported that an acceptable vaccine could be produced with rickettsiae grown in tissue cultures. Her technique was shortly eclipsed by Herald R. Cox's simpler method of cultivating rickettsiae in fertile hens' eggs. (Courtesy of the National Library of Medicine.)

the vaccine process required much more luxuriant growth of the rickettsiae than the developing technique was able to produce.

A much simpler technique for cultivating the filterable viruses was discovered in 1931 by Alice Miles Woodruff and Earnest Goodpasture at Vanderbilt University. They found that the chorioallantoic membrane of the developing chick embryo provided an ideal medium for the growth of the fowl pox virus. This membrane is one of several in chick embryos; the amniotic and yolk sac membranes are two others. The chorioallantoic membrane is located just beneath the shell of the egg, hence it was easy to inoculate and to observe any growth of the pathogen that occurred. Soon after Woodruff and Goodpasture announced their method, other researchers identified a number of viruses that flourished on this membrane.[4]

At the National Institute of Health, a senior bacteriologist, Ida A. Bengtson, joined the typhus unit specifically to explore various methods of cultivating Rocky Mountain spotted fever organisms. Having become the first woman on the staff of the Hygienic Laboratory in 1916, Bengtson completed work for a Ph.D. in bacteriology in 1919 at the University of Chicago.[5] Before taking up work on the spotted fever problem, she had distinguished herself in studies of anaerobic bacteria and the toxins they produced. She also identified a new variety of *Clostridium botulinum,* which caused a disease known as "limberneck" in chickens, and studied the etiology of trachoma, an eye disease whose causative agent was then suspected to be a rickettsia. In 1935, Bengtson and Rolla E. Dyer began experimenting with the Woodruff and Goodpasture technique. They eventually managed to cultivate spotted fever rickettsiae on the chorioallantoic membrane of chick embryos, but the stubborn organisms refused to grow in the quantities necessary for vaccine preparation.[6]

After these disappointing results, Bengtson turned back to standard tissue culture techniques, studying the results other investigators had achieved with a variety of tissue types. The combination that worked best, she found, contained modified Maitland media, minced chorioallantoic membrane, and guinea pig tunica vaginalis, the scrotal membrane in which rickettsiae were concentrated. Shortly thereafter, she reported that a vaccine could be made from spotted fever rickettsiae cultivated in this manner. "The amount of vaccine which may be prepared is sufficient to suggest this method of preparation as practicable."[7]

Bengtson's method, although not ideal, might have supplanted the tick tissue method, had not a serendipitous discovery intervened to revolutionize the preparation of all types of rickettsial vaccines. Before this scientific breakthrough is discussed, however, a digression is necessary to examine the political context in which it occurred, because this particular discovery might not have come so soon, if ever, without the beneficial stimulation of President Franklin D. Roosevelt's New Deal program. In 1935, just as Bengtson was beginning her work, Roosevelt's activist social planners were guiding the wide-ranging Social Security Act through Congress. Signed into law in August, the act not only provided for old age assistance and other welfare measures but also authorized the expenditure of large sums for public health work.[8] Title VI provided $2 million annually for health research in the U.S. Public Health Service. This intersection of public policy and medical research stimulated the work of federal investigators. They could purchase new equipment, undertake new projects, and, perhaps most importantly, hire young researchers for the first time since the Great Depression began.

Passage of Social Security was anticipated with relish in the U.S. Public Health Service for some months before Congress voted on it. Inviting suggestions for ways to expand research must have been pleasant indeed for Service leaders, who had endured years of diminished budgets. In March 1935 Assistant Surgeon General Lewis R. Thompson, director of the Division of Scientific Research, received from Ralph R. Parker a long list of research projects that would be worthy of funding at the Spotted Fever Laboratory. An ambitious $17,540 comparative study of typhus-like diseases was first on Parker's "wish list," followed by an allocation of $9,000 to "study methods of improving the present spotted fever vaccine and to seek some simpler method of vaccine production."[9]

Enactment of Social Security also presaged major changes in the U.S. Public Health Service. Hugh S. Cumming, who had served as surgeon general since 1920, found President Roosevelt's New Deal more liberal than his personal conservative philosophy could support. In 1936 he retired and was replaced by Thomas Parran, who, during Roosevelt's tenure as governor of New York, had been granted leave from the Service to become New York state health officer. In 1937, Parran reorganized the research program of the Service, consolidating the Division of Scientific Research with the National Institute of Health. As a result, NIH's longtime director, George W. McCoy, who, like Cumming, was a conservative, was replaced by Lewis R. Thompson, director of the Division of Scientific Research and a strong New Deal supporter.[10]

In Montana the most noticeable change during this period was the laboratory's new name. Through January 1936 the facility was known popularly as the Spotted Fever Laboratory and officially as the Hamilton Station of the U.S. Public Health Service. In February it became the Rocky Mountain Laboratory (RML).[11] Soon other traditional customs also disappeared. Parker had always prefaced his monthly reports to the surgeon general with the phrase "I have the honor of submitting," after which he surveyed general topics, often commented on personnel and on additions to the physical plant, and finally focused on specific research activities. By 1938 the older formalities and the highly personal form of monthly reports gave way. Personnel and facilities reports were filed separately, and the monthly reports contained streamlined summaries of research projects.

Most importantly for the spotted fever research program, the Title VI provisions of the Social Security Act enabled the Service to hire Herald R. Cox, a microbiologist whose primary duty was to search for a less dangerous, more efficient means to produce spotted fever vaccine. Born on 28 February 1907 in Rosedale, Indiana, Cox took his undergraduate degree at Indiana State College in 1928 and earned a Doctor of Science degree in 1931 at Johns Hopkins University with research in the filterable viruses.[12] From 1932 to 1936 he was an assistant in Peter K. Olitsky's laboratory at the Rockefeller Institute, where, according to one eminent virologist, Cox "got a wonderful

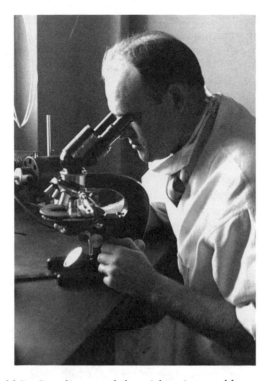

In 1937 Herald R. Cox discovered that rickettsiae would grown luxuriantly in the yolk sacs of fertile hens' eggs. This discovery revolutionized the production of Rocky Mountain spotted fever vaccine. It also provided a means to produce vaccines against epidemic typhus and other rickettsial diseases. (Courtesy of the Rocky Mountain Laboratories, NIAID.)

training in doing experimental work with various viruses." He reported for duty at Hamilton on 31 May 1936.[13]

For "the better part of two years," Cox experimented with flask cultures of tissues derived from chicken embryos and chorioallantoic membranes. He used a variety of nutrient media, "without a bit of worthwhile success." After offering his resignation to Parker and being told to keep trying, Cox had one of those happy accidents of science that solved the problem. In late February 1938 he temporarily ran out of the chorioallantoic membrane and embryonic chicken tissues needed to conduct one experiment properly. What he had immediately available, however, was yolk sac membrane tissue, aseptically removed and stored in an Erlenmeyer flask. In order to proceed with his plans, he inoculated the yolk sac tissue with rickettsiae. Within a week, Cox found "literally thousands" of rickettsiae growing in the yolk sac cultures. "That night I was too excited to sleep," he recalled in a later memoir. His mind racing, he realized that flask culture was unnecessary. "It would be so much simpler to inoculate fertile hens' eggs directly into the yolk sac area, through the air sac end of the egg," he reasoned. Since he lived close to the laboratory, Cox decided to try this new idea immediately. At four o'clock that morning, he went back to the laboratory and inoculated the first yolk sacs directly through the egg shell.[14]

After several repetitions of the experiment with uniformly successful results, Cox reported the breakthrough via the laboratory's April monthly report. When the news reached the NIH in Bethesda, however, Rolla E. Dyer was apparently not convinced. With some relish, Cox recounted Dyer's trip to Montana to inspect the new procedure.

Dr. Dyer came into the lab at about 1:30 P.M. It was the first time we had ever met, and I soon learned that he was one that came immediately to the point in his speech and did not stand for any monkey business. The first thing that Dr. Dyer said to me was, "Cox, I don't believe a damned word in that recent monthly report of yours, in which you state that you are able to cultivate rickettsiae in great numbers in fertile hens' eggs, because Dr. Ida Bengtson and I tried for about 3 years to grow rickettsiae in fertile hens' eggs and we didn't have a bit of luck." I said, "Dr. Dyer, did you ever examine the yolk sac membrane tissue in those eggs to see if any rickettsiae were there?" He said, "No, we didn't." I said, "Well, that was your mistake, because that is where you would find the rickettsiae. Now, let's quit arguing and you sit down and look at these representative slides of spotted fever, epidemic typhus and Nine Mile fever, and then tell me what you think of them." Well, Dr. Dyer sat down and looked at slides for about 10–15 minutes. Then he turned around and said, "Well, I'll be, but you've convinced me. You surely have done what you stated you did." Then he stood up and shook my hand, as if to seal the bargain.[15]

It is difficult to overstate the impact of Cox's discovery on every area of rickettsial disease research during the next decade. As soon as he published his method, it was apparent that the long-sought means had been found to cultivate all types of rickettsial organisms not only easily but cheaply. Almost immediately, with two technicians, E. John Bell and Lyndahl Hughes, Cox went to work making experimental vaccines against spotted fever, epidemic typhus, and Q fever. They found that even the earliest ones satisfactorily protected guinea pigs. Since production required eggs instead of ticks, vaccine manufacture would no longer be tied to a geographical location where ticks were widely available. Further, the cost of production would drop dramatically, so commercial firms could be expected to take over production of the Cox vaccine, as it came to be called. The cultivation of rickettsiae in eggs also made it unnecessary to stock thousands of laboratory animals in which strains of the diseases were previously maintained. Many other lines of research suddenly became fruitful, including metabolic studies and the concentration of antigens for diagnostic tests and for the production of improved therapeutic immune sera. "The features that make the yolk sac technique of particular value," Cox himself noted in 1941, when he accepted the American Association for the Advancement of Science's Theobald Smith Award, "are its extreme simplicity and the ease with which cultures may be maintained with a minimal risk of contamination."[16]

At the same time that Cox was developing his yolk sac method, Hans Zinsser and his associates in the department of bacteriology and immunology at Harvard University School of Medicine were developing an alternative method to culture rickettsiae. Like Ida Bengtson's attempts with modified Maitland media, the Harvard group sought to utilize tissue cultures, but they chose spleen tissue on agar slants. By 1939 they reported some success with the method and described their vaccine production technique.[17] Thus by the end of the decade, three new methods were available in the United States for the culture of rickettsiae: Bengtson's modified Maitland media technique, Cox's yolk sac method, and Zinsser's agar slant approach.

Over the next two years, Cox compared the practicality of his method with Bengtson's, and researchers at the Lederle Laboratories, a division of the American Cyanamid Company, measured the immunizing values and ease of preparation of the Cox vaccine against the agar slant tissue culture vaccine. With Bengtson's method, Cox pointed out, it was difficult to produce a vaccine of consistent potency. Technical difficulties with the Maitland method, moreover, would make large-scale production difficult. The Lederle group arrived at a similar conclusion about agar slant culture. In low doses, they found, the Cox vaccine protected guinea pigs better. "We have made large volumes of vaccine by both methods and are convinced that under the conditions necessary to produce vaccine in large amounts the yolk sac technic [sic] is also easier to carry out and much less costly in time and materials."[18]

By 1940, Cox's Rocky Mountain spotted fever vaccine was ready to be used experimentally in humans. Ralph R. Parker cheerfully informed the surgeon general that the vaccine appeared safe and that "likely" it would "soon replace the tick-tissue product now employed." After September 1939, however, when war broke out in Europe, the peacetime focus on indigenous spotted fever gave way to concern about

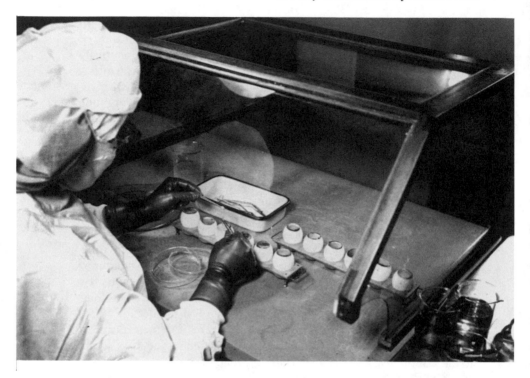

A technician in the 1940s is shown harvesting yolk sacs from eggs infected with rickettsial organisms. (Courtesy of the Rocky Mountain Laboratories, NIAID.)

the international wartime threat of epidemic, louse-borne typhus. Outbreaks of typhus were expected in Hungary and Romania, where thousands of Polish refugees had fled the German invasion. In order to test the efficacy of Cox's experimental typhus vaccine, forty liters were forwarded to five isolated Hungarian villages. A portion of the refugees received the vaccine while others were left unvaccinated as controls. When Germany invaded the Balkans, Hungary was absorbed into the Axis bloc, and, unfortunately, all records of the test were lost.[19]

Although the threat of war loomed large in 1940 and 1941, the United States remained neutral in the conflict. Public health officials could make only contingency plans for dealing with what Surgeon General Thomas Parran called the "national defense emergency."[20] Among those plans was a concentrated effort to improve the epidemic typhus vaccine prepared by Cox's technique, for any involvement in the hostilities would place U.S. military forces at risk of contracting the classic scourge of armies. Military strategists who evaluated possible sites for a second front in Europe carefully weighed the danger of typhus in their deliberations. The disease certainly militated against the Balkans as an invasion site. "Typhus was accordingly looked upon as one of the great disease threats that must be nullified if the Army was going to achieve its aim of reducing disease incidence to a point at which it would finally become a minor casualty producer," wrote a U.S. Army physician in a postwar retrospective article. World War I delousing techniques—bathing and steam or chemical treatment of clothing—had proved at best to be only temporary. The magnitude of the perceived typhus threat, therefore, provided great impetus to research on the promising but unproven Cox vaccine.[21]

At the NIH in Bethesda, Maryland, Norman H. Topping, the new chief of the typhus unit, directed an intensive research program to this end. The son of an obstetrician, Topping had grown up in Los Angeles, where his family moved after his birth on 12 January 1908 in Flat River, Missouri.[22] After taking his M.D. in 1936 from the University of Southern California and deciding against going into private practice, the young physician chose to pursue a career in the U.S. Public Health Service. An internship in San Francisco was followed by duty rotations before Topping was assigned to the NIH in July 1937. He arrived just before the September class of young officers—the first new group to receive research training since the beginning of the Depression. For a short period, Topping worked on dental research, but when Rolla E. Dyer invited him to join the typhus unit, he enthusiastically took up the study of spotted fever and Q fever. In 1938, Topping's interest in combating these diseases became somewhat more than just an intellectual challenge. On 30 December he was admitted to Walter Reed General Hospital "because of his own diagnosis of Rocky Mountain spotted fever." Described by the attending physician as "a dejected man with a 'hangover' appearance" and a temperature of 103.8° F, Topping suffered with spotted fever for nineteen days but eventually made a complete recovery.[23]

Beginning in 1939, Topping and his colleagues in the NIH typhus unit focused on evaluating and improving the Cox vaccine. They believed that Cox's technique offered the most cost-effective method, but in initial tests the experimental vaccine proved insufficiently concentrated to protect guinea pigs against large doses of virulent typhus rickettsiae. Because of this setback, the typhus unit felt impelled to evaluate vaccines made by techniques developed outside the United States. In 1930 a Polish investigator, Rudolf Weigl, had produced the first of these vaccines, which was similar to the Spencer-Parker tick tissue vaccine for spotted fever. Weigl isolated individual lice under a microscope and, with a tiny needle, inoculated them intrarectally with typhus-infected blood. Batches of these lice were then fed for a week or more on human volunteers who had recovered from typhus. Finally, Weigl excised the infective gut tissue of each louse and treated it with phenol. Tissue from fifty to one hundred lice was required to immunize a single individual. Although Weigl's vaccine was efficacious, it was hardly adaptable to large-scale production.[24]

Another approach to preparing a vaccine against the endemic form of typhus transmitted by fleas had been pursued by Hans Zinsser's long-time Mexican collaborator, M. Ruiz Castaneda. Announced a year before Zinsser's untimely death from leukemia in 1940, this vaccine was made from the lungs of rats that had been infected intranasally with murine typhus rickettsiae.[25] Ruiz Castaneda's method of growing rickettsiae was simple, but it was suitable only for murine typhus vaccines. The rickettsiae of epidemic typhus did not multiply to any extent in rats. In 1940, however, two French researchers prepared a mouse lung vaccine against epidemic typhus fever that protected guinea pigs. Even this promising vaccine, wrote Norman H. Topping, had "several disadvantages when compared to cultivation of the rickettsiae in fertile hens' eggs." In most localities, animals were more expensive, the intranasal inoculation of animals with viable rickettsiae was an extremely dangerous procedure, and possible contamination of the vaccine with naturally occurring rodent diseases could not be eliminated as a hazard.[26]

Herald R. Cox's method, even with its limitations, thus appeared more promising than others available, especially after a Canadian investigator developed a technique that improved it significantly. James Craigie, a researcher in the Connaught Laboratories of the University of Toronto School of Hygiene, employed ethyl ether to promote separation of rickettsiae from the tissue in which they were cultivated. His method depended on the fact that rickettsiae, like a number of viruses, such as poliomyelitis and vaccinia, and like many pathogenic bacteria, were repelled from the interface of ether-water mixtures, while insoluble tissue or medium constituents were selectively attracted to the interface. Ethyl ether had the additional advantage of being bactericidal and capable of rendering rickettsiae noninfective with great rapidity.[27]

When the Japanese bombed Pearl Harbor on 7 December 1941, and the United States entered the war, bringing the vaccine into production for military use became imperative. On 11 December, Dyer and Topping, along with officials of the U.S. Army, U.S. Navy, and Division of Biologics Control at NIH, traveled to Toronto to study Craigie's ether separation technique. Thus was launched an intensive research effort to improve the vaccine by Cox in Montana, by the NIH typhus team in Bethesda, and by Harry Plotz's group at the Division of Virus and Rickettsial Diseases at the U.S. Army Medical School in Washington, D.C.

Cox had little luck, but the Washington and Bethesda groups made progress. Ida A. Bengtson found a way to increase the yield of rickettsiae from yolk sacs, and, with Topping, discovered that alum precipitation increased the vaccine's ability to produce complement fixing antibodies. Topping and M. J. Shear discovered that a soluble antigen, which had previously been discarded, could be added to the vaccine to enhance protective power. Plotz and his colleagues at the U.S. Army Medical School also identified this antigen, almost simultaneously. Bengtson, Topping, and Richard G. Henderson demonstrated a toxin produced by the epidemic typhus organism in yolk sac cultures, an observation that permitted development of a mouse neutralization test for the vaccine.[28]

As the United States mobilized for war, the NIH typhus unit was pressed to define standard vaccine production methods, even though research was incomplete and the early experiments revealed that several approaches produced equally effective protection. In August 1942, Topping outlined the best method then known for producing epidemic typhus vaccine in a directive prepared for restricted circulation. He cautioned that further refinements might be forthcoming. With regard to the Craigie ether extraction method, Topping observed that it had "already been modified several times" and that as work progressed, further modifications would probably be necessary.[29]

The tight control exercised over this and all other scientific publications relating to typhus during the war clearly reflected the strategic importance of the research. At the NIH investigators were assigned publication dates in the *Public Health Reports* in order to provide documentation of their research for later peacetime career considerations. Virtually no paper on matters relating to military medicine was published openly; most were circulated in mimeographed form to Allied researchers working in the same field.

Additional human trials of the improved vaccine were needed, and Topping worked with Rolla E. Dyer to locate an area in which typhus epidemics occurred frequently but which was less volatile than war-torn Hungary. In August 1941 they arranged through the Pan American Sanitary Bureau, headed by former Surgeon General Hugh S. Cumming, to test the vaccine on Indian miners in isolated villages in Bolivia. Unfortunately, the follow-up by an official of the Bolivian health department was inconclusive.[30] Another test of the vaccine was undertaken by Rockefeller Foundation researchers working in Spain, where an epidemic had struck ten thousand people. John H. Janney and John C. Snyder of the foundation hoped for a controlled study in Spanish prisons, but turnover in the prison population thwarted their plans. When Pearl Harbor was bombed, moreover, they were forced to interrupt their work to return home. On the basis of limited evidence, Spanish observers believed that the vaccine did help to control the spread of the disease. Further evidence was gained when Snyder and four laboratory assistants, who had been vaccinated with the Cox material, contracted typhus in the laboratory and suffered exceptionally mild cases.[31]

With suggestive but not conclusive proof of efficacy, epidemic typhus vaccine prepared by Cox's method with various modifications went into wartime production. Spotted fever vaccine also continued to be manufactured with rickettsiae propagated in yolk sacs, and it benefited from the improved methods. Because Cox's spotted fever vaccine was so much simpler and cheaper to produce—and apparently at least as effective as the tick tissue product—the Rocky Mountain Laboratory ceased production of the Spencer-Parker vaccine in 1942 as an economy measure. Later, small lots of tick tissue vaccine were again produced because of reports that some recipients were allergic to egg proteins in the Cox vaccines. The number of people at risk of contracting spotted fever was small, however, when compared to the threat of typhus in military and civilian populations. Research on Rocky Mountain spotted fever thus "drifted to the side lines of activity" at the RML. Within the year, representatives of commercial firms were visiting the laboratory, seeking to learn how to produce typhus vaccine, and two national magazines featured the work in reviews of wartime diseases. Cox himself left Montana at the end of 1942 to accept the position of associate director, later director, of viral research at Lederle Laboratories.[32]

During the war, the Rocky Mountain Laboratory, established in the remote Bitterroot Valley to produce a vaccine against what was considered to be a local disease, literally became a national vaccine factory. In addition to typhus and spotted fever vaccines, the facility also produced yellow fever vaccine for the military.[33] The laboratory's strategic importance was reflected in the extraordinary security mounted to protect it. Immediately after the Japanese attack on Pearl Harbor, two night watchmen were ordered deputized and additional ones were

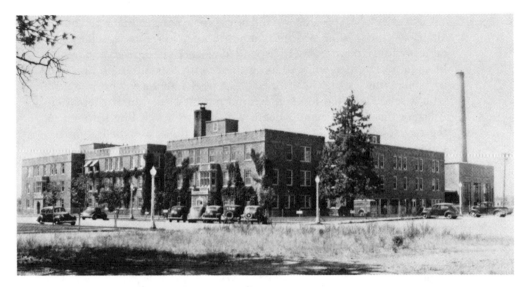

By the 1940s, the Rocky Mountain Laboratory had grown through the addition of several new wings and buildings. During World War II, the laboratory produced vaccines against typhus, yellow fever, and Rocky Mountain spotted fever. (Courtesy of the Rocky Mountain Laboratories, NIAID.)

armed. Beginning on 1 January 1942, armed guards were placed on duty at all times.[34]

Rocky Mountain spotted fever proved to be a minimal problem for the military during the war. Only eighty-one cases occurred among U.S. Army personnel, and more than half of these were recorded during 1943, when large numbers of troops were in training camps around the United States. Thirteen deaths among these cases produced a mortality rate of 16.05 percent—lower than the 18.89 percent national average recorded between 1931 and 1946. Early in the war the army adopted a policy of limited vaccination, targeting only those personnel such as patrols and guards who routinely worked in tick-infested, endemic areas. In 1942 the RML provided enough vaccine to vaccinate twenty thousand military personnel. Because this amount appeared to be excessive, the quantity was reduced. Only ten thousand people were vaccinated in 1943 and just thirty-five hundred in 1944. In 1945, however, the U.S. Army required vaccine for sixteen thousand people because of the large number of prisoners of war housed in endemic areas.[35]

Casualties from spotted fever did not occur among military personnel alone, of course. One wartime domestic infection was especially notable because it contributed to expanded worker's compensation rights. In 1942 a Utah man engaged in outdoor work was bitten on his hand by "something," which he brushed off. A week later he was hospitalized with a severe spotted fever infection, and he died shortly thereafter. Alleging that her husband's death was due to a tick bite suffered in the course of his work, the widow sued and was awarded compensation. His employer appealed this decision to the Utah Supreme Court, arguing that ticks almost never bit humans on the hand, hence the infection was more likely contracted during the victim's leisure time. The court, however, observed that the victim worked in or near tick-infested brush areas and that the sequence of events was consistent with the pattern of fulminating spotted fever. Because of this it could be inferred "that the deceased picked up the tick in the course of his employment," hence the compensation award to the widow was sustained.[36]

The nation's attention and principal rickettsial research effort, however, was focused not on spotted fever but rather against epidemic typhus, the greatest direct threat to Allied troops. Without attempting to do justice to the story of typhus in World War II—a subject that deserves its own fuller treatment—a brief survey of the administrative machinery and major results of typhus control efforts is in order. Most of the leading postwar investigators in spotted fever and other rickettsial diseases established contacts and gained experience in the crucible of war, and the focus of their efforts was this close relative of Rocky Mountain spotted fever. Many preventive and therapeutic measures developed for typhus, moreover, were adapted for application against spotted fever.

The threat of classic, epidemic typhus to U.S. military forces was first addressed in 1942 as the invasion of North Africa was being planned. There were reports of typhus cases among the populations of Algeria and Morocco and of increasing numbers of cases in Egypt. Because of this, leaders of the U.S. Army, U.S. Navy, and U.S. Public Health Service promoted the formation of a special commission to coordinate efforts for combatting it. On Christmas eve 1942, President Franklin D. Roosevelt signed the extraordinary Executive Order 9285, establishing the United States of America Typhus Commission. Separate from other committees created to deal with the multiple medical and scientific problems of the war, the Typhus Commission was granted wide-ranging powers to protect U.S. troops against typhus wherever it occurred or even, in the words of the order, where it "may become a threat." In addition, it was empowered to prevent the introduction of typhus into the United States. Composed of representatives of the U.S. Army, U.S. Navy, and U.S. Public Health Service, the commission was originally headed by Charles S. Stephenson, chief of the Preventive Medicine Service in the Bureau of Medicine and Surgery of the U.S. Navy, who reported directly to the secretary of war. Stephenson resigned in February 1943 because of illness, and in August 1943 his successor, Leon A. Fox of the U.S. Army Medical Corps requested transfer to a position as field director. Stanhope Bayne-Jones, also of the U.S. Army Medical Corps, then assumed the directorship, which he held until 1946, when the commission was dissolved.[37]

Because epidemic, louse-borne typhus occurred rarely in the United States, most military physicians had never seen a case of the disease. In February 1943 the U.S. Army Surgeon General's Office sent a group of medical officers to Guatemala to observe an outbreak of suspected epidemic typhus. Since murine typhus was known to be present in Guatemala, and since it could be spread epidemically by lice as well as by fleas, it was originally unclear which type of typhus had stricken the area. Eugene P. Campbell and Robert Vought, physicians working for the Institute of Inter-American Affairs, another extraordinary wartime government organization, believed from epidemiological and clinical information that this was, indeed, classic, louse-borne typhus. Blood samples from several villages were sent to the U.S. Army Medical School, where both the Weil-Felix test and the newly developed complement fixation test confirmed their clinical diagnosis. "With war coming on," Campbell observed, "the lack of clarity and reliability in distinguishing endemic—mild, or flea-transmitted—typhus from the serious, epidemic, louse-borne infection was a great concern to us in the field."[38] With such abbreviated experiences, U.S. military physicians prepared to deal with expected epidemics, for much military action was anticipated in known typhus foci.

By the time U.S. troops went into North Africa, all had received the Cox vaccine against typhus. During the course of the war, the U.S.A. Typhus Commission distributed vaccine to some 30 million people. Much was funneled through British organizations and through the health division of the United Nations Relief and Rehabilitation Administration, which combated epidemic diseases among civilians.[39] Although typhus did attack civilians in war-torn areas, in prisons, and in the concentration camps in German-occupied areas, it proved to be of little consequence to the U.S. military effort. Between 1942 and 1945 there were only 104 cases of epidemic typhus among U.S. military personnel and no deaths.[40]

Although this record might imply that the Cox vaccine had succeeded admirably, British and U.S. studies were inconclusive about whether the vaccine actually reduced incidence of naturally acquired typhus. On the other hand, all observers agreed that it was highly effective in reducing the case fatality rate.[41] A principal reason that typhus never seriously challenged vaccinated U.S. troops was the development of an effective insecticide, the widespread use of which stopped nascent epidemics among civilian populations before they began. This chemical was dichloro-diphenyl-trichloroethane, more commonly called DDT.

First produced in 1874, DDT was not discovered to have insect-killing powers until 1939, after which a wave of research was conducted on its potential as a means to kill disease-carrying lice and mosquitoes. Major federal agencies involved in this work included the Bureaus of Entomology and Plant Quarantine of the U.S. Department of Agriculture, the Division of Pharmacology of the U.S. Food and Drug Administration, and the National Institute of Health. The International Health Division of the Rockefeller Foundation also contributed to the effort, and all research was coordinated by the National Research Council and the Committee on Medical Research of the Office of Scientific Research and Development. Two earlier powders lethal to lice—MYL in the United States and AL-63 in England—had been used with some success, but neither proved to be as effective as DDT. When short-term preliminary tests, conducted primarily in an Orlando, Florida, laboratory and at U.S. Department of Agriculture laboratories in Beltsville, Maryland, indicated that DDT was nontoxic for humans or animals, the chemical was ruled safe—despite warnings from the Audubon Society—and adopted by the U.S. Army in 1943 as the standard agent to be used against lice.[42]

Before the advent of DDT, the application of insecticide to individuals was a cumbersome, awkward, and time-consuming process. People had to remove their clothes, which were then dusted by hand, with great care taken to apply the insecticide to the seams where lice often hid. The Rockefeller Foundation's typhus team, however, found that the new powder could be applied with a "blowing machine" to puff it under clothes without their wearers having to remove them. Not only was the method faster, but it was also accepted by even the most modest civilians. A curious side effect of the new chemical was its sale on the black market in many countries because it was thought to be an opiate. "These people could sleep after they got deloused," remarked

Stanhope Bayne-Jones. "They thought that this was the best sleep producing drug that they had ever come across."[43]

Three months after Allied forces landed in Italy in September 1943, an epidemic of typhus in Naples provided the first true test of DDT's effectiveness. U.S. Army medical officers cooperated with officials of the U.S.A. Typhus Commission and with representatives of the Rockefeller Foundation. They identified and isolated cases and dusted as many members of the civilian population as possible with DDT. A Rockefeller Foundation report on the dusting operation observed: "This system of rapid dusting without disrobing enabled the mass dusters to care for as many as 66,000 patrons a day. More than 1,300,000 were treated in January [1944] alone—and Naples has a population of less than 1,000,000, which shows that some people came for more than one treatment. . . . The epidemic in Naples which might have taken thousands of lives collapsed with astonishing rapidity."[44]

The very success of DDT in controlling epidemics of typhus forestalled a large-scale evaluation of the Cox vaccine's preventive powers under wartime conditions. In contrast, the yolk sac technique for cultivating rickettsiae clearly proved itself as a means to produce the concentrated antigens necessary for developing a more sensitive diagnostic tool for typhus and for Rocky Mountain spotted fever. Constructing a useful laboratory test for any infectious disease depended on the availability of strong antigens that would react with antibodies in a patient's serum to cause clumping or some other visible reaction in a test tube. The necessary antigens were obtained by growing large quantities of a pathogenic organism. Before Cox discovered that rickettsiae would multiply luxuriantly in yolk sacs of the developing chick embryo, researchers were hampered by the limitations of cultivating them in their arthropod vectors. Laboratory diagnosis was thus restricted to the guinea pig infection test first pioneered by Howard Taylor Ricketts or to the Weil-Felix test developed in 1916.

Before the mid 1920s, the need for more sensitive tests had not appeared acute, because the geographical location of typhus-like symptoms seemed to define their nature. Spotted fever was believed to be confined to the northwestern states. Typhus, initially viewed exclusively as a louse-borne disease, was thought to be absent from the United States, except for occasional outbreaks around New York, which were attributed to importation of the disease from Europe and thought to be self-limiting. Brill's disease, viewed as a peculiar, little-understood manifestation of typhus in New York City, conformed to the larger pattern. In 1926, however, when Kenneth F. Maxcy described the endemic form of typhus existing in the eastern United States, this geographical scheme was disrupted. A second type of typhus required some means to differentiate it from the classic epidemic form. In 1931, when the NIH typhus unit reported the existence of spotted fever in east-coast states, further impetus was given to the search for better diagnostic techniques for the rickettsial diseases.[45]

Throughout the 1930s, the Weil-Felix reaction remained the only serological test available to confirm clinical observations. Initially developed as a means to detect epidemic typhus, the test was examined in 1923 by F. L. Kelly for its possible use as a diagnostic tool for spotted fever. Kelly's research indicated that no reaction was obtained with the sera of spotted fever patients. In 1928, however, LeRoy Kerlee and Roscoe R. Spencer reported in a paper published shortly after Kerlee died that the Weil-Felix test was indeed useful in spotted fever. Noting that Kelly had made only a few titrations and studied only nine cases, early in the disease, Kerlee and Spencer used the OX-19 strain of *B. proteus* to test sera taken at intervals from seven days to one year after disease onset. Their research showed that agglutination became more complete as the diseases progressed and that agglutinins persisted longer in patients suffering from spotted fever than in those with typhus.[46]

Two years later, Spencer and Maxcy, who had used the Weil-Felix test extensively for diagnosis in typhus cases, repeated Kelly's earlier experiments with a larger number of spotted fever and endemic typhus cases, using sera taken late in the disease. They found that the agglutination reaction was different in spotted fever and typhus. Spotted fever produced agglutinins of broader affinities and greater variability than those produced by typhus. Although the two diseases were closely related antigenically, typhus and spotted fever were immunologically distinct. Neither disease afforded protection to recovered animals against inoculation by the other.[47]

Since the serum of typhus patients agglutinated the OX-19 strain of *B. proteus* at high titers and that of spotted fever patients at low titers, the Weil-Felix test provided a rough mechanism to differentiate between the two diseases. As the only laboratory technique available, by the early 1930s it has been widely adopted in the United States to confirm clinical diagnoses. It was of no value early in the disease, of course, because the reaction depended on the increase of antibodies as the body fought off the invading organisms. It was also useless if the patient died before sufficient antibodies had been produced.[48] Another major drawback was its ambiguity in mild or atypical rickettsial infections, those cases most difficult to diagnose clinically as well.

Curiously, although guinea pigs were the principal animal model used in rickettsial disease research, their sera did not agglutinate in the Weil-Felix test.[49] Other signs of infection in these animals had therefore been studied for their uniqueness in particular diseases. Until the mid 1920s, swelling of the scrotum in male guinea pigs had been considered diagnostic for infection with spotted fever, and lesions formed in the brains of guinea pigs indicated infection with epidemic typhus. After the identification of murine typhus in 1926, however, this simple scheme no longer sufficed. Murine typhus had also been shown to cause scrotal swelling in guinea pigs, and in 1933, Lucius F. Badger of the NIH typhus unit demonstrated that brain lesions in this laboratory animal were not limited to typhus infections but also occurred in Rocky Mountain spotted fever. To complicate the picture further, Badger reported that other infectious agents could produce similar signs as well. "The identification in the laboratory of an unknown strain of virus as one of endemic typhus or as one of spotted fever," he told a meeting of the American Society of Tropical Medicine, finally depended on the production of definite and complete cross-immunity with a known strain of the virus suspected.[50]

During the 1930s, Henry Pinkerton and George M. Haas in the Department of Pathology at Harvard University Medical School contributed one new tool to assist laboratory diagnosis of rickettsial diseases. Beginning with S. Burt Wolbach's observation that spotted fever rickettsiae were found in the nuclei of tick tissues, Pinkerton and Haas reported from their own studies that typhus rickettsiae multiplied in the cytoplasm of the cells but never invaded the nuclei. Spotted fever rickettsiae, regardless of how atypically the disease was manifest, grew sparsely in the cytoplasm but formed compact spherical colonies in the nuclei of infected cells. The Pinkerton-Haas criteria proved useful for laboratory studies and at autopsies of typhus or spotted fever victims. They were, of course, not applicable in clinical diagnosis.[51]

By the early 1940s, Herald R. Cox's yolk sac cultivation method provided a means to produce the concentrated antigens necessary for developing a new test based on the phenomenon known as complement fixation. It had first been described in 1901, when Jules Bordet, a Belgian scientist, had observed that an ingredient in the blood, which he called "alexine" but is now known as complement, was used up or fixed to cells in antigen-antibody reactions.[52] In 1911, Benjamin F. Davis and William F. Petersen, associates of Howard Taylor Ricketts, studied the complement fixing capability of spotted fever serum. They used tick eggs as well as the serum and macerated organs of infected guinea pigs as sources of antigens, but their results were inconclusive.[53]

Over the next two decades, European researchers used alcoholic extracts of organs from fatal cases of epidemic typhus as antigens to study complement fixation in that disease, but again, the results were unsatisfactory.[54] In 1936 M. Ruiz Castaneda first reported positive complement fixation for typhus fever serum mixed with suspensions of endemic rickettsiae obtained from the peritoneal washings of infected x-rayed rats.[55]

With the advent of Cox's easy method of growing rickettsiae, a sensitive complement fixation test was soon developed.[56] At the NIH, Ida A. Bengtson and Norman H. Topping developed the test and evaluated its usefulness for differentiating rickettsial diseases at the same time that they were attempting to improve the Cox vaccine. "The question of differentiation is of special importance," they noted in a 1942 paper, "in those sections of the country where both endemic typhus and Rocky Mountain spotted fever occur, as in the eastern and southeastern sections of the country." Their studies showed that the complement fixation test was superior to the Weil-Felix test according to four key criteria. First, the complement fixation test furnished evidence of rickettsial infection earlier than the Weil-Felix test in 23.9 percent of human sera tested. Second, it was superior because the complement fixation reaction persisted longer than did the Weil-Felix reaction. Third, low titers were significant in the complement fixation procedure. Finally, spotted fever sera tested negative nearly all the time against typhus antigens in the complement fixation test, while they often gave a false positive Weil-Felix reading.[57]

Harry Plotz, Kenneth Wertman, and their collaborators at the Division of Virus and Rickettsial Diseases of the U.S. Army Medical School in Washington, D.C., confirmed the NIH group's findings, using rickettsial antigens made by the agar slant method. Sera from two patients whose symptoms were confusing tested clearly positive for spotted fever and clearly negative for typhus. Further studies comparing the complement fixation test to the standard method of observing guinea pig reactions also produced evidence of the test's superiority. "Irrespective as to whether the guinea pig develops evidence of disease as expressed by a febrile reaction or scrotal swelling, or an inapparent disease without these reactions," they wrote in a 1946 paper, "specific complement fixing antibodies develop in early convalescence. The use of the complement fixation reaction, likewise, permits the detection of those animals that represent missed infections or those that develop fever from nonspecific causes. The use of the complement fixation method for strain identification is specific, rapid and inexpensive."[58]

By the end of the decade, the complement fixation test had joined, if not supplanted, the Weil-Felix test as a major diagnostic tool in rickettsial disease studies. Unfortunately, reagents for both tests were available only from a handful of laboratories, principally those of the NIH, the RML, and the Division of Viral and Rickettsial Diseases of the U.S. Army Medical School. Joseph E. Smadel, who was on the staff of the last-named institution, observed in 1948 that, even with the new tests, it still took ten days to three weeks to identify rickettsia and that such work required the maintenance of a "museum of infectious agents" as well as "stocks of known antigens, antiserums and immune animals."[59] Physicians or public health workers mailed samples of blood to the laboratories and waited the requisite time for the results.

Furthermore, scientific efficiency could be thwarted by nature or by human error at any link in the chain from patient to laboratory. The harsh Montana winter, for instance, occasionally interfered with analyses of blood samples sent to the RML. "The post office sometimes left mail sacks out on the platforms in minus thirty degree weather," recalled David B. Lackman, former chief serologist at the RML. "Blood specimens in the sacks froze at that temperature," producing an unusable "syrupy mess." Physicians were encouraged to centrifuge blood specimens to remove the solid cells before mailing, he also noted, but many lacked the equipment or expertise to prepare the specimens in this manner. By the 1950s, however, commercial firms were manufacturing rickettsial antigens, which facilitated the establishment of additional state or regional diagnostic laboratories.[60]

The development of the complement fixation test, coupled with decades of experience with rickettsial diseases, made short work of identifying a completely new rickettsial disease that appeared in February 1946. This malady was first described as a separate clinical entity among residents of an apartment complex in Kew Gardens, New York. It was named rickettsialpox to indicate that it was caused by a rickettsial organism and that it had initially been misdiagnosed as mild chickenpox. Charles Pomeranz, a local exterminator and amateur entomologist, alerted New York health authorities to the possibility of some sort of arthropod-borne disease after he found mite-infested mice in the apartment-complex basement. When New York investigators called on the U.S. Public Health Service for assistance, Robert J. Huebner and his colleagues in the Division of Infectious Diseases at the NIH and William L. Jellison, entomologist from the RML, joined in the collaborative effort. They isolated, described, and classified the etiologic agent as a hitherto unknown rickettsia of the spotted fever group. Because the organism was found to inhabit the mite *Allodermanyssus sanguineus*, a parasite of the house mouse, they named it *Rickettsia akari*, *akari* meaning "mite." Epidemiological research determined that the disease was contracted wherever mites had access to human living areas. In the case of the original apartment complex, the mites climbed up a central incinerator chute and infested the carpeting in apartments, thus rendering young children especially susceptible. In sharp contrast to the decades it took to understand spotted fever and the centuries during which epidemic typhus remained a mystery, the complete picture of rickettsialpox was elucidated within eight months.[61]

Shortly before this triumph of laboratory investigation, however, another mysterious disease had eluded clarification. In 1942 and 1943 there were "mass outbreaks of an apparently new clinical syndrome" at Fort Bullis in Texas that came to be called Bullis fever. It resembled a rickettsial disease, especially Q fever, and it was linked to a tick vector, but no immunological relationship between it and any known rickettsiosis could be conclusively demonstrated. Since no further cases occurred, investigation was halted, and, to the present, Bullis fever remains an unexplained mystery.[62]

Herald R. Cox's spectacularly successful method of growing rickettsiae in yolk sacs had been discovered in the search for a better vaccine against Rocky Mountain spotted fever. Two of its most important consequences were the epidemic typhus vaccine that protected U.S. troops during World War II and the development of the complement fixation test. Although it was clearly an advance over the culture of rickettsiae in ticks and in lice, Cox's technique was not without its limitations. Yolk sac vaccines did not provide complete protection against contracting rickettsial diseases, although, like the Spencer-Parker vaccine, they did mitigate the course of the diseases. The more sensitive complement fixation test, moreover, shared one major weakness with the Weil-Felix test: both were diagnostic only when antibody levels rose during the course of the illness. Neither was of value at the time a patient first became ill. For more than three decades after Cox's discovery, however, his method remained the standard procedure for producing spotted fever vaccine, and the complement fixation test stood as the diagnostic tool of choice for rickettsial diseases. With the versatile egg, Cox accomplished his goal, freeing vaccine production from the danger and expense entailed in the tick tissue method and opening wide new horizons for research on rickettsiae when World War II ended.

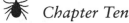 *Chapter Ten*

Spotted Fever Therapy, from Sage Tea to Tetracycline

Many methods of treatment have been advised and employed in the attempt to cure this disease. They run the gamut of the Pharmacopoeia from sage tea to quinine and they have returned to that tacit admission of ignorance, "good nursing and symptomatic medication."

William Colby Rucker, 1912

"The desire to take medicine," wrote William Osler of the Johns Hopkins University School of Medicine, "is perhaps the greatest feature which distinguishes man from animals."[1] Whether folk remedies, patent medicines, or compounds from orthodox pharmacopeias, all sorts of pills, powders, liquids, and potions have been ingested by victims of disease in their quest to cure their sufferings. They have also submitted to being bled, purged, vomited, and sweated. They have extolled water, hot or cold, placed their trust in injections or faith healers, and succumbed to the promises of quacks. Those people unlucky enough to contract Rocky Mountain spotted fever were no different. Because this disease was not identified until after the bacteriological revolution, however, the search for an effective therapy against it was infused with the positivism that has characterized twentieth-century medical science. Early spotted fever investigators were inspired by the dramatic cures discovered for diphtheria and tetanus and hoped for a similar breakthrough. None expressed hopelessness even as therapy after therapy failed to elicit a response.

Unlike many diseases known for centuries, spotted fever was never generally viewed as a manifestation of God's wrath against sinners.[2] Even before the tick-borne nature of spotted fever had been established, the disease was not considered contagious, and its victims were thus spared long quarantines like those that confined diphtheria and smallpox patients. The history of spotted fever is different in this sense from air- or water-borne diseases, which often inspired widespread fear of frequenting public places and generated antagonism against groups rumored to be the source of the disease. Falling property values in infected areas and agitation against the establishment of a laboratory in the noninfected district did indeed cause unrest in the Bitterroot Valley. Spotted fever's geographical limitation to specific areas and its certain link to ticks, however, precluded a sense of national peril against an unknown terror. Unlike the disease itself, the optimism of scientific medicine was contagious—from the beginning of scientific investigations in 1902, people at risk in the Bitterroot Valley were convinced that research would eventually produce a therapy for their dread disease.[3]

Like the researchers who had preceded him, Thomas B. McClintic, the U.S. Public Health Service investigator who lost his life to spotted fever in August 1912, examined potential cures for the disease. During the fall and winter of 1911–1912, while he worked in Washington at the Hygienic Laboratory, McClintic decided to investigate the therapeutic potential of arsenical compounds. Treatment with these substances had received a boost in 1910, when Paul Ehrlich introduced the arsenical he called Salvarsan as the first effective specific against the trypanosome of syphilis. Not surprisingly, arsenic compounds soon were widely employed by physicians hoping that they might also be a "magic bullet" against other diseases. McClintic, moreover, had recently learned from a Stevensville, Montana, physician that two spotted fever victims recovered after receiving sodium cacodylate, an antimalarial arsenical. His research with arsenicals, he noted, was theoretically based on "some indications pointing to the infection of spotted fever being protozoal in character." He thus chose to treat guinea pigs and rhesus monkeys with those arsenicals known to have a toxic effect on protozoan organisms.[4]

In addition to sodium cacodylate, he tried Salvarsan itself and hexamethylenamine, a urinary tract bactericide known by its trade name, Urotropin. In order to test both the therapeutic and prophylactic powers of the drugs, he administered doses to some of his experimental animals at the time they were inoculated with spotted fever. Usually, however, treatment began when the temperature of the animal began to rise. His results were "by no means" encouraging. "In fact," he wrote, "the administration of the drugs seems, on the whole . . . to have hastened the death of most of the animals that were treated."[5]

McClintic's successors experienced similar frustrations. In 1918, S. Burt Wolbach reported to the chairmen of the Montana State Boards of Health and Entomology that he had conducted experiments on the therapeutic value of an antimony compound with negative results. Like McClintic, he observed that the hoped-for therapy actually had "a deleterious influence" and accented the vascular lesions in experimental animals. During the 1920s, Roscoe R. Spencer worked with salts of bismuth. In his 1923 annual report, he likewise concluded that these "chemotherapy experiments . . . have yielded no striking results."[6]

If these researchers sought a magic bullet that would selectively kill spotted fever organisms, others adopted what might be described as the shotgun approach of internal antiseptics. In 1924, H. P. Greeley, a physician from Madison, Wisconsin, speculated that "tick fever" might be more responsive to intravenous medications "because of its pathology." Greeley's logic, based on his knowledge that spotted fever attacked the capillaries, led him to treat a twenty-eight-year-old woman by injecting 20 cc of a 1 percent solution of Mercurochrome-220 soluble intravenously. "Within an hour," he noted, "there was a severe chill, and following it the temperature rose to 104.8° F. Within six hours, the muscular pains and soreness began to leave." Although he admitted that one case did not prove his argument, he called for further trials of the chemical.[7]

Greeley's logic was characteristic of the type that underlay many spotted fever drug tests. If a drug was known to be efficacious for a disease having some symptoms in common with spotted fever, it seemed reasonable to test it. Such was the case in 1926, when a Dr. Henline suggested that Ralph R. Parker try Caprokol, the trade name for hexylresorcinol, another urinary tract antiseptic also used against hookworms and roundworms. Since kidney failure sometimes accompanied spotted fever, Parker observed that it might "be worth while to try this out." Similarly, L. C. Fisher of the Department of Medicine of the University of Minnesota reasoned that the nature of the vascular lesions and the localization of the virus in the endothelium suggested that spotted fever might respond to intravenous chemotherapy. Impressed by British reports that "various colloidal substances" effectively modified the course of experimental typhus if given early, Fisher tested new drugs of this type: "Germanin (Bayer 205), metaphen, triphal (organic gold compound), and tryparsamide." None proved any better than earlier drugs in protecting guinea pigs against spotted fever.[8]

Whenever scientific progress seems thwarted at every turn by the mysteries of disease, folk and quack remedies enjoy a surge of popularity.[9] The failure of medical science to uncover an effective cure for Rocky Mountain spotted fever encouraged many people to take therapy into their own hands. Unorthodox and quack treatments, based primarily on the *post hoc, ergo propter hoc* fallacy, abetted by the fear of an uncontrollable danger, and nearly always promoted with bold promises backed up with the mere pretense of evidence, took many forms. In 1916, for instance, a Dr. Fox of Arco, Idaho, claimed to have discovered a "mixture of medicines which thru actual tests already made shows that it will abrupt a case of Rocky Mountain tick fever in five days." Dr. Fox based his claim to efficacy on the fact that five spotted fever victims recovered after taking his unnamed mixture. Patient number six may not have been so lucky, for nothing further was heard of Dr. Fox and his remedy.[10]

Advocates of other proposed therapies clothed their claims in the findings of bacteriology, promoting their products as "germ killers." In 1941, one such product, manufactured by a family in Forest Grove, Montana, and known only as "the remedy," was sent to the Rocky Mountain Laboratory for testing. "The remedy is a liquid," wrote Martin J. Elam in his accompanying letter. Because it contained "several ingredients, one being a poison," he instructed, it was "to be applied externally." Claiming that his nostrum was "an efficient germ killer," Elam asserted that it had cured his friends and neighbors of "blood poisoning, pink eye, insect stings and bites, infected tick bites," while having "no harsh effect on sores or the mucus membrane."[11]

An even longer list of diseases was purportedly cured by a patent medicine similarly marketed as an external germ killer. Sold by the Triangle Drug Company in Edgerton, Wyoming, the C.Y.T. Tick Bite and Blood Poison Remedy was certified as effective for blood poison, snake bite, tick bite, toothache, gout, eczema, bunions, frostbite and chilblains, barbers' itch, ringworms, carbuncles, boils and warts, ingrowing toenails, rusty nail punctures, and bee and insect bites. Such a wonder drug deserved exceptional advertising, and its handbill unabashedly proclaimed C.Y.T. to be "The Greatest Discovery of the Twentieth Century for Men, Women, and Children." A separate page was required for the large number of testimonials from happy customers. Adopting the cautionary style of orthodox medicine, C.Y.T.'s handbill writers featured the word *poison* in large letters, gave directions for the user "to rub in some vaseline or some good grade cold cream" after applying, and included this admonition in boldface type: "Do not apply after the inflammation and pain has been stopped." John A. Anderson, president of Triangle Drug Company, sent a bottle of the remedy to the RML for testing. Anderson believed that laboratory tests would show that C.Y.T. would "kill the virus of Rocky Mountain Spotted Fever, if used in time. We advise applying the med-

icine as soon as the patient has been bit by a tick, not waiting to see
if he has been bit by an infected or a non-poisonous tick and in such
cases results have been excellent."[12]

Older beliefs in the commonality of all diseases also contributed to
therapies proposed for spotted fever. Humoral theory, for example,
held that an imbalance in body humors caused disease. Blood was one
essential body humor. Since spotted fever rickettsiae had been demonstrated in blood, and since syphilis was widely known as "bad
blood," it is not surprising that the two might be linked. In 1938 an
Idaho man who styled himself a "Dr of Naturapthie" and a twelve-
year veteran cowboy in Wyoming, Colorado, and Idaho, claimed that
"Spoted [sic] Fever is the (3rd) stage of Syples [sic] No Person who is
free from Syphlectic Blood will Take Spoted Fever."[13]

A Wyoming woman, who claimed she had "the right to M.D." but
did not practice, combined humoral theory and folk wisdom with
some simple chemistry. Arguing that the tick "is not more poisonous
than others of its nature, except when it has been feeding on the carrion
of sheep or other decayed flesh," she advocated treatment for a tick
bite more commonly recommended for snake bites: "By saturating the
saliva with tobacco, any friend may with impunity make suction over
the wound by the mouth." She also recommended that the victim
follow this treatment by using ammonia both externally and internally,
since "we find the bite acts as an acid in the blood." Her main concern
was the education of mountaineers and sheepherders, for whom spotted fever was an occupational hazard. Opining that sheepherders especially needed her advice because of their "slothful nature," she stated:
"In isolated places I have proposed the application of freshly prepared
mud, frequently changed, and much bathing if near streams. Also a
free cathartic, with alkaline potions. Much fruit of a very acid nature
and light diet with plenty of rest. The nightly removal of all clothing
and the running of the hand over the body would warn us of the tick's
presence in ample time for quick treatment and save many lives."[14]

Occasionally, unorthodox remedies were bizarre. One married couple who contracted the disease in Idaho attributed their recoveries to
the ministrations of a Chinese doctor. The doctor, wrote the wife,
"didn't come near the bed" but prescribed that they steep the teeth
and toenails of a Chinaman in water to produce a curative brew. "I
was to take ½ cup at 10 o'clock each day for 3 days," she stated,
"and after 10 days or more I got up, but was never so weak in my
life."[15]

The exaltation of the common man with common sense contributed
to another line of therapy in spotted fever. Representing one basic

commonsense approach was Knute F. Turnquist, who suffered from the disease in Lo Lo, Montana, in 1906. Turnquist's self-designed treatment was direct and simple: he stayed drunk for two days. More often the commonsense approach was reflected in hope that an effective cure might lie in some familiar substance simply overlooked by the scientific community. And indeed, for a brief time in Montana, bicarbonate of soda — ordinary baking soda — was thought to be the simple, surprise cure for spotted fever that no one had thought to investigate, because a number of patients recovered after being treated with it. During the devastating 1921 tick season, however, when all eleven victims of spotted fever died, earlier hopes were dashed. A dejected Robert A. Cooley wrote in response to an inquiry about the treatment from a University of Nevada professor who had earlier visited Montana: "At the time you were here the matter of bicarbonate of soda as a treatment for spotted fever was very much in our minds because of some recent experiences. It so happened that we had an unusual number of cases this year and this treatment was tried in a number of instances. The further experience we had was quite discouraging. The best we can say now is that there is a possibility that it may be of some value."[16]

Many people relied on folk remedies when they or their relatives fell ill with spotted fever. Far and away the most widely recommended was tea made from sagebrush. The use of sage tea, a woman from Washington State wrote to the RML, "is so simple you perhaps will think it a joke but I'm very sure it will work."[17] As proof of efficacy she cited the successful recovery of her sister and husband at different times. From Nebraska came a similar letter hailing the medicinal qualities of sage tea: "Have you found a cure for the Rocky Mountain spotted fever? If not will you try this tea: take the bark from the Idaho sage brush and make a medium strong tea. . . . The tea cured an uncle of mine in Idaho."[18] So many letters suggesting the use of sage tea arrived at the laboratory, in fact, that Ralph R. Parker, whose duties included answering each letter, commented to a friend: "Of course, it has been laughed at, but actually I know of no attempt to determine if it does have value. Personally, I doubt it but my doubt is not backed by any evidence. I may get reckless some time and try it on a few guinea pigs. If spotted fever shouldn't kill them, perhaps the tea will."[19]

Most advocates of sage tea pressed their cases on humanitarian grounds. "I just won't feel right keeping it to myself in case it would help some one," stated one correspondent.[20] Many other people, however, sought compensation from the federal government for their assistance. Especially during the Great Depression, people seemed to feel justified in asking for a portion of New Deal largess. In 1936, Thomas C. Cooper of Helena, Montana, offered to tell the laboratory a secret about the origins of wood ticks. "I just happen to stumble upon the original insect that turns into a wood tick last fall and this spring, I have positive proof that I am correct."[21] Having answered Cooper's letter in appropriately noncommittal but respectful language, Parker received a second missive requesting money.

If I was financially situated so that it was possible, I would only be too glad to divulge this secret just for humaritarian [*sic*] sake, however, inasmuch as the government is spending money with its boondoggling ideas for much less important things than this, and also inasmuch as I am in my declining years now I see no reason why the government should not pay me for something that will benefit its citizens in health the most important of all things. . . . Awaiting further word from you.[22]

Although Parker always explained that the government would not pay for information or treatments, he often offered to subject proposed therapies to analysis and testing at the RML. Many such offers were refused, but a number of preparations were indeed tested. In 1941, James Sproat, a physician in Portland, Oregon, sent one hundred ampules of a solution he claimed would cure spotted fever and a variety of other maladies. "Should the solution turn amber in color," stated his accompanying letter, "there is no cause for alarm as its efficacy is not effected [*sic*] in the least." Sproat commented that "the normal adult dose is 30 c.c. daily," injected intravenously, but he observed that a physician should exercise his own judgment about the efficacious dosage. "In treating chronic conditions, i.e., osteomyelitis and some forms of arthritis, over a long period of time, I have found the best dosage to be 30 c.c. every twenty-four hours. But in acute infections, i.e., carbuncles, infected wounds, erysipilis [*sic*] and similar acute infections, . . . I have given . . . as high as 4 or 5 doses of 30 c.c. each in twenty-four hours."[23] Presumably the liquid failed to stand up under the laboratory's controlled tests, for nothing further was heard of it.

Parker gathered two large files of folk, quack, freak, and mercenary letters relating to spotted fever therapy. It is significant, however, that the disease generated no major therapeutic scandal. Spotted fever's geographical isolation and relatively low incidence militated against widespread exploitation of victims. Furthermore, unlike chronic diseases in which the placebo effect often fooled patients into believing that quack therapies were efficacious, spotted fever ran a severe and unmitigated course from onset to recovery or to death.

By the early 1930s nearly all investigators were disheartened about the prospects for discovering new chemical agents against infectious diseases. Not since the introduction of Paul Erhlich's Salvarsan had a chemical magic bullet been found that was effective against infectious diseases. One bright ray of hope broke into the dismal therapeutic situation during the late 1930s: the discovery of the powerful sulfonamide drugs.[24] In 1935, Gerhardt Domagk, director of research in experimental pathology and bacteriology at the research laboratories of the I. G. Farben Industrie in Elberfeld, Germany, announced that a red dye called Prontosil would cure mice of a lethal infection with hemolytic streptococci. The following year a British team got dramatic results with the drug in the treatment of streptococcal childbed fever. The active agent of the trademarked drug was soon found to be sulfanilamide, and shortly afterward other sulfa derivatives were manufactured. The new sulfa drugs were hailed widely as wonder drugs, and even the editors of the generally restrained *Science* magazine echoed public optimism when they headlined a story on sulfas "Hope of Curing Tuberculosis, Influenza, and Leprosy."[25]

At the National Institute of Health in Bethesda, Maryland, Norman H. Topping set about testing the effectiveness of Prontosil and sulfapyridine against spotted fever and endemic typhus. "Since chemotherapy is being used so extensively in the treatment of a wide variety of infectious diseases, it was believed advisable to test in the laboratory the action of two of the most popular chemotherapeutic agents," he observed. His hopes, as well as those of people living in areas where spotted fever was prevalent, were dashed by the results of the experiments. Not only did the drugs have no positive effect on the course of either disease, but experimental animals treated with the sulfa drugs died sooner than control animals. "These experiments indicate," Topping wrote after his research, "that these two drugs should not be used in the treatment of typhus and Rocky Mountain spotted fever." As new varieties of the sulfa drugs were synthesized in the early 1940s, Ralph R. Parker and his colleagues at the RML tested them all— sulfathiazole, sodium sulfathiazole, sulfaguanidine, and sulfadiazine— with equally disappointing results. During this same period, Parker also tested two other drugs developed for wartime uses. Unfortunately, neither the antimalarial agent atabrine nor a promising antibiotic substance tyrothricin protected guinea pigs from spotted fever.[26]

The results of such experiments, however, did not always affect the way practicing physicians treated their patients. Responding to the public's fascination with and insistence on taking medicine, some physicians continued to administer sulfa drugs and other medications that had been demonstrated to be worthless in treating spotted fever. Topping himself noted this fact a few years later when he cooperated with practicing physicians in conducting a clinical trial of an improved antiserum. "Several of the cases," he noted, had "received one of the sulfonamides; one case received intravenous metaphen; at least one case received large doses of quinine; several had intravenous fluids; several had blood transfusions; and one had intravenous immune human serum."[27]

Because of the failure of known drugs to alter the course of Rocky Mountain spotted fever, the Spencer-Parker vaccine, introduced in the mid 1920s, provided the only efficacious medical strategy against the disease for more than two decades. As dependence on the vaccine increased in infected areas, it became almost mythologically venerated. In 1937, Hollywood film makers seized upon this American success story and catapulted the tale of vaccine development into celluloid immortality. One of the genre of 1930s and 1940s medical triumph films, *The Green Light* was produced by Warner Brothers Studios and based loosely on a Lloyd C. Douglas novel in which scientists sought permission—a "green light"—to proceed with vaccine development. Starring Errol Flynn and Anita Louise, the film was spiced with a love triangle and a dramatic denouement when Flynn became a "human guinea pig" for the sake of science. Although the film apparently did well at the box office, reviews were mixed. One critic judged it a "pretty good picture," but another wished that it had been given a red light before production.[28]

In the Bitterroot Valley, where spotted fever was especially virulent, residents took extraordinary precautions in addition to their annual vaccinations with the Spencer-Parker vaccine. "Every spring the folks would shave the boys' hair so they could be sure no ticks were attached to us," recalled a native Bitterroot Valley resident, Nick Kramis, who lost an aunt to spotted fever and suffered a bout with it himself shortly after he began working in the tick-rearing room at the RML. Parents also issued stern warnings to their children against straying into infected areas. "We were strictly enjoined not to go on the west side of the Bitterroot River," stated Richard A. Ormsbee, another native Bitterrooter. "My father enforced this with me, but I did not try to escape his interdiction, either!"[29]

Throughout endemic areas across the country, spotted fever and its prevention became a regular spring public education feature in many newspapers.[30] By 1939, moreover, Nick Kramis, then the photographer at the RML, had produced a film entitled *The Life History of the Rocky Mountain Wood Tick* that enjoyed wide popularity among civic clubs and other groups who wished to educate their members about how to avoid the disease.[31] Lending support to this campaign, Parker occasionally published articles or provided information to science writers. In 1933 he summarized much information in a *Special Bulletin* issued by the Montana State Board of Health. Infected people, he cautioned, should take no drugs without the advice of their physician. "Certain drugs, such as aspirin, which uninformed persons are likely to use, are deleterious in their effects and should be avoided."[32] Parker also noted that the Spencer-Parker vaccine was widely used as a treatment for spotted fever, "in spite of the fact that it is not recommended for this purpose."[33]

In 1944, just over a decade later, the American Medical Association's popular health journal *Hygeia* offered nearly the same advice. Its informational spotted fever article was adorned with a cartoon of a frantic mother calling her physician for information after finding a tick on one of her children. Having captured the reader's attention, the author listed facts "parents should know about ticks and spotted fever to protect their children and spare themselves anxiety." The article provided detailed information about the epidemiology of spotted fever, how to remove and dispose of ticks properly, and how residents of a "woody section of a tick-infested area," could obtain the vaccine.[34]

Reviews of spotted fever written for medical audiences in the late 1930s emphasized that the recommended treatment was "purely symptomatic and supportive." In such a paper written for the *Rocky Mountain Medical Journal*, George E. Baker admonished physicians against "an attitude of helplessness or hopeless inactivity." Carefully directed symptomatic care and supportive measures, he believed, aided patients in eliminating toxins from their bodies and in fighting against the invading organism. In addition, Baker recommended from his own experience—for it was not, he noted, mentioned in the literature—the administration of neosalvarsan dissolved in metaphen. The recoveries witnessed using these drugs, he speculated, might have been caused by "the bactericidal action of metaphen together with the spirocheticidal action of neosalvarsan upon a micro-organism which is bacterium-like in character, but which has staining properties at least resembling that of spirochetes."[35] Plainly the same logic that motivated administration of Mercurochrome in the 1920s continued to inspire physicians in the early 1940s.

Although chemotherapy appeared valueless against spotted fever, the development of Cox's yolk sac method to cultivate rickettsiae in large quantities rekindled interest in producing an antiserum against the disease. The medical crisis presented by World War II provided further impetus for research on this long-abandoned therapeutic strategy. In 1940, Norman H. Topping announced a hyperimmune rabbit

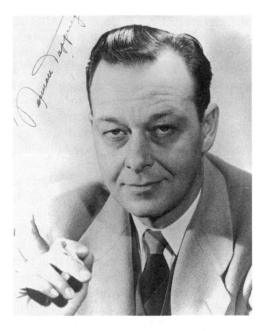

Norman H. Topping's research on spotted fever at the NIH was launched in 1938 when he fell ill with a laboratory-acquired infection. He recovered and made significant contributions to understanding the disease, including key epidemiological studies, work on the role of dogs as carriers of infected ticks, and development of an immune serum that lowered mortality considerably. (Courtesy of the National Library of Medicine.)

serum against Rocky Mountain spotted fever that gave positive results in preliminary tests with guinea pigs and monkeys.[36] Over the next three years, with the cooperation of practicing physicians, he tested the new therapy on seventy-one unvaccinated, naturally infected patients in both the eastern and western United States. From the beginning, results appeared promising. The antiserum reduced deaths from an expected rate of 18.8 percent to 3.8 percent.[37]

In 1941, Topping's antiserum received widespread publicity when it was used against the case of spotted fever suffered by J. Frederick Bell, a twenty-six-year-old student in bacteriology who visited the Rocky Mountain Laboratory in May to discuss cooperative work planned for the coming year. Because of a change in the timing of his visit, Bell was not inoculated before his arrival, as was customary. "As soon as I thought to ask him about spotted fever vaccination," Ralph

R. Parker noted, "he received one injection."[38] Although Bell was not exposed to potentially dangerous areas of the laboratory, Parker was uneasy about the breach of routine requiring immunization of all visitors. Subsequent events underscored the reason for Parker's caution.

On 16 May, Bell started east in the company of his brother-in-law Carl Larson, who later became director of the Rocky Mountain Laboratory. When they reached Rapid City, South Dakota, Bell entered the hospital with high fever, severe headache, general aching, and photophobia.[39] Since he had no rash, Q fever or typhus was originally suspected. "One day a beautiful young nurse came in and gave me a sponge bath," Bell recalled in a later interview. "After she left I looked down at my wrists and arms and there I could see the spots." He rang the bell to summon her back, whereupon he pronounced his own diagnosis: "I know what I've got at last—I've got Rocky Mountain spotted fever."[40] When the RML was informed of Bell's condition, Parker rushed 60 cc of Topping's experimental antiserum to the attending physician. Bell responded well, and newspapers in South Dakota, Minnesota, and Iowa picked up the medical news, hailing the "New Serum" that rendered a "speedy cure" of Bell's illness. As a result, inquiries poured into the laboratory.[41]

Because epidemic typhus was of such great concern in 1941, a similar antiserum was soon prepared to combat it as well. During the 1943 typhus epidemic in Egypt, described as one of the most severe that the country had experienced, this typhus antiserum was among the therapies studied by members of the U.S.A. Typhus Commission. Results of this test were similar to those in the spotted fever trials.[42] Both spotted fever and typhus antisera were limited by the requirement that they be administered early in the course of a disease, preferably before the third day. Even so, they were the first therapeutic agents to make a clear difference in the prognosis of patients.

While these studies were taking place, a new rickettsial menace, long known to the Japanese as tsutsugamushi but called scrub typhus by U.S. troops, threatened the Allied countermove to stem the Japanese advance in the Pacific. James J. Sapero and Fred A. Butler of the U.S. Navy described the situation early in 1942, when U.S. forces began to occupy "numerous widely separated tropical islands throughout a vast subequatorial region." Although the area was known to be a hyperendemic focus of disease, most medical officers were unfamiliar with scrub typhus and other exotic tropical maladies such as malaria, dengue, dysentery, yaws, filariasis, and leprosy. "There followed, as a consequence," observed Sapero and Butler, "a series of outbreaks of tropical diseases in epidemic proportions of a magnitude and potential threat seldom if ever exceeded in American military history."[43]

Scrub typhus, one of the most serious of these diseases, disabled some 18,000 Allied troops, including 6,685 U.S. servicemen between January 1943 and August 1945. Fatality rates varied from a low of 0.6 percent in some regions to as high as 35 percent in others; there were 234 deaths among U.S. troops.[44] Japanese military forces suffered less from tsutsugamushi, doubtless because the endemic disease was familiar to Japanese physicians and public health workers. Except for the 1908 comparative study between Rocky Mountain spotted fever and tsutsugamushi made by U.S. Army physicians Percy M. Ashburn and Charles F. Craig, few western studies on the disease had been pursued. In contrast, Japanese investigators had continued to study the two diseases into the 1930s, even though two of them died from laboratory-acquired spotted fever infections during their research. The two Japanese who succumbed were Kokyo Sugata, an assistant of Norio Ogata of the Chiba Medical College, who died on 4 July 1931; and Masajiro Nishibe, a professor at the Niigata Medical College, who died on 13 August 1932.[45]

Usually scrub typhus was diagnosed by clinical observation of typical typhus-like symptoms: high fever, headache, muscle and joint pain, and a rash. For laboratory confirmation, a Weil-Felix test had been developed during the 1920s and 1930s by British researchers and their colleagues at the Institute of Medical Research in Kuala Lumpur, Federated Malay States. They had observed that the sera of tsutsu-gamushi patients reacted positively to the OX-K strain of *B. proteus* and negatively to the OX-19 strain.[46]

The U.S.A. Typhus Commission began to study scrub typhus, noted its director, Stanhope Bayne-Jones, "because of its last name. . . . When we took in scrub typhus, no one stopped to ask whether the Executive Order applied or not." Because it caused so many disabilities and deaths among Allied troops, the Typhus Commission brought in a variety of experts to attack this capricious malady, which often struck one group of soldiers while leaving others nearby untouched. Cornelius B. Philip and Glen Kohls, entomologists who had left the RML to join the military after war broke out, sought to identify arthropod vectors of the disease, which had been suspected because victims exhibited an eschar, or initial lesion, a characteristic of the more familiar European tick-borne disease, boutonneuse fever. Francis G. Blake, dean of the Yale University School of Medicine, and Kenneth F. Maxcy, professor of epidemiology at Johns Hopkins School of Hygiene and Public Health, investigated the epidemiology and medical treatment of the disease.[47]

By the end of the war, two major lines of defense against scrub typhus had been developed. First, the U.S. Army launched preventive education efforts, including posters describing the mite, where it was likely to be found, and how soldiers should prepare their campsites to avoid it. Second, investigators funded by the Medical Research Committee of the Office of Scientific Research and Development developed chemicals to impregnate clothing that would repel the tsutsugamushi mite. Dimethyl phthalate was initially chosen, but in 1945 the War Department replaced it with benzyl benzoate, because it would withstand more launderings before having to be reapplied. Even so, soldiers' clothing had to be retreated every two weeks.[48]

Military physicians who cared for scrub typhus victims adopted supportive therapy like that used for years against Rocky Mountain spotted fever. Norman H. Topping believed that an antiserum should be effective for treatment and perhaps even for prophylaxis of scrub typhus. With the eschar as an early diagnostic feature, Topping reasoned, antiserum could be given earlier and with greater benefit. By 1945 he had prepared one that gave promising results in mice. Research by the U.S. Army, U.S. Navy, and U.S. Public Health Service also focused on the development of a vaccine against the disease. Before either vaccine or antiserum could be tested, however, the war ended.[49]

A similar situation occurred in the Mediterranean theater with yet another rickettsial disease. During the winter of 1944 and spring of 1945, Allied troops in this region fell ill with a malady first termed the Balkan grippe but soon shown to be Q fever. The sudden appearance of this disease in the Mediterranean area foreshadowed later findings that it was widespread around the globe, rather than confined to Australia and to the western United States, as had been believed when it was first discovered.[50]

Experience with all the rickettsial diseases during World War II led to a much more specific understanding of their pathologic mechanisms. In contrast to earlier observations, which were generally limited to descriptions of damage to particular tissues, wartime physiological research illuminated the dynamic biological mechanisms involved. In 1944, Theodore E. Woodward and Edward F. Bland, members of the U.S.A. Typhus Commission, reported that studies of typhus in French Morocco had revealed the "overwhelming generalized involvement" of the peripheral circulatory system. Rickettsiae invaded the entire circulatory tree, causing swelling of the endothelial cells. By occluding blood flow, they gave rise to the formation of clots in the smaller and occasionally even the larger blood vessels. This damage produced "an increase of capillary permeability," which altered the electrolytic composition of the blood and lowered the osmotic pressure as plasma proteins escaped into the tissues. These phenomena further starved the capillaries of needed oxygen and nutrients, thus setting up a vicious cycle that culminated in circulatory failure.[51]

To combat this widespread damage, aggressive supportive therapy was indicated. The same year that Woodward and Bland published their prescription for typhus therapy, a North Carolina physician, George T. Harrell, and his colleagues outlined a similar program for the treatment of Rocky Mountain spotted fever. Unlike the undifferentiated "good nursing" recommendations of earlier decades, the supportive therapies advocated by both groups were highly specific: adequate fluid intake, blood plasma transfusions if necessary, ammonium or sodium salts to improve hypochloremia, a nourishing protein and carbohydrate diet, and abandonment of the common practice of administering digitalis to stimulate the heart except to treat critical heart problems.[52]

Such a program was unfortunately necessary because the most stunning medical triumph of the war years—the development of penicillin—had proved valueless against the rickettsial diseases. Discovered in 1928 by Alexander Fleming, the mold *Penicillium notatum* had been largely ignored until an expensive cooperative effort between pharmaceutical firms and the U.S. government made large-scale production possible.[53] By 1943 tests in several civilian hospitals had demonstrated penicillin's potency against a host of infections. Not a chemical compound like the sulfa drugs, this *antibiotic* was a substance produced by living organisms that was antagonistic to the growth of many bacteria. Here, at last, was the long-sought "magic bullet" that cured staphylococcal infections, pneumococcal pneumonia, rheumatic fever, syphilis, and gonorrhea.

Tests of the effectiveness of penicillin against Rocky Mountain spotted fever and other rickettsial diseases were conducted in 1945 at the Rocky Mountain Laboratory and in the research laboratories of the Sharp and Dohme pharmaceutical house. At Sharp and Dohme, Florence K. Fitzpatrick treated spotted-fever-infected guinea pigs within forty-eight hours after the onset of fever. All the animals died. Blood plasma levels of the drug, she noted, were sufficient to expect recovery had penicillin been of any value.[54]

Even though penicillin had proved to be of no use against rickettsial diseases, its example spurred further research for a chemical or antibiotic agent that would supplant the limited value of antisera. Early efforts followed a lead suggested in 1937 by Hans Zinsser and E. B. Schoenbach at Harvard Medical School. They had demonstrated that the rate of intracellular multiplication of rickettsiae in tissue cultures was determined by the metabolic rate of the host cells. Under conditions of high metabolic activity, little or no multiplication of the intracellular parasites took place. Only under conditions of reduced metabolic activity was active multiplication noted.[55] This information set investigators searching for a nontoxic substance that would increase cellular metabolism and thereby inhibit rickettsial multiplication.

In 1942 para-aminobenzoic acid, commonly called PABA and generally considered to be a vitamin, was identified as a promising antirickettsial agent. In a classified report to the Division of Medical Sciences of the National Research Council, John C. Snyder, John Maier, and C. R. Anderson described its effectiveness in reducing mortality from experimental murine typhus in white mice.[56] A year later, H. L. Hamilton, Harry Plotz, and Joseph E. Smadel reported to the director of the U.S.A. Typhus Commission on PABA's effect on the growth of typhus rickettsiae in the yolk sac of the infected chick embryo.[57]

The first large-scale test of PABA was conducted in 1943, a part of the therapeutic trials made during the typhus epidemic in Egypt. The results indicated that PABA ameliorated the clinical course of the disease if it was started during the first week of illness. The drug produced no unfavorable effects with the exception of a tendency to develop a low white blood cell count, which could be monitored. When Andrew Yeomans and his colleagues published these findings in the *Journal of the American Medical Association*, its editors wondered, "What effect will para-aminobenzoic acid and related compounds have on Rocky Mountain spotted fever and other rickettsial diseases?" That question was soon answered. In 1945, Ludwik Anigstein and Madero N. Bader reported that PABA was indeed efficacious against spotted fever in guinea pigs. Shortly thereafter, Harry M. Rose and his colleagues at Columbia University College of Physicians and Surgeons reported the first clinical results of a single human case of Rocky Mountain spotted fever treated with PABA. The patient, a woman, improved rapidly after twenty-four hours of therapy.[58]

Additional evidence for the efficacy of PABA therapy was soon amassed. The cases of spotted fever suffered by a Fairfax, Virginia, couple were cured with PABA after they failed to respond to immune rabbit serum therapy. A group of cases studied by physicians in Wilmington, Delaware, indicated that spotted fever responded even more sensitively to PABA than did typhus. They also, however, noted the limitations of the drug as reflected in its failure to cure a sixty-seven-year-old man with long-standing renal disease and a history of heart attack. This case, they stated, "may serve to illustrate the point . . .

that *p*-aminobenzoic acid retards or prevents the spread and prolif-eration of the rickettsias in the body but is not an antidote for any toxin already released and does not repair damage already done."[59]

PABA was rickettsiostatic, not rickettsiocidal—that is, it inhibited further growth of rickettsiae but did not kill them outright. Because of this, it was essential that treatment begin as soon as possible. Once the organisms had damaged the tissues and multiplied to large numbers, the drug could not stop them. The giant step in therapy represented by PABA, however, inspired greater confidence than ever before among physicians. A review of spotted fever written in 1947 by Samuel F. Ravenel reflected this greater sense of knowledge about and control over the disease gained during the war years. "In the early days, the treatment of this disease was symptomatic, which simply enabled the patient to die or recover somewhat more comfortably." In contrast, Ravenel was able to outline a comprehensive treatment plan that should enable any physician to do battle with confidence against Rocky Moun-tain spotted fever.[60]

Although PABA therapy enriched the physician's armamentarium in the fight against spotted fever, it was soon eclipsed by more powerful drugs. Unlike the development of the Spencer-Parker or Cox vaccines, a cure for spotted fever did not emerge from a direct attack on the disease in isolation. Rather, it resulted from planned, persistent, and expensive empirical searches for antibiotics undertaken by pharma-ceutical companies. The example of penicillin research, with its large investment and larger profits, was the stimulus for the effort to find antibiotics against other diseases. Not yet knowing the structure, much less the physiology, of rickettsiae or viruses, investigators proceeded without benefit of detailed knowledge about the organisms they were combating.

Even so, by the late 1940s, Harry F. Dowling noted in his compre-hensive study of infectious disease therapy, *Fighting Infection*, "at least half a dozen companies had teams of investigators actively looking for antibiotics."[61] One of them, Parke, Davis and Company, established a research grant at Yale University to enable Paul Burkholder, a bot-anist, to search soil samples for microorganisms with antibiotic po-tentialities. He isolated a promising mold from Venezuelan soil, which was subsequently named *Streptomyces venezuela*. Parke, Davis scien-tists extracted a substance from it that inhibited the growth of a number of pathogenic bacteria. The new antibiotic was named chloramphenicol and given the trade name Chloromycetin.[62]

In their publication announcing the discovery of the drug, Parke, Davis scientists noted that Chloromycetin was more effective than

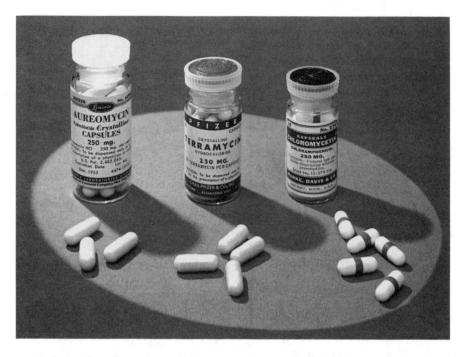

With the discovery of broad-spectrum antibiotics, Rocky Mountain spotted
fever became a curable disease. Aureomycin and Terramycin were trade
names for the tetracycline drugs. Chloramphenicol was sold under the
name Chloromycetin. Potentially toxic side effects of the drugs were not
recognized for nearly a decade after they were introduced. (Courtesy of the
Rocky Mountain Laboratories, NIAID.)

PABA against *Rickettsia prowazekii*, the organism that caused epidemic
typhus, in experiments on chicken embryos and mice.[63] They sent
samples of the promising drug to Joseph E. Smadel, then scientific
director of the Walter Reed Army Institute of Research, who had a
"working arrangement" with Parke, Davis to test "any new antimicrobial drugs which exerted even the slightest inhibitory effect for
viral and rickettsial agents."[64] When he got similar results in his laboratory, Smadel enthusiastically recommended immediate trials in humans.[65]

Shortly thereafter, Eugene H. Payne of Parke, Davis took a team of
scientists to Bolivia, where an epidemic of typhus was raging. The
power of this new drug against typhus was dramatically confirmed.
An anecdote recounted by Dowling bears repeating here as an illus-

tration: "In collaboration with local doctors, . . . [Payne] treated 22 of the sickest patients, five of whom had been listed as certain to die. All recovered, including one for whom the death certificate had already been filled out and signed, awaiting only the insertion of the hour of death." Smadel's tests of Chloromycetin on typhus patients in Mexico were equally successful. He then arranged with Raymond Lewthwaite, director of the Institute for Medical Research at Kuala Lumpur, Malaya, to conduct field trials of the new antibiotic on scrub typhus cases. All ninety-four patients treated with it recovered.[66]

On the basis of these spectacular results, Maurice C. Pincoffs and his colleagues of the University of Maryland School of Medicine in Baltimore cooperated with Joseph E. Smadel of the Army Medical School to test Chloromycetin furnished by Parke, Davis against spotted fever. Patients were given tablets of the drug in dosages based on body weight that had proved effective against scrub typhus—an initial large dose followed by smaller doses every three hours. No toxicity was observed, but the researchers noted that the drug had not been used over a long period of time. The results of the therapy were indisputably positive. Irrespective of the height of the preceding fever or the age of the patient, body temperature fell to normal within seventy-six hours after the initial dose. The average duration of fever was a mere 2.2 days. Shortly thereafter, other researchers confirmed these results and the popular press acclaimed Chloromycetin as the "greatest drug since penicillin."[67]

Almost simultaneously with the development of chloramphenicol, researchers at Lederle Laboratories announced the development of an antibiotic from *Streptomyces aureofaciens*, which, because of its gold color, was named Aureomycin. In June 1948 a research group at Children's Hospital in Washington, D.C., collaborated with members of the Department of Preventive Medicine at Johns Hopkins University School of Medicine to test Aureomycin in thirteen patients suffering from Rocky Mountain spotted fever. "The response of these patients has been impressive," the researchers wrote, "and it is apparent that Aureomycin is an effective therapeutic agent."[68] Shortly thereafter, researchers at a third pharmaceutical house, Charles Pfizer and Company, produced another antibiotic effective against rickettsial diseases. Isolated from *Streptomyces rimosus*, this drug was called Terramycin. When the chemical structures of Aureomycin and Terramycin were elucidated, they were found to be nearly identical. Together they became known as the tetracyclines, and, with later analogues and with chloramphenicol, they were termed broad-spectrum antibiotics. These drugs were effective not only against rickettsial infections and those diseases that had yielded already to penicillin but also against diseases whose stubborn bacterial agents had resisted all earlier therapies, including typhoid fever, brucellosis, mycoplasma pneumonias, and chlamydial infections.[69]

The advent of antibiotics effective against rickettsial diseases crowned the awesome achievements of scientific and medical research during the 1940s. Through research on the atomic bomb, physicists had opened a qualitatively new field that held great promise in medicine and in world energy production while simultaneously threatening worldwide destruction. Atomic power and antibiotics symbolized the power of research that had also produced a host of less-publicized discoveries, from improved blood transfusion techniques to radar. These achievements led many leaders of the scientific and medical communities to argue forcefully for expanded federal funding of research, especially in basic studies that formed a broad body of knowledge from which specific applications might emerge.[70] This effort, according to Charles V. Kidd, was "the loudest, most expensive, most persistent, most calculating, most emotional, most effective and socially useful propaganda campaign" ever mounted on behalf of science.[71]

Of many proposals, none was more far-reaching than that promulgated by the Committee on Science and Society of the American Association for the Advancement of Science. Twelve points for a national research policy emerged from a symposium held in December 1944. Point 2 called for "extending systematic research into every field or activity of life, as a considered policy of critically examining whatever we believe and do, and proceeding to a revision of established assumptions and practices wherever research reveals they are required or desirable." Point 9 went so far as to assert that research should be a coordinate function of the U. S. government equal to the legislative, executive, and judiciary.[72]

During the next decade, Congress and both Democratic and Republican presidents supported the expansion of federally sponsored scientific and medical research—even if they declined to grant science coequal status under the Constitution. The National Science Foundation was created, and the NIH flourished with the establishment of a program of grants to university researchers and the creation of several new institutes.[73] Discussions about basic and applied research, moreover, produced a new agenda for research at the NIH. Its traditional public health responsibility of assisting states with on-site disease problems, such as the Rocky Mountain spotted fever work in Montana, was transferred to the newly created Communicable Disease Center, later called the Centers for Disease Control, in Atlanta, Georgia. An enlarged and reorganized NIH claimed basic studies as its mission, utilizing a document on postwar science policy widely known as the Steelman Report to articulate the distinctions between basic and applied research.[74] Laboratory studies to uncover new information were generally regarded as basic research. Gathering statistics on the incidence of disease fairly clearly fell in the applied category. These distinctions, of course, were somewhat subject to interpretation. Much epidemiological research and field studies of vector-borne diseases were often difficult to classify.

The NIH director, Rolla E. Dyer, set about applying the terms of the new mandate to the programs of the several institutes that comprised the now plural National *Institutes* of Health. Among these was the National Microbiological Institute, comprised of the agency's historic research programs in infectious and tropical diseases and its work in biologics standards.[75] Although the Rocky Mountain Laboratory was made a coequal branch of the new institute, the focus on basic research presented a somewhat awkward problem for RML, which had served during the war years principally as a vaccine factory — clearly an applied rather than a basic function. Furthermore, applied research was conducted by its staff of entomologists, who enjoyed a worldwide reputation as authorities on tick taxonomy, and by its serologists, who performed laboratory tests for physicians and public health agencies throughout the northwestern states. These duties, however, overlapped with other, more basic studies, such as identifying tick vectors of diseases and studying the antigenic relationships among disease organisms. As discussions about the laboratory's postwar research program continued, NIH administrators moved rapidly to transfer production of yellow fever and rickettsial vaccines to the private sector. The last batches of Spencer-Parker vaccine made from tick tissues were produced in 1948. The chief vaccine maker, Earl Malone, who had supervised production since the mid 1920s, turned to other assignments until his retirement in 1958.[76]

In January 1949 Victor H. Haas, first director of the National Microbiological Institute, traveled to Montana to discuss with Ralph R. Parker how RML should redirect its research in light of the new NIH emphasis.[77] The ambiguity of the Steelman distinctions between basic and applied research was clearly revealed in the interchanges between Haas and Parker at the conference. "It is especially important," Haas stated to Parker,

that we shall conform to the policy decisions made by higher levels that the function of the N.I.H. is basic research. . . . I think many things that were fundamental research a year ago or a month ago or 10 years ago are not fundamental research today. Let us say, for example, that when the natural history of spotted fever was unknown, investigation of that problem was fundamental research, just as I think the investigation of equine encephalomyelitis is fundamental research today.

Parker took issue: "I would disagree that we know the natural history of spotted fever—we know very little about it." Haas replied, "That is right. I only used that as an illustration."[78]

Although Parker was prepared to redirect the RML's research in accordance with NIH policy, he was never able to implement the new plans. On 4 September 1949 he suffered a heart attack and died.[79] In the history of Rocky Mountain spotted fever, Parker's death may be viewed as a watershed. He had investigated the ecology of spotted fever, participated in the development of the tick tissue vaccine, supervised the production of the Cox vaccine, personally tested the efficacy of numerous drugs, and witnessed the introduction of effective broad-spectrum antibiotics. Parker probably possessed a broader knowledge of spotted fever than did any other single person. After his death the history of spotted fever became less directly tied to western Montana and to the Rocky Mountain Laboratory, although that facility continued to serve as a major center for rickettsial research.

In the late 1940s the wartime vocabulary of conquest, triumph, and victory seemed particularly appropriate to describe the half-century struggle to prevent and cure the most severe rickettsial disease in the western hemisphere. And indeed, in 1949 the first of a genre of "conquest" articles appeared. It was the first Howard Taylor Ricketts Award Lecture at the University of Chicago. The speaker was Russell M. Wilder, then on the staff of the Mayo Clinic, who had assisted Ricketts in the 1910 research on typhus fever that took his life. Entitling his lecture "The Rickettsial Diseases: Discovery and Conquest," Wilder proclaimed, "This discovery of a cure . . . represents the final chapter of an epic."[80] His choice of the word *final* may have been premature, but without doubt the impact of antibiotics was of epic proportion. By fulfilling the promise of medical research, these "miracle drugs" justified the persistent faith and optimism of investigators and laymen alike.

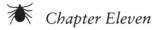 *Chapter Eleven*

Spotted Fever after Antibiotics

Experience has shown that success may be temporary when all the answers are not known.

Mack I. Shanholtz, Virginia State Health Commissioner, 1961

During the 1950s, Rocky Mountain spotted fever seemed nearly to disappear in the United States. The number of reported cases fell from 570 in 1949 to 301 in 1953. Throughout the remainder of the decade, the incidence of the disease hovered at 250–300 cases with fewer than two dozen deaths per year.[1] Except for the families and friends of the victims, most people could argue with conviction that antibiotics and insecticides had eliminated spotted fever as a threat to modern society. Because *Rickettsia rickettsii* had not been eradicated, however, the history of Rocky Mountain spotted fever did not end with antibiotics. The period between the late 1940s and the early 1970s may be characterized as a time of little drama in the story, yet it was during these years that much of the morphology, ecology, and physiology of *R. rickettsii* was elucidated.

One significant portion of the ecology of spotted fever was defined between 1935 and 1950. During this period the disease was shown to be widespread throughout—and apparently exclusive to—the western hemisphere.[2] In South America by the early 1940s spotted fever was known to exist in Tobia, Colombia, and in rural areas of São Paulo, Minas Gerais, and Rio de Janeiro, Brazil.[3] In 1938 the first figures on spotted fever in Canada revealed that, although the disease had been known since 1923, only eight cases were officially documented.[4] During the next decade, a project to amass data on spotted fever and bubonic plague in Canada revealed that cases of spotted fever were known in British Columbia, Alberta, and Saskatchewan, with most cases occurring in southeastern Alberta. Three species of spotted fever tick vectors were identified, but only *D. andersoni*, abun-

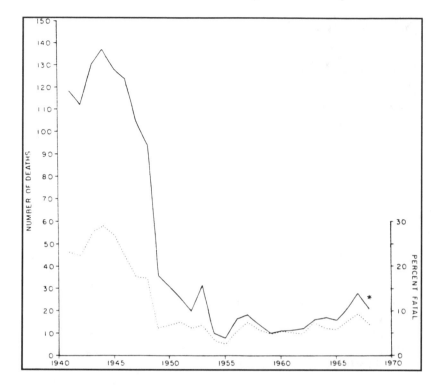

Deaths and ratios of cases to fatalities of Rocky Mountain spotted fever in
the United States, 1940–70. The solid line represents the number of deaths;
the dotted line tracks the ratio of cases to fatalities—that is, the mortality
percentage. The data for 1968 were provisional. The impact of broad
spectrum antibiotics, introduced in 1948, is dramatically apparent.
(Reproduced from Michael A. W. Hattwick, "Rocky Mountain Spotted
Fever in the U.S., 1920–1970," *Journal of Infectious Diseases* 124 [1971]:
112–14.)

dant in the southern part of the three western provinces, was known
to harbor virulent strains of *R. rickettsii.* The small number of infected
ticks in nature and the tedious work of surveying them were underscored by the Canadian report: only 5 of 72,227 ticks collected in
British Columbia and only 10 of 49,201 collected in Alberta were
demonstrated to be infective.[5]

For some time, spotted fever seemed curiously absent from Mexico
and other Central American countries. Writing in 1943, Gordon E.
Davis of the Rocky Mountain Laboratory observed that it hardly
seemed "credible that a disease present in southwestern Canada,

throughout the United States, in Colombia, and Brazil should be entirely absent" from the Central American region.[6] Indeed, the following year "an acute petechial fever with a high death rate," was reported from the districts of Choix and Fuerte de Sinaloa in Mexico. Local residents, who called the affliction *fiebre de Choix* or *fiebre manchada*, reported to Miguel E. Bustamante and Gerardo Varela of the Instituto de Salubridad y Enfermedades Tropicales in Mexico City that the affliction appeared each year. A 75 percent mortality, typical rickettsial symptoms, and the presence of ticks strongly suggested Rocky Mountain spotted fever.[7] Subsequent studies confirmed that spotted fever existed alongside murine typhus in the Mexican states of Durango and Sinaloa, and that it occurred with epidemic typhus in San Luis Potosi and Veracruz. All three rickettsial diseases occurred in Coahuila. Only in Sonora did spotted fever exist in isolation. Arthropod vectors found naturally infected were *R. sanguineus* in the north and northeast regions and *A. cajennense* on the east Mexican coast.[8]

In 1950 spotted fever was first reported in Panama. Although the diagnosis of the first Panamanian case was made upon autopsy, the next two reported victims were treated with antibiotics and recovered. Carlos Calero and José M. Nuñez of the Panama Hospital and Santo Thomás Hospital in Panama and Roberto Silva-Goytia of the Instituto de Salubridad y Enfermedades Tropicales in Mexico City found that infections occurred in both rural and urban settings across the isthmus. By 1953, Enid C. de Rodaniche at Gorgas Memorial Hospital had recovered *Rickettsia rickettsii* from naturally infected *Amblyomma cajennense* ticks, already known as a vector of spotted fever in Colombia, Mexico, and Brazil. Because this tick was abundant and attacked humans "readily" in all stages, Rodaniche wondered why clinical spotted fever had not been encountered across the isthmus with greater frequency in the past.[9]

Since spotted fever had been identified in North, South, and Central America, Mexican investigators Bustamante and Varela proposed that its name be changed to American spotted fever to eliminate its misleading exclusive association with the Rocky Mountain area of North America. A Brazilian investigator argued that all geographical adjectives should be abandoned and the disease called simply spotted fever. U.S. investigators W. M. Kelsey and G. T. Harrell suggested that tick-borne typhus was the most appropriate scientific designation. None of these proposals, however, gained widespread support. The popular name Rocky Mountain spotted fever simply could not be dislodged.[10]

Complacency about spotted fever, of course, was abetted by a plethora of popular articles that emphasized the miraculous properties of antibiotics and insecticides in controlling infectious diseases.[11] A federally funded flea control project begun in 1945 demonstrated beyond cavil DDT's power against the vectors of murine typhus. In nine southeastern states and in Texas—where 92 percent of all cases of murine typhus occurred—DDT dusting produced a 62 percent decline in cases. "Barrier spraying" against ticks along roadsides, the dusting of dogs with DDT, and the development of more effective tick repellents played a similar role in the containment of spotted fever. Confidence in the efficacy of insecticides ran so high, in fact, that some scientists joked that these chemicals might render their positions obsolete.[12]

Control of rickettsial diseases with chemical pesticides, however, lasted for less than two decades. By the 1960s irrefutable evidence had been amassed that mosquitoes, lice, mites, and other arthropod vectors could develop resistance to insecticides. In *Silent Spring*, her celebrated book on the dangers of the indiscriminate use of such chemicals, Rachel Carson recorded the declining power of DDT against typhus after its initial success during World War II.

The control of body lice in Naples was one of the earliest and most publicized achievements of DDT. During the next few years its success in Italy was matched by the successful control of lice affecting some two million people in Japan and Korea in the winter of 1945–46. Some premonition of trouble ahead might have been gained by the failure to control a typhus epidemic in Spain in 1948. Despite this failure in actual practice, encouraging laboratory experiments led entomologists to believe lice were unlikely to develop resistance. Events in Korea in the winter of 1950–51 were therefore startling. When DDT powder was applied to a group of Korean soldiers the extraordinary result was an actual increase in the infestation of lice. When lice were collected and tested, it was found that 5 per cent DDT powder caused no increase in their natural mortality. Similar results among lice collected from vagrants in Tokyo, from an asylum in Itabashi, and from refugee camps in Syria, Jordan, and eastern Egypt, confirmed the ineffectiveness of DDT for the control of lice and typhus. When by 1957 the list of countries in which lice had become resistant to DDT was extended to include Iran, Turkey, Ethiopia, West Africa, South Africa, Peru, Chile, France, Yugoslavia, Afghanistan, Uganda, Mexico, and Tanganyika, the initial triumph in Italy seemed dim indeed.[13]

As with insecticides, broad-spectrum antibiotics were used widely, even indiscriminately, during the 1950s. Among those investigators who monitored the incidence of spotted fever during this decade, it was apparent that the popular drugs masked its true incidence in the United States. "It is probably safe to say," wrote the authors of a 1955 review paper, "that a relatively small percentage of Rocky Mountain spotted fever and typhus infections now develop to the point of complete diagnosis and reporting." Further complicating the picture was the influence of antibiotics on diagnostic tests. Studies at the Rocky

Mountain Laboratory revealed that the appearance of antibodies in both the Weil-Felix and the complement fixation tests was altered if the patient had received antibiotics. It also became increasingly hard to obtain blood samples that showed a change in antibody level. Patients receiving antibiotics rarely returned to their physicians for a follow-up blood test. It thus became virtually impossible to confirm suspected cases.[14]

The popularity of the "miracle drugs," moreover, deflected early reports about their toxic side effects. Chloramphenicol, which had passed toxicity tests in animals and appeared to have no adverse effects other than causing temporary anemia, was in wide use before its dangers came to public attention. Evidence gathered as early as 1950 that the drug could cause a dangerous depression of the blood marrow resulting in fatal aplastic anemia at first attracted little attention. Because death often occurred two or more months after treatment had stopped, it was often difficult to relate it to the earlier administration of chloramphenicol. In 1952, however, accounts of an entire series of such cases temporarily restricted the use of the drug. Soothing pharmaceutical propaganda, however, soon restored the use of chloramphenicol to a high level. Further evidence of the drug's hazards appeared some years later, when it was often administered to newborn babies prophylactically. Many of these infants developed the so-called grey syndrome, named for the ashen grey pallor that accompanied circulatory collapse and death. It was not until 1959, however, that a therapeutic experiment at the Los Angeles County Hospital demonstrated chloramphenicol's causative connection to this condition.[15]

By the early 1960s medical texts began recommending against the use of chloramphenicol for rickettsial infections, usually noting the tetracyclines as effective alternatives. Even as these texts came off the presses, additional reports appeared, suggesting that the tetracyclines might also be hazardous, especially to patients' teeth. Since 1957 the tetracyclines had been known to have an affinity for bone tissue. Because the drugs fluoresced under ultraviolet light, scientists could identify the sites in the body where they lodged after treatment.[16] In 1962, I. S. Walton and H. B. Hilton at the King Edward Memorial Hospital for Women in Perth, Australia, published the results of a study on fifty babies who had received the drugs during their first few weeks of life. Forty-six of the children suffered stains on their primary teeth. As with those children treated with chloramphenicol, nearly half of these babies had been given tetracyclines prophylactically rather than for any medical problem. In 1963 investigators at the National Institute of Dental Research published a review article alerting the medical community to the dangers of these drugs. "Tetracycline is the drug of choice in many infections in which the consequences of the infection outweigh the possible damage to the teeth," they concluded, but they warned about the hazards of injudicious use.[17]

With a death rate of over 20 percent in untreated persons, Rocky Mountain spotted fever was one of those diseases in which the risks of the tetracyclines or even chloramphenicol seemed worth taking. When the 1950s enthusiasm for antibiotics gave way by the 1970s to extreme caution in prescribing such drugs, those physicians who frequently treated spotted fever cases had no hesitation about their use. Thus a 1977 paper in the *Journal of the American Medical Association* suggesting that the tetracyclines should be virtually abandoned drew sharp criticism from southeastern physicians located in endemic spotted fever areas. Noting that a single, short course of oxytetracycline or doxycycline caused the least staining of teeth, they were clearly willing to subject their patients to the risk of a nonfatal condition in order to save them from potentially fatal spotted fever.[18]

Antibiotics proved to be double-edged swords, but their advent at the end of World War II had signaled a decline in concern about many infectious diseases, especially those, such as Rocky Mountain spotted fever, that struck so few victims each year. To be sure, people continued to die from spotted fever as well as from other infectious diseases, but the American animus against death was largely redirected after World War II toward the chronic diseases, especially cancer and heart disease, which had been growing as foci of public concern since the 1920s. As a result, the 1950s witnessed a dramatic plunge in federal funding for research on infectious diseases relative to the rising rate for research on chronic diseases. In a 1957 study, for example, Charles V. Kidd observed that between 1948 and 1954 the study of communicable diseases had dropped from first to eighth place in terms of federal and foundation monies allocated for their support. Studies of the endocrine system, in contrast, had risen from fifteenth to fourth. Although Kidd noted that such classifications of research might be somewhat arbitrary and at times influenced by fads, he concluded that the figures confirmed "the general opinion that the substance of medical research" had "indeed shifted remarkably over the last decade."[19]

In spite of the facts that more patients visited physicians because of infections than for any other group of illnesses and that infections in the United States were the primary cause of death in 6 percent of all deaths, investigators found funding agencies, whether Congress or private foundations, more inclined to support research on chronic diseases. Dorland J. Davis, director of the National Institute of Allergy

and Infectious Diseases from 1964 to 1975, articulated the often un-
thinking assumptions that plagued infectious disease research. "I recall
becoming terribly annoyed at a chart that was proposed for showing
to some influential group—I don't know whether it was Congress or
another group—which showed the death rates for cancer and heart
disease going up steeply and the death rate for infectious disease going
down sharply. I think I got it stopped all right, but . . . it took quite
an effort to get people to think of infectious diseases as still a serious
health problem."[20]

The National Institute of Allergy and Infectious Diseases was the
categorical incarnation of the former National Microbiological Institute. One story, probably apocryphal but nonetheless revealing, held
that the new name enhanced Congress's willingness to grant the institute funds because people continued to die of infectious diseases and
suffer from allergies, but "nobody ever died of microbiology."[21] Despite
the new name, a 1965 analysis of federal support for research in
microbiology found that the field remained significantly undersup-
ported. Prepared for President Lyndon Johnson as a part of a larger
review of the NIH, and popularly known as the Wooldridge Committee
report, the study attributed the situation to several factors, including
the perception that antibiotics had solved the problem of infectious
diseases. Another, more difficult problem to attack was the overshad-
owing of traditional microbiological research by the "glamour and
scientific status of the flowering field of molecular biology." Although
agreeing that this new field was undeniably important, the review panel
believed that its attraction had retarded more traditional studies of
"host-parasite relationships," the whole field of tropical medicine, and
medical entomology.[22]

For rickettsial diseases in particular, major federal funding was provided by two agencies. The smaller of the two was the Commission
on Rickettsial Diseases of the Armed Forces Epidemiological Board,
one of several commissions supported by the board to maintain expertise in particular diseases of military importance, especially in the
event of atomic warfare. "Despite its name," wrote Paul B. Beeson,
the board was "primarily a civilian agency." Its Commission on Rickettsial Diseases, headed first by Joseph E. Smadel and subsequently by
Charles L. Wisseman, Jr., supported university research on rickettsiae
through three or four U.S. Army or U.S. Navy contracts each year,
ranging from $30,000 to $250,000. According to Wisseman, during
the 1960s these contracts resembled grant awards in support of respected research programs rather than the more usual military mechanism of quid pro quo service contracts. Meetings of the commission,

furthermore, provided a scientific forum for U.S. rickettsiologists and a national meeting at which promising young investigators could be recruited.[23]

The second source of federal funds for rickettsial research was the grants program of the National Institutes of Health, especially the National Microbiological Institute and its successor institute, the National Institute of Allergy and Infectious Diseases. Between 1946, when the grants mechanism began to function, and 1971, when the situation began to change somewhat, slightly less than $6 million in grants was awarded for research on rickettsial diseases compared to more than $526 million awarded by the National Microbiological Institute and NIAID for all types of extramural research in microbiology, parasitology, virology, and immunology.[24] This relatively low level of funding was due in part to the small number of new researchers coming into the field of rickettsiology and in part to a growing emphasis on viral and immunological research. New techniques made virology and immunology fruitful fields, and many of the diseases caused by viruses and immunological deficiencies had no known treatment.

Those young investigators who did enter the field of rickettsiology generally came from a relatively small number of institutions whose interest in rickettsial diseases was historic or had developed during World War II. Initially most rickettsial investigators were housed at the National Institutes of Health, with rickettsial units at Bethesda, Maryland, and at the Rocky Mountain Laboratory in Hamilton, Montana; at the military viral and rickettsial unit at Walter Reed Army Institute for Research in Washington, D.C.; and at Harvard University Medical School in Cambridge, Massachusetts, site of the investigations of S. Burt Wolbach and Hans Zinsser. The University of Chicago, home of Howard Taylor Ricketts, also fostered some rickettsial research, as did the Rockefeller Institute for Medical Research in New York, the locale of Hideyo Noguchi's early work. Investigators trained in these centers had also established satellite programs in several universities. Henry Pinkerton, for example, studied with Wolbach at Harvard and later moved to Saint Louis University School of Medicine. One center of clinical research on Rocky Mountain spotted fever grew up in North Carolina, a site of high spotted fever incidence in the east. Another became established at the University of Maryland School of Medicine in Baltimore, largely as a result of collaboration with the unit at Walter Reed in Washington, D.C. Once Q fever had been identified as a major problem across the western states, several western universities and public health agencies, especially in Texas, Kansas, and California, developed expertise in this rickettsial disease. Most of the rickettsial investigators who directed these programs during the 1950s had been trained, of course, in the crucible of wartime work with the U.S.A. Typhus Commission.[25]

NIH grants for rickettsial diseases were inaugurated in 1946, with a $7,240 grant to J. A. Montoya of the Pan American Sanitary Bureau for an immunological comparison of the Cox and Castaneda typhus vaccines. Throughout the 1950s and 1960s, investigators were funded for studies of rickettsial epidemiology, for research on immunology and serological tests, for the maintenance of rickettsiae in cell lines, and for the investigation of arthropod vectors.[26] This work was complemented by the intramural NIAID rickettsial diseases program, located at the RML. With its ever-growing collection of ticks from around the world, the RML became an official tick reference center for the World Health Organization.

Basic laboratory research on rickettsiae also prospered. With technical advances pioneered during the 1930s and 1940s, investigators were able to define the morphology and physiology of rickettsiae more precisely. One of the most dramatic new instruments of the early 1940s was the electron microscope, which permitted scientists to go beyond their limitations under light microscopes in understanding the structure of tiny microorganisms.[27] "It is a well recognized principle in natural science that understanding of structure is basic to analysis of function," wrote Stuart Mudd and Thomas F. Anderson of the University of Pennsylvania in a paper on the implications of electron microscopy. With the light microscope, researchers had not been able to resolve the fine structure of bacterial cells or rickettsiae, nor could they visualize at all most of the viruses. "Bacteria and rickettsias as examined by ordinary bacteriologic methods appear to be simple and structureless," Mudd observed in a companion paper, and he cautioned, "The long habit of observing such minute and apparently simple objects is often reflected in methods of dealing with bacteria in practice as though they were much simpler than they actually are."[28]

The electron microscope provided the first clues to the complex structure of rickettsiae, which generally had been grouped with the viruses because of their common requirement of intracellular existence. In 1943, Harry Plotz and his colleagues published the first electron micrographs of rickettsiae in the *Journal of Experimental Medicine*. Comparing the organisms of epidemic and murine typhus, Rocky Mountain spotted fever, and Q fever, they found striking similarity in the morphological structure of the four types of organisms. The new instrument clearly showed that rickettsiae, like bacteria, had a limiting cell wall distinct from the inner protoplasm.[29]

Furthermore, the electron microscope not only revealed the larger rickettsial forms previously studied with the light microscope but also rendered visible "smaller coccoidal forms of rickettsiae" identified by their limiting membrane and internal structure. These small oval forms were of considerable interest, Plotz and his associates stated, because they could not be differentiated with certainty from tissue particles by ordinary microscopy. "The occurrence of such organisms may throw light on the concept of 'invisible forms' of rickettsiae which has been brought forward to explain certain experiments in which rickettsiae have not been demonstrated in material of known infectivity." The detection of rickettsiae invisible under ordinary methods apparently elucidated one of the mysteries that had hindered acceptance of the organisms as the etiological agents of the typhus-like diseases. Both Roscoe R. Spencer and Ralph R. Parker must have welcomed the vindication of their findings. In the margin of one copy of their initial paper reporting the existence of apparently invisible forms of rickettsiae, one anonymous skeptic had written, "Can't see it, can't measure it—it doesn't exist."[30]

Stuart Mudd's prophecy that knowledge about the structure of organisms would enhance understanding of their function was soon realized in the case of the rickettsiae. "Since electron microscopy shows that the cell walls of bacteria and rickettsias form a relatively small fraction of the mass of the cells and since the inner protoplasm may be toxic, these facts have practical implications," he observed. "It is perhaps not too rash to predict that purified surface antigens will increasingly come into use as diagnostic reagents and even as vaccines for active immunization."[31] Because there was little impetus to produce improved rickettsial vaccines during the 1950s and 1960s, however, the use of purified surface antigens—the proteins on the outer cell membrane—as laboratory reagents was the most immediate outcome of the new knowledge.

One fruitful line of research, for example, was the more specific characterization of rickettsiae. Since 1916 the Weil-Felix test had provided a means for crude distinctions among members of the typhus-like disease group, after which cross-protection tests in guinea pigs were employed for more precise differentiation. In the 1930s boutonneuse fever had been distinguished from Rocky Mountain spotted fever in this way. More sensitive techniques such as the complement fixation test, which had been made possible by purified surface antigens, soon thereafter revealed that a close immunological relationship existed among the rickettsial diseases.[32]

Information gleaned in such studies eventually generated a new classification system that replaced the earlier schemes based on place names, geography, or vectors. Regarding the awkwardness of these systems, two South African investigators, Adrianus Pijper and C. G. Crocker had observed in 1938: "A wit once divided botanical scientists into two classes, the lumpers and the splitters. In 1920 the number of Rickettsioses for which a separate entity was claimed was three or four, and in 1936 the number had risen to well over twenty. Has there been too much splitting, and is lumping indicated?"[33]

Complement fixation studies permitted rickettsial diseases to be lumped into discrete groups displaying similar antigenic properties: the typhus group, the tsutsugamushi group, and the spotted fever group. The organisms that caused Q fever and trench fever proved so antigenically different that each was classified in a wholly separate genus. Within the rickettsial genus, the spotted fever group was distinguished by a soluble antigen that was group specific and fixed complement in the presence of antibodies induced by any other member of the group. On this basis the group included all the tick-borne rickettsial diseases but also rickettsialpox, which had a mite as its vector. Once the soluble antigen had been removed from a specific culture of rickettsia by repeated washings, the species-specific antigens could be detected.[34]

This technique also demonstrated that several rickettsiae isolated from ticks but apparently nonpathogenic for humans belonged in the spotted fever group. The earliest of these "organisms in search of a disease," as they were sometimes called, was named *Maculatum agent* in 1939 by Ralph R. Parker, when he and his colleagues first isolated it in *Amblyomma maculatum* ticks.[35] In 1965 this organism was renamed *Rickettsia parkeri* in honor of Parker.[36] Two other nonpathogenic rickettsiae were identified as members of the spotted fever group: *Rickettsia montana* and the Western Montana *U* strain of *Rickettsia rickettsii*.[37]

Comparative studies between *Rickettsia rickettsii* and other pathogenic spotted fever group rickettsiae around the world revealed surprising relationships. The only one that closely resembled *Rickettsia rickettsii* was *Rickettsia sibirica*, the agent of North Asian tick typhus, a disease first described in the 1930s and found throughout Siberia in the Soviet Union, in some localities of China, and in the Mongolian Peoples Republic.[38] Another member of the spotted fever group, *Rickettsia australis*, caused a disease known as Queensland tick typhus, which was first described in 1946 in North Queensland, Australia.

This organism responded immunologically like *Rickettsia akari,* the agent of rickettsialpox.[39]

In 1965, David B. Lackman, E. John Bell, Herbert G. Stoenner, and Edgar G. Pickens at the Rocky Mountain Laboratory proposed that the spotted fever group organisms be divided into four subgroups:

A—*Rickettsia rickettsii,* and *Rickettsia sibirica*
B—*Rickettsia conorii* and *Rickettsia parkeri*
C—*Rickettsia akari* and *Rickettsia australis*
D—*Rickettsia montana* and Western Montana U rickettsia[40]

More recent studies, however, based on comparative analyses of the genetic composition of rickettsial organisms, suggest that some taxonomic modifications may be necessary. *R. sibirica* may be sufficiently different from other spotted fever group organisms to occupy a separate category, and the genomes of *R. rickettsii* and *R. conorii* appear to be more closely related than previously believed.[41]

This line of research has also revealed the existence of other rickettsial organisms, whose properties have not been explored completely. In India, a number of reports between 1943 and 1981 identified variant spotted fever group rickettsiae as causes of Indian tick typhus.[42] Because of this disease's mild clinical manifestations, however, most cases go unreported, and additional research is needed for more accurate identification of the specific rickettsiae involved. In 1985 a possibly new, clearly pathogenic rickettsia of the spotted fever group was identified in Japan when it caused three cases of exanthemous fever in women from a farm area in Anan-shi. Laboratory study ruled out tsutsugamushi and confirmed instead an infection of the spotted fever group.[43] Variant spotted fever group rickettsiae have also been described in Israel, in Southeast Asia, and in Czechoslovakia.[44] They may also exist in Africa, but, as in India, because most cases go unreported, information is more difficult to gather.[45] New nonpathogenic spotted fever group rickettsiae also continue to be identified, including one in Switzerland and another in the southeast United States.[46]

By the late 1960s another body of work that utilized new instruments and techniques had resolved the ambivalent characterization of rickettsiae as organisms midway between bacteria and viruses. Within ten years after Wendell Stanley crystallized the tobacco mosaic virus in 1935, other scientists had discovered that viruses were not, as Stanley had originally believed, "autocatalytic proteins." Nucleic acids—deoxyribonucleic acid (DNA) and ribonucleic acid (RNA)—were identified as the components of cells that governed life processes, not only of viruses but of all living things. Bacteria contained DNA in their nuclei and RNA in their cytoplasm. Viruses were shown to contain either DNA or RNA but not both. Although initial research on rickettsiae had not detected RNA in these organisms, Hans Ris and John P. Fox at the Rockefeller Institute demonstrated in 1949 that washing procedures used to purify rickettsiae in the early studies had destroyed or greatly reduced the RNA in rickettsial cells. Including electron micrographs showing distinct nuclear structures in rickettsiae, they reported that both DNA and RNA were indeed present in these organisms.[47]

Further buttressing this position was a 1949 study by Marianna R. Bovarnick and her mentor John C. Snyder at Harvard University that demonstrated independent metabolic activity in rickettsiae—a characteristic not shared by viruses. Using the Warburg respirometer, a device developed in the 1920s by Nobel prize winner Otto Warburg for measuring metabolic activity, Bovarnick and Snyder established that purified suspensions of epidemic and murine typhus rickettsiae exhibited a distinctive respiratory activity, glutamate oxidation. Their work provided the impetus to other workers, who further clarified the process of rickettsial metabolism and verified that rickettsiae, unlike viruses, were also able to perform some reactions necessary for their own proliferation.[48]

Improved tissue culture methods in the 1950s also enhanced studies on the morphology and physiology of rickettsiae under controlled conditions. The mechanism by which rickettsiae invaded cells was studied by Zanvil A. Cohn and his colleagues at Walter Reed Army Institute of Research. They concluded that rickettsiae attacked only living cells and described conditions necessary for entry to occur. Building on Cohn's work, Herbert H. Winkler and Elizabeth T. Miller of the University of South Alabama College of Medicine later observed that an organism attaches itself to a host cell membrane and "tickles" the cell to induce phagocytosis, the process of being taken into a cell. Once inside the host cell, rickettsiae grow and multiply with little detectable damage to the parasitized cell until it finally ruptures.[49]

The Walter Reed rickettsial team showed that single cells of *Rickettsia rickettsii* divided by transverse binary fission, a bacterial but not viral phenomenon. In the course of their work, they had also noted that the spotted fever organism sometimes emerged from infected cells "by way of long, filamentous microfibrillar structures protruding from the edge or surface of the cell." Although the number of rickettsiae lost from cells via microfibrils was small, they believed that this mechanism deserved "careful consideration" since it might "play an important role in dissemination of pathogens, particularly between adjacent cells."[50]

By 1969 the body of knowledge so carefully built in these studies led to the overwhelming conclusion that rickettsiae were not akin to viruses but were instead "highly fastidious bacteria," as Richard A. Ormsbee, a specialist in Q fever rickettsiae at the Rocky Mountain Laboratory, described them in a review paper. "The importance of this conceptual advance" could not be "stressed too strongly," Charles L. Wisseman, Jr., of the University of Maryland School of Medicine observed some years later, because "it brought to bear on rickettsiology the enormous conceptual framework of the science of bacteriology." During the 1970s and 1980s, moreover, rapid strides in technology unshackled the study of rickettsiae in the laboratory. Improved purification methods, simple methods for counting the organisms, and better methods for cloning rickettsiae were among the many new techniques available.[51]

Unfortunately, even as these new techniques were being developed, it appeared that research interest in rickettsiae and rickettsial diseases would not be sustained in the United States. Throughout the 1950s and 1960s the numbers of rickettsial investigators had declined steadily.[52] By 1967 they had become so scarce in the United States that, one scientist observed, they had "trouble having a meeting other than dinner together."[53] In 1971, moreover, the number of NIH grants for rickettsial disease research reached a nadir of between two and five, depending on how one counted related subjects.[54] This problem often became the focus of discussions at meetings of the Commission on Rickettsial Diseases, and two participants in these deliberations summarized the situation in published articles. Theodore E. Woodward of the University of Maryland School of Medicine lamented the lack of young people attracted to the field, observing that those researchers who still thought about rickettsiae almost every day had "a generous display of gray hair." Richard A. Ormsbee cited figures showing that when grouped by age, the largest group of rickettsial researchers averaged 55 years old; the next largest group, 65 years of age. "Only four scientists under 40 years of age were in career jobs as rickettsiologists in 1971."[55]

The preservation of rickettsiology as a separate field of inquiry was further jeopardized when the military services began reevaluating their programs in this area. In 1973 the Armed Forces Epidemiological Board disbanded all its commissions, including the Commission on Rickettsial Diseases. Because this organization had served as the major national forum for rickettsiologists, its demise came as a blow to many in the field. The U.S. Army, moreover, shifted its research priorities away from rickettsial diseases in general to focus on developing a vaccine against scrub typhus, because of that disease's potential military importance. Likewise, U.S. Navy research emphasis was directed toward preparing new vaccines against murine and epidemic typhus. This left the National Institute of Allergy and Infectious Diseases in the "awkward spot," as its deputy director, John R. Seal, later noted, "of being the principal Government supporter of rickettsial research but not having been given any extra funds to meet this responsibility."[56]

At NIAID, furthermore, the historic debate over the inclusion of medical entomology in the research program had been revived in the late 1960s when U.S. involvement in the Vietnam War led to tighter budgets for medical research. Institute administrators and the Board of Scientific Counselors, an advisory group of distinguished nongovernmental scientists, intensively examined existing programs as they struggled with questions of research priorities in a period of restricted growth. The merit of traditional epidemiological and microbiological studies of vector-borne diseases also came under scrutiny during this period. Because intramural rickettsial and entomological research sponsored by NIAID was located at the Rocky Mountain Laboratory, the future of this facility became the focus of debate.

Those who believed that research in medical entomology should be abandoned argued that it was more properly supported by the military or by the National Science Foundation. In addition, they believed that if the institute sought to maintain leadership in medical research, it should support promising studies in immunology and in molecular biology more substantially than traditional microbiological and epidemiological research. Supporters of the opposing position argued that medical entomologists afforded expertise nowhere else available to physicians around the world who needed aid in identifying vectors of unknown diseases. Time and again, the U.S. experience with scrub typhus during World War II was cited as an example of the kind of unknown arthropod-borne diseases that the country might encounter if drawn into a war in tropical regions.[57]

By the late 1970s tight budgets and staff reductions impelled NIAID administrators to revise institute priorities for the intramural program. At the end of the decade, medical entomology was discontinued at the Rocky Mountain Laboratory and the historic tick collection shipped to the Smithsonian Institution. The RML was reorganized into three laboratories, only one of which continued the traditional research program, and the facility was renamed the Rocky Mountain Labo-

ratories. Under the auspices of the NIAID extramural program, however, a variety of grants and contracts for rickettsial disease research
continued to be funded, and, indeed, virtually all university research
on rickettsiae received NIAID support.[58]

In addition to these changes, in the early 1970s commercial biologics
houses in the United States had discontinued production of specific
rickettsial antigens for diagnostic tests. Although the Centers for Disease Control continued to supply these antigens to state health laboratories and to other designated diagnostic centers, the decline in
demand for such services was reflected in the relatively few institutions
equipped to make the tests. Reliance on the broad-spectrum antibiotics
had virtually halted efforts to improve laboratory tests. Routine laboratory diagnosis, Richard A. Ormsbee noted, was "no better in 1972
than it was at the close of World War II in 1945." He warned that
"biomedical competency in rickettsial diseases" in the United States
would be "largely lost within the next 10 years if these trends continue." Ormsbee also described a parallel situation in Western Europe.
"Laboratories in Brussels, Paris, Rome, London, and Zurich, which
once maintained vigorous programs of rickettsial research stimulated
by the occurrence during World War II of Balkan grippe (Q fever) in
Yugoslavia and Greece and by epidemic typhus in Egypt and Italy,
now are mainly devoted to other subjects." Conversely, the well-staffed
laboratories of "Bratislava, Bucharest, and Moscow" continued to
support research on rickettsial diseases vigorously.[59]

Given the steady erosion in the numbers of young investigators and
a persistent sense that rickettsial diseases posed little threat to the
United States, it is doubtful whether any individual could have swayed
institutional priorities on behalf of rickettsiology by virtue of rhetoric
alone. What did help to reinvigorate the state of rickettsial research
in the United States was an unexplained natural phenomenon: in the
1970s the incidence of Rocky Mountain spotted fever in the United
States began to rise inexorably.

In 1959, Joseph E. Smadel had warned that changing population
patterns, especially the creation of suburban housing developments
near large east coast cities, might generate a rise in the incidence of
spotted fever. Noting that this region was an endemic area of the
disease, Smadel cautioned prospective suburbanites not to forget the
existence of "islands of infection" of *Rickettsia rickettsii*, which or-
dinarily were maintained in "silence" between ticks and the small
animals on which they fed. "Maryland provides an example in point
through its projected urbanization of the countryside around Baltimore
and Washington." Even before the upturn in cases was documented,

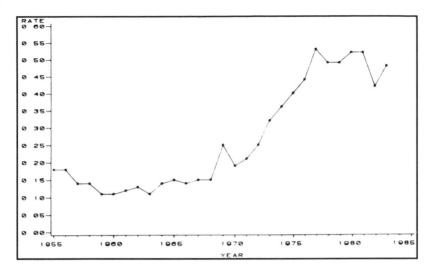

Reported cases of Rocky Mountain spotted fever per 100,000 population, by year, in the United States, 1955–83. This graph reveals the surprising increase in Rocky Mountain spotted fever that was first observed in 1969. (Reproduced from D. B. Fishbein, J. E. Kaplan, K. W. Bernard, and W. G. Winkler, "Surveillance of Rocky Mountain Spotted Fever, United States, 1981–1983," *Morbidity and Mortality Weekly Report, CDC Surveillance Summaries* 33 [1984]: 15SS–18SS.)

Smadel's prediction appeared prescient to many who monitored the incidence of the disease. In 1965 a group of researchers concluded that the true incidence of Rocky Mountain spotted fever was actually "much greater than the number of reported cases." By 1970 the numbers were clearer. Michael A. W. Hattwick at the Centers for Disease Control noted that reported cases in the United States had increased from 200–300 per year during the 1950s to 498 in 1969. The case fatality ratio also showed "a small but definite rise" since 1960. Most of these cases were identified in the southeast, while the number of cases in the west remained low. By 1977, 1,115 cases were reported in the United States, 42 of which were fatal. Among the states most afflicted, North Carolina, Virginia, Tennessee, Maryland, and Oklahoma headed the list.[60]

In 1970 the rise in spotted fever cases stimulated the Centers for Disease Control to initiate a surveillance program that reexamined the epidemiology and clinical features of spotted fever. The first five years' data gathered from this study confirmed that, although a problem existed, it had not yet reached the proportions of the pre-antibiotic era. In the southeast the incidence of spotted fever reached 12 per million in 1974, one-sixth of the 76 per million recorded in the Rocky Mountain states in 1935. The death-to-case ratio, moreover, remained between 5 and 10 percent, less than half the national average before antibiotics were introduced. Epidemiologists at the Centers for Disease Control reported that, since 1960, spotted fever cases had been reported from every state except Alaska, Hawaii, Wisconsin, Maine, and Vermont. Suggesting that a change in population patterns might account for the increase, they also speculated that physicians might be recognizing the disease more frequently than in the past, and they postulated that a cyclic change in the tick vector or the microorganism itself could be involved.[61]

Coming after a period of complacency about infectious diseases, the increasing incidence of spotted fever seemed unusual to many epidemiologists. Some attributed it to a gradual invasion of the eastern United States by *Rickettsia rickettsii* from the Rocky Mountain regions. Others postulated that the western *R. rickettsii* had gradually, and for unknown reasons, become avirulent for humans. In 1977, Willy Burgdorfer at the Rocky Mountain Laboratory dismissed these theories as having no scientific merit. Historically, he pointed out, spotted fever in the Rocky Mountain regions was "an occupational disease among people settling in enzootic areas." Once the land was cleared and cultivated, tick infestation decreased, and with it, the incidence of spotted fever. In uncultivated western territories that remained heavily populated with tick-infested rodents, Burgdorfer observed, people continued to contract the disease when, during a short pleasure or business outing, they became "part of the ecologic cycle of *R. rickettsii*." In contrast, spotted fever in the east had traditionally been "characterized by high incidence among children and women—a phenomenon related to infestations of household pets, particularly dogs, with the vector tick." The shift of eastern populations into natural foci of spotted fever and the creation of wooded recreational areas out of previously cultivated land, Burgdorfer concluded, adequately explained the increasing incidence of the disease in the eastern United States.[62]

Ecological factors might account for the increase in incidence of spotted fever, but as new studies charted the epidemiology of the disease, a few surprises emerged. Overall figures were consistent with earlier patterns. Nearly two-thirds of the cases occurred in children under fifteen years old, and 61 percent of the patients were male. Only 52 percent of fatal cases were in young people, but 74 percent were in male patients. The lower death-to-case ratio in female patients, especially in those aged fifteen through forty-four, was not explained by differing rates of rash or tick bite—an unexpected finding. It suggested that "a degree of protection against fatal Rocky Mountain spotted fever" might be afforded women "during their reproductive years."[63] Most peculiar was the relatively high 13.9 percent mortality among black male victims. It was more than double the 5.8 percent recorded for white males. This racial difference, CDC epidemiologists found, was not a function of age. They believed that this "very high" death-to-case ratio in black males, especially in those younger than ten, could be explained in part by the difficulty of observing a rash in dark-skinned patients. Another factor, they suggested, might be the more limited access to medical care available to poorer blacks in the United States.[64] This analysis was consonant with the social concerns of the early 1970s, but, as we shall see in chapter 12, a more basic physiological process was involved.

In 1981 the number of cases of Rocky Mountain spotted fever in the United States peaked at 1,192, a national incidence of 51 cases per million people. Beginning in that year, Oklahoma became the state having the highest incidence of cases in relation to its population, 410 per million, and its neighbors Texas and Arkansas also reported an increased incidence of cases. Despite the high incidence, Oklahoma recorded only 397 cases between 1981 and 1983, while heavily populated North Carolina, the state with the greatest number of cases, reported 736 during this period. South Carolina with 288 cases and Virginia with 238 cases were the third and fourth most infected states in the early 1980s. The entire "cycle" of increased cases appeared to be limited to the United States, for no reports were received of this phenomenon in other western hemisphere countries.[65]

Across the Atlantic Ocean, however, a similar increase in tick-borne rickettsioses was also observed and first reported in 1981 by Vittorio Scaffidi, an Italian rickettsial researcher located in Palermo, Sicily. Between World War II and the mid 1970s, he noted, cases of rickettsioses of all kinds had been reduced to "mere sporadic episodes." Since 1975, however, several regions of Italy, including Lazio, Liguria, Sicily, and Sardinia, had registered "an extraordinary epidemiological event." Boutonneuse fever, the spotted fever group disease prevalent throughout the Mediterranean basin, had increased from about 30 cases per year to 864 cases in 1979. Scaffidi believed, moreover, that the actual number of cases was underreported in the region. He speculated that ecological changes involving the tick vectors of boutonneuse fever "must be presumed."[66]

Although Scaffidi noted that this phenomenon had not been reported elsewhere in the Mediterranean basin, investigators in other Mediterranean countries soon published additional accounts of the unusual increase. From Israel came reports that from six cases documented in 1973, the numbers had swelled to sixty-three by 1978.[67] In July 1982, Ferran Segura and Bernat Font wrote to the editor of *Lancet* to report an increase in Spain of the disease, which was known there as Mediterranean spotted fever. A total of seventeen cases had met their clinical and serological criteria; case distribution had increased from two in 1978 to six in 1981. The increase had been confirmed by other hospitals in the same area, and most cases came from urban areas. Perhaps, they speculated, this reflected a known increase in the number of pet animals among city dwellers. "Clearly the resurgence in Mediterranean Spotted Fever seen in Italy is also happening in Spain," they wrote, and they suggested that indeed it was "a pattern common to the whole geographical area in which this disease is endemic."[68]

This unusual increase in tick-borne rickettsial disease stimulated renewed research in the Mediterranean countries and led as well to fruitful international collaborations.[69] The Sicilian group, for example, led by Scaffidi's colleagues Serafino Mansueto and Giuseppe Tringali, began studying boutonneuse fever's epidemiology in western Sicily and the persistence of antibodies to *R. conorii* in humans and in dogs. In the 1930s dogs had been shown susceptible to infection with tick-borne rickettsial diseases. They also, of course, could bring infected ticks into the homes of their human owners.[70] All of this research revealed that although the basic pathological physiology of the tick-borne rickettsial diseases had been described, much remained unknown in the last decades of the twentieth century about their natural histories.

Diagnosis of Rocky Mountain spotted fever also continued to be difficult in atypical cases, a situation underscored in a 1977 tragedy at the Centers for Disease Control in Atlanta, Georgia. In mid February Robert Dubington, a building custodian, and George Flowers, a warehouseman, both of whom worked in the same building at the CDC, were hospitalized with symptoms of high fever, nausea, diarrhea, and vomiting. Mental confusion and convulsions followed, but no rash was observed. Flowers died on 27 February, and Dubington died two days later, on 1 March. Initially, Legionnaires' disease, the mysterious bacterial malady that had struck unexpectedly in 1976 and was under investigation at the CDC, was suspected in these deaths. Post-mortem studies, however, revealed that both men had died from Rocky Mountain spotted fever. It remained unclear how they contracted the disease, for neither had routine access to laboratory areas.[71]

Plainly this disease, thought "conquered" in 1948, retained the ability to wreak misery and death. The resurgence of Rocky Mountain spotted fever in the United States thus accomplished what rickettsial investigators had been unable to achieve by exhorting their colleagues. A new generation of investigators, many of whom were too young to recall the pre-antibiotic era, were challenged to apply their training in immunology, in molecular biology, and in other new fields to the problem of Rocky Mountain spotted fever. By 1980 a new professional organization, the American Society of Rickettsiology and Rickettsial Diseases, had been formed.[72] Junior and senior rickettsiologists collaborated in reexamining diagnostic tests, vaccines, clinical knowledge, and therapy. In this task, they could draw on the body of basic research accumulated since World War II that provided information about rickettsial organisms essential to formulating new strategies against the disease.

Chapter Twelve

Mysteries Explained, Mysteries Remaining

All interest in disease and death is only another expression of interest in life.

Thomas Mann, *The Magic Mountain*

"The easiest way to lose ground in the fight against infectious diseases," wrote Harry Dowling in 1977, "is to assume that they have been conquered and nothing more needs to be done."[1] The dangers of such neglect became obvious in relation to Rocky Mountain spotted fever during its surprising upsurge in the 1970s. Although a number of advances in understanding the basic biology of rickettsiae had been made since World War II, virtually no new methods of diagnosis, prevention, or therapy had been developed. This situation suggests that, in the United States, active programs of research on any disease are difficult to sustain without the stimulus of an imminent disease threat. In examining the recent history of spotted fever, however, it is also clear that rapid advancement in applied fields since 1970 largely depended upon the advances in basic research fields made during spotted fever's quiescent decades between 1950 and 1970. Efforts to control and combat this disease of nature are still under way, and any definitive evaluation of these endeavors will require a longer historical perspective. Several long standing mysteries raised by spotted fever have been solved, however, and those that remain suggest directions for future inquiry.

When spotted fever began to increase during the 1970s, renewed clinical studies of the disease confirmed older assessments of the grave danger posed by infections with *Rickettsia rickettsii*. Circulatory collapse, kidney failure, and neurological damage were all potential threats. Since 1919, when S. Burt Wolbach published his major review of the disease, spotted fever had been understood as an affliction of the circulatory system. From the 1940s through the 1960s, occasional papers had discussed specific cardiac complications of spotted fever and their treatment. At the end of the 1970s, however, new research indicated that the disease did not cause significant loss of heart function. The greater danger appeared to be the threat to the circulatory tree, as had been suggested in World War II.[2]

In contrast to an early appreciation of spotted fever's effect on the circulatory system, it was not until the 1950s that its full potential impact on the brain was appreciated. In 1947 a physician in Ann Arbor, Michigan, had queried the editor of the *Journal of the American Medical Association* about long-term neurological effects from spotted fever. The *Journal's* editor had restated the position taken at that time by most textbook authors. Headache, hearing loss, lethargy or restlessness, mental confusion, and sometimes delirium characterized the disease during the acute course, but these afflictions were expected to last only a few weeks.[3] Later studies disputed this conclusion, noting that infection with *Rickettsia rickettsii* could destroy the myelin sheath around nerves and cause the formation of granulomatous tissue in the brain.[4] "Pathologic examination reveals greater damage to the brain in spotted fever than in any other rickettsial disease," concluded one group of investigators in 1952.[5]

In its most severe form, spotted fever may mimic other diseases, especially acute appendicitis. The pathological physiology of these abdominal symptoms is not yet understood, but, as the authors of another recent paper noted, they "underscore the protean manifestations" of spotted fever.[6] The mechanism by which the organism damages human cells is also just beginning to be understood. "Evidence is accumulating," wrote David H. Walker of the University of North Carolina School of Medicine at Chapel Hill in 1982, "that injury occurs to the cell membrane on penetration into and release from the host cell by rickettsiae."[7]

During the 1970s, Walker and his colleagues initiated a variety of studies on Rocky Mountain spotted fever because of their location in North Carolina, an endemic spotted fever area reporting a large number of cases each year. During and after World War II, the state's high incidence had spurred George T. Harrell, Jerry K. Aikawa, and their colleagues at the Bowman Gray School of Medicine of Wake Forest University in Winston-Salem to conduct studies on clinical problems associated with the disease, especially capillary permeability and fluid loss. A clinical review paper written by Harrell in 1949 stood for decades as definitive in clinical practice, and in 1966, Aikawa published a monograph on spotted fever that summarized much of this work.[8]

Walker's group continued this North Carolina tradition, focusing especially on clinical and epidemiological studies.

One problem they solved, for example, was the mystery of high spotted fever mortality in black males, a phenomenon noted in 1976 by epidemiologists at the Centers for Disease Control. Two tentative explanations had been offered at that time: the difficulty of identifying a typical spotted fever rash on dark skin and diminished access to medical care, a problem common to lower socioeconomic groups. Neither rationale proved satisfactory, because black females, who shared both criteria, exhibited a mortality rate no higher than did white females. The figures instead suggested, Walker and his colleagues believed, the existence of some sex-linked genetic condition that occurred primarily among blacks and rendered males more vulnerable. It was known that about 12 percent of American black males suffered from a glucose-6-phosphate dehydrogenase (G6PD) deficiency, a genetic-linked metabolic disorder much less common in whites and in black females. The North Carolina group therefore studied the frequency of G6PD deficiency among black males who died from spotted fever and, indeed, found that the incidence was much higher than expected. "Ultimately," they concluded, "G6PD-deficient persons may represent a target population for an effective vaccine against Rocky Mountain spotted fever."[9]

In addition to black males with a G6PD deficiency, several other groups of people at high risk were identified as potential candidates for vaccination against spotted fever. One large cluster was comprised of children and adults living in highly infected districts, especially those with existing medical problems that might become life-threatening under the strain of a severe infection. Army recruits training in "tick belt" states made up another population at risk.[10] Laboratory personnel, although a relatively small group, were often exposed to highly virulent strains of spotted fever, as the fatal cases sustained by many early laboratory martyrs attested (see Table 4). The two 1977 deaths at the Centers for Disease Control, moreover, prompted a letter to the editor of the *New England Journal of Medicine* in support of vaccine development for the protection of laboratory workers. Even before this tragedy, other concerned scientists had published a number of studies on the risks of laboratory infection.[11]

When the 1970s increase in spotted fever cases renewed interest in protective vaccination, however, the only vaccine available was the Cox yolk sac product, which had been produced virtually unchanged by Lederle Laboratories since the 1940s. The first clear indication that the state of spotted fever prophylaxis was unacceptable came in 1973,

TABLE 4. *Deaths from Laboratory-Acquired Spotted Fever Infections*

Year	Name	Position
1912	Thomas B. McClintic	Passed Assistant Surgeon, U.S. Public Health Service
1918	Stephen Molinscek	Laboratory assistant to Hideyo Noguchi, Rockefeller Institute for Medical Research
1919	Arthur H. McCray	Bacteriologist, Montana State Board of Health
1922	William E. Gettinger	Student assistant, U.S. Public Health Service
1924	George Henry Cowan	Field assistant, Montana State Board of Entomology and U.S. Public Health Service
1928	Albert LeRoy Kerlee	Student assistant, U.S. Public Health Service
1927	Elisabeth Brandt	Laboratory technician for Max Kuczynski, Berlin
1931	Kokyo Sugata	Assistant to Norio Ogata, Chiba Medical College, Japan
1932	Masajiro Nishibe	Professor, Niigata Medical College, Japan
1935	Jose Lemos Monteiro	Brazilian investigator, Butantan Institute, São Paulo, Brazil
1935	Edison de Andrade Dias	Monteiro's assistant
1942	Héctor Calderón Cuervo	Investigator in Bogota, Colombia
1977	Robert Dubington	Building custodian, U.S. Centers for Disease Control
1977	George Flowers	Warehouseman, U.S. Centers for Disease Control

when a seven-member team of researchers led by Herbert L. DuPont at the University of Maryland School of Medicine in Baltimore tested stored samples of the Spencer-Parker tick tissue vaccine and commercially produced Cox yolk sac vaccine. Groups of volunteers from the Maryland House of Correction in Jessup, Maryland, who had been informed of the risks involved and advised that they could withdraw from the study at any time, were inoculated with one of the vaccines or left unvaccinated as controls. Subsequently each was injected with a large dose of virulent *R. rickettsii.* All developed cases of Rocky

Mountain spotted fever and were treated. The results of this test were unequivocal: neither type of spotted fever vaccine prevented the disease.[12]

This finding would not have been surprising to the original producers of those vaccines, whose own studies revealed that they lessened the severity of infection rather than preventing it. In the 1920s and 1930s when the Spencer-Parker and Cox vaccines were developed, human trials with virulent organisms were unthinkable, because no therapy existed that could cure a severe case of the disease. Instead, the vaccines had been tested in experimental animals for efficacy, purity, and potency.[13] After the development of broad-spectrum antibiotics, the need for any vaccine seemed minimal, and no work had been done to improve the existing product.

About the time the DuPont study was published, Richard H. Kenyon, William M. Acree, George G. Wright, and Fred W. Melchoir, Jr., members of the U.S. Army Medical Research Institute of Infectious Diseases at Fort Detrick in Frederick, Maryland, reported that they had prepared a new candidate vaccine against Rocky Mountain spotted fever. Using *R. rickettsii* propagated in tissue cultures of chick embryo cells rather than in the chick embryos themselves, the group prepared two vaccines for testing in guinea pigs. The first was irradiated to kill the rickettsiae, a procedure based on recent studies with tularemia and psittacosis organisms indicating that vaccines killed by ionizing radiation retained greater antigenicity than those killed by heat or chemicals. The second vaccine was treated with formaldehyde to kill rickettsiae. Initial tests on guinea pigs demonstrated that both cell culture vaccines were more than nine hundred times as active as the old yolk sac vaccine. Surprisingly, the vaccine prepared with formaldehyde proved superior to the irradiated vaccine in protecting guinea pigs from direct challenge with *R. rickettsii*. Over the next few years, the army group worked to improve the formaldehyde cell culture vaccine by various techniques and to conduct initial tests of its efficacy in animals and safety for humans.[14]

In October 1976, however, Congress withdrew all funds for the army's spotted fever vaccine program, arguing that it duplicated research efforts at the National Institute of Allergy and Infectious Diseases. Shortly thereafter, William S. Augerson, commanding general of the U.S. Army Medical Research and Development Command, wrote to the NIAID director, Richard Krause, requesting that "NIAID assume responsibility for completion of qualifications necessary to license this RMSF vaccine for human use." After reviewing the proposed vaccine's promise, the potential population that would benefit from vaccine development, and the program's cost, Robert Edelman, chief of the Clinical Studies Branch in NIAID's Microbiology and Infectious Diseases Program, won concurrence from the director of the program, William Jordan, to recommend that the institute sponsor the work.[15]

On 30 October 1978 the NIAID Microbiology and Infectious Diseases Advisory Committee considered plans for testing the candidate vaccine. Samuel L. Katz, chairman of the Department of Pediatrics at Duke University Medical Center, urged the committee to go forward with clinical trials of the candidate army vaccine. "Because our state reports the largest number of cases each year of any throughout the nation," Katz stated, "we have come to speak of the disease as North Carolina Tick Typhus." Buttressing the case that a large potential population for the vaccine existed, Katz noted that North Carolina physicians actually treated 1,524 cases of suspected spotted fever each year, in contrast to the 200 cases they reported to the CDC.[16]

The advisory committee agreed that the program should continue, but it recommended that before any direct human trials were conducted, two other studies should be done. "A careful and intense epidemiologic study was needed to clearly determine the incidence and importance of the disease and to define populations in which the usefulness of the vaccine in preventing disease in humans might later be determined." In addition, the committee recommended that a primate model be developed in order to study "the nature of the disease, the immune response to infection and the safety, immunogenicity and efficacy of candidate vaccines."[17]

Reasons for such a cautious approach were articulated by John R. Seal, NIAID deputy director. Noting the relatively small size of the population that would seek protection from a new spotted fever vaccine, Seal noted that few commercial laboratories were likely to be interested in producing it. "Here we seem to be on a track of a limited use vaccine which, under present law, would have to be dispensed by the CDC under IND [investigational new drug] regulations." More importantly, Seal was concerned about whether the new vaccine would be any more effective than the old Cox vaccine, which lessened the severity of the disease but did not prevent it.[18]

The recommended preliminary studies were implemented, and the epidemiologic data provided somewhat surprising results. Catherine M. Wilfert at Duke University Medical Center led a team of researchers in identifying cases of spotted fever that could be serologically confirmed in two North Carolina counties. In contrast to the estimates by physicians that many more cases occurred than were reported, Wilfert and colleagues found that only one of three reported cases exhibited antibodies in the blood. Although no primate model was developed for broad studies on the nature of spotted fever infection, the candidate vaccine was tested in guinea pigs. Results indicated that it protected them only partially from infection with virulent *R. rickettsii*. As with the older vaccines, higher doses and frequent booster injections increased protection.[19]

The ambiguities in these findings raised questions about the vaccine's probable efficacy as well as the number of people who might benefit from it. Ten years of research had been invested in the product, however, and in 1983 a placebo-controlled double-blind study in humans was conducted by a group led by Mary L. Clements at the Center for Vaccine Development of the University of Maryland School of Medicine in Baltimore. Of the fifty-two volunteers vaccinated, sixteen were challenged with virulent *R. rickettsii* one month after vaccination. Six unvaccinated volunteers also received the challenge dose as controls. The results of this test were only marginally better than in the DuPont study. Twelve of the sixteen vaccinated volunteers developed typical Rocky Mountain spotted fever, as did all the controls. As with the earlier vaccines, the incubation period was longer, the duration of constitutional symptoms shorter, and the height of fever lower in the vaccinated volunteers. "The vaccine provided only partial protection against Rocky Mountain spotted fever," concluded the investigators.[20]

The failure of this new vaccine to provide complete protection against spotted fever dashed the hopes of anyone seeking vaccination against the disease. In 1980, while the army vaccine was still being developed, a U.S. Food and Drug Administration panel comprised of leading rickettsiologists, pediatricians, and virologists had evaluated the efficacy and safety of Lederle Laboratories's yolk sac vaccine. Citing the 1973 DuPont study, the members of the Food and Drug Administration panel expressed little confidence in the product's efficacy. They noted that between 1969 and 1972 there had been no complaints about its safety; however, they observed, this "probably indicated more the failure to report complaints than inherent safety." The panel awarded the vaccine "an unfavorable benefit/risk ratio," and assigned it category III-A status, which meant that it could remain commercially available pending completion of additional tests. The decision, however, was moot. On 11 June 1979, even before the panel met, Lederle Laboratories had requested that its license to produce spotted fever vaccine by the yolk sac method be revoked and had withdrawn the product from the market.[21]

It is likely that both the caution of the Food and Drug Administration panel and the decision of Lederle Laboratories were influenced by more than dispassionate scientific inquiry. By the 1970s the public had become more willing to sue commercial producers of vaccines when products failed or caused toxic side effects. Because U.S. law placed financial responsibility on vaccine producers for the statistically predictable number of injuries and deaths that occur from widespread vaccination programs, firms such as Lederle often reduced their liability by halting production of products considered risky. When the number of potential vaccine recipients was small, as in the case of Rocky Mountain spotted fever, commercial advantage was completely overshadowed by considerations of liability. Even though no suit had been brought over Lederle's spotted fever vaccine, the company's swift action reflected a larger problem that has yet to be resolved.

The groups involved in assessing the failure of the old yolk sac and new tissue culture vaccines arrived at the same conclusion about why neither provided full protection. Basing their evaluations on new discoveries in immunology made during the preceding decades, the FDA panel, the DuPont group, and the Clements group speculated that the humoral immunity stimulated by the vaccines was insufficient to provide full protection against the disease. Although additional research on the immune response in spotted fever infections must be done before conclusive proof can be presented, they suggested that recovery from a frank spotted fever infection probably produced immunity mediated by cellular rather than by humoral mechanisms, because there was no correlation between the presence of antibodies in serum and protection from the disease.[22]

Although these two types of immunity had been known since the late nineteenth century, detailed knowledge about their components, mechanisms, and interactions had only begun to be elucidated in the 1960s. The humoral immune system, named from the historic usage of the word *humors* for body fluids, was shown to function through the actions of specialized white blood cells, called B cells, which produce antibodies against foreign antigens on the surface of invading organisms. Circulated throughout the blood and other body fluids, these antibodies are most effective against bacteria, their toxins, and viruses present in body fluids. The cell-mediated immune system, comprised of other white blood cells, especially those known as T cells, works in addition to the humoral system. The T cells do not produce antibodies, but they coordinate attacks by several other types of white cells against cancer cells, transplanted tissue, and intracellular bacteria and viruses. *Rickettsia rickettsii*, of course, falls into the last category.[23]

These concepts helped to explain another longstanding mystery of spotted fever and possibly pointed the way toward a more successful vaccine. Howard Taylor Ricketts had first attempted to treat spotted fever victims with immune serum taken from people or animals that had recovered from a spotted fever infection. All such immune sera failed to effect the dramatic cures possible when diphtheria patients were treated similarly. Diphtheria, of course, is caused by the action of a toxin, which is rapidly rendered harmless by the antibodies present in immune sera. Spotted fever rickettsiae, in contrast, inhabit the cells of the host, where they are protected from antibody attack.

Because both the Spencer-Parker and the Cox spotted fever vaccines had utilized killed rickettsiae, furthermore, they may not have stimulated cell-mediated immunity as did recovery from an active case of the disease. In contrast, a number of vaccines against viral diseases such as rabies, yellow fever, and polio were prepared from attenuated—that is, weakened but not killed—strains of virus. Such products mimicked active infection and produced cell-mediated immunity without the risk of severe disease. Howard Taylor Ricketts had attempted without luck to attenuate the spotted fever organism early in the century, and after the development of the Spencer-Parker vaccine, further efforts to attenuate the organism had been abandoned.

Between 1974 and the mid 1980s, several groups of investigators launched projects aimed at designing a vaccine to produce the complete protection stimulated only by frank infection with the disease or by a successful attenuated vaccine.[24] Using a variety of techniques developed by molecular biologists, they first focused on identifying individual surface proteins of *Rickettsia rickettsii* that might serve as antigens in an improved vaccine. In reviewing this work, Hui Min Feng, Celia Kirkman, and David H. Walker at the University of North Carolina School of Medicine observed that one series of these studies produced a "reasonable catalogue" of approximately thirty-five rickettsial proteins. Another group of studies utilized monoclonal antibodies and the methods of immunoblotting and radioimmunoprecipitation to analyze these proteins as antigens.[25]

Gregory A. McDonald, Robert L. Anacker, and Kareen Garjian at the Rocky Mountain Laboratories cloned the gene for one of these antigens in *Escherichia coli* bacteria and tested the effectiveness of the recombinant-DNA product as a vaccine against Rocky Mountain spotted fever. They reported that the material protected mice from a lethal dose of virulent *R. rickettsii*. Although this candidate vaccine faces years of refinement and testing, it may prove to be the hoped-for effective and safe preventative against spotted fever.[26]

Since no vaccine is available at present, and since relatively few people at occasional risk of contracting spotted fever would be vaccinated in any case, the key to effective therapy is rapid diagnosis. The increase in spotted fever incidence during the 1970s also stimulated a renewed interest in diagnostic tests, which, like the vaccine, had not been significantly improved since World War II. As late as 1976, for example, Charles C. Shepard and his associates at the Centers for Disease Control stated flatly, "No laboratory diagnostic procedure is now available that will provide a specific laboratory diagnosis in time to help the physician in his decision about therapy" in suspected spotted fever cases.[27]

In 1978 another CDC study—this one on the characteristics most frequently associated with fatal Rocky Mountain spotted fever—reiterated the need for more accurate diagnostic tests. Delay in seeking treatment proved not to be an important factor associated with dying from spotted fever. The high fever and debility accompanying the disease sent most patients to a physician at about the same time. The average amount of time that elapsed between the onset of illness and the initiation of appropriate therapy, however, was more than two days longer for fatal than for nonfatal cases. When patients who later died first visited a physician, the study noted, they rarely displayed the classic diagnostic triad of fever, rash, and history of tick bite. Instead, they presented nonspecific symptoms, such as fever, headache, and malaise, which were characteristic of several diseases. Gastrointestinal complaints, including nausea, vomiting, abdominal pain, and diarrhea, were also prominent symptoms in approximately one-third of the fatal cases and were present in only 4 percent of those who recovered. Because of these puzzling initial symptoms, the critical history of whether the patient had been bitten by a tick was obtained three days later among fatal cases than it was from those who recovered. In short, those patients who were treated with an antirickettsial broad-spectrum antibiotic within the first five days of illness usually recovered, while all but two of the fatal cases studied were not treated before the sixth day of illness. "The major problem in diagnosis appears to be the presence of nonspecific or misleading symptoms occurring before onset of rash," the authors concluded.[28]

What was clearly needed was a laboratory test that, no matter what symptoms were present, could rapidly demonstrate whether the patient was infected with *R. rickettsii*.[29] In their search for such a test, investigators in the 1970s first reviewed the research of previous decades, hoping to find leads to exploit. In the early 1950s, R. Shin-man Chang, Edward S. Murray, and John C. Snyder at the Harvard University School of Public Health had discovered that sera from spotted fever patients as early as six days after the onset of illness agglutinated human group O erythrocytes, or red blood cells, after the erythrocytes were sensitized with substances extracted by ether from suspensions of infected yolk sac membranes. This diagnostic test, called the indirect hemagglutination (IHA) test, proved more sensitive and technically simpler than the complement fixation test. Very little active material was required—enough could be prepared from one infected yolk sac to test at least five hundred sera. This procedure, however, had never been developed commercially. It had not been found superior to the complement fixation test, and because of the generally low level of interest in spotted fever during the 1950s, the older technique had remained the standard laboratory procedure.[30]

Nearly two decades later, with spotted fever on the rise, several investigators sought to improve the IHA test. One group introduced the use of stabilized sheep erythrocytes so that the test could be performed under field conditions. Another team adapted the test to microtiter plates and employed the technique known as sucrose density gradient centrifugation to purify antigen from *R. rickettsii*. With these changes, the IHA test provided positive results in a greater percentage of cases than did the complement fixation test.[31] The microagglutination test, developed in 1969, and the latex agglutination test, developed in 1980, provided two additional variations on this technique. The microagglutination test is sensitive, but because it requires large amounts of rickettsial antigen, it has remained primarily a research tool. The latex agglutination test, which is simple, quick, and requires no elaborate instrumentation, is now commercially available.[32]

Another promising approach to diagnosis took advantage of the ability to "label" antibodies with fluorescent or radioactive material or with enzymes. To test for the presence of *R. rickettsii*, antibodies labeled with fluorescent dye are added to a patient's serum on a glass slide and allowed to react. After being washed to remove any unattached antibodies, the slide is examined under an ultraviolet light, which renders visible any labeled antibodies attached to the rickettsiae. If no rickettsiae are present, all the labeled antibodies are washed away, and no fluorescence is seen. Before this technique was adapted for diagnosis of spotted fever, it had been widely used in research laboratories. As early as 1950, A. H. Coons and his colleagues used a fluorescence technique to describe rickettsiae in the human body louse. In 1960 and 1961, Willy Burgdorfer and David B. Lackman adapted the technique to identify *Rickettsia rickettsii* in tissues of infected ticks and guinea pigs.[33] In the mid 1970s, antibody labeling was employed for laboratory diagnosis of spotted fever. Variations of the technique have produced direct and indirect immunofluorescence tests, a microimmunofluorescence test, and an enzyme-linked immunoabsorbent assay.[34] Studies of the new tests have demonstrated that their sensitivity is significantly greater than the old Weil-Felix and complement fixation tests.[35]

In the late 1970s, two groups reported the development of the most rapid diagnostic test yet available. A team from Fort Detrick and the University of Maryland led by Theodore E. Woodward found that as early as the fourth day of illness, a skin biopsy of any suspect rash could be tested within four hours by the indirect immunofluorescence test. David H. Walker and his associates at the University of North Carolina School of Medicine adapted the direct fluorescent antibody technique for the skin biopsy method. Both techniques were demonstrated useful in diagnosing suspected cases of spotted fever.[36]

Although all of these new tests promised quicker, more sensitive, and more reliable results than the old complement fixation test, none of them, Walker observed in a 1982 review paper, could be relied on by the practicing physician for the diagnosis of acute spotted fever. Unless a rash had already developed from which a skin biopsy could be taken—and many fatal cases of spotted fever showed no rash in the early stages—patients usually lacked sufficient antibody levels for laboratory tests to be useful. Just the previous year, however, Walker and his colleagues had identified eschars in spotted fever patients. These small, dark scabs covering the site where an infected tick had attached were characteristic of many rickettsial infections, but they had been considered notably absent in Rocky Mountain spotted fever. Although eschars in spotted fever might continue to be unusual events, the researchers noted, their potential existence could prove helpful in diagnosis. In addition to assisting clinical diagnosis, a biopsy of the eschar might reveal the presence of rickettsiae before the skin rash appeared.[37]

At present, rapid diagnosis of Rocky Mountain spotted fever depends primarily on a physician's awareness that a patient might be at risk to contract the disease. Especially in geographic areas where spotted fever is rarely seen, a medical history that includes questions about recent travel in areas where ticks are prevalent may be the principal clue. To alert both physicians and the public to the dangers of the disease, a variety of media has been utilized by state health agencies in highly infected areas. In Virginia, for example, a public education program keyed to the theme "Virginia's Hidden Enemy" includes newspaper articles, television and radio announcements, brochures aimed at practicing physicians, and posters located in schools and other public places.[38] Such efforts are especially useful to visitors from

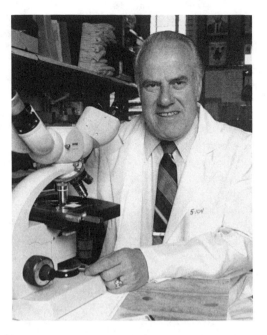

Willy Burgdorfer of the Rocky Mountain Laboratories became one of the
leading investigators of spotted fever during its surprising upsurge in the
1970s. His contributions included an explanation of why the disease had
been limited to the west side of the Bitterroot River and the discovery of
the organism that causes Lyme disease—a serendipitous offshoot of spotted
fever research. (Courtesy of the Rocky Mountain Laboratories, NIAID.)

noninfected areas, who are often unaware that a disease known as
Rocky Mountain spotted fever might pose a threat outside the western
states.

Another widespread misconception about spotted fever is that children are the only group likely to contract it. Having more contact
through outdoor play with wooded areas and with dogs harboring
ticks, children between the ages of five and nine certainly incur the
largest number of cases. As a group from the Bureau of Epidemiology
of the Centers for Disease Control noted in 1982, however, it is adult
victims between the ages of forty and fifty-nine who are the most likely
to die, once infected. Again, the key to recovery is rapid diagnosis,
and, unfortunately, physicians who treat adults are less likely to recognize symptoms as rapidly as pediatricians, most of whom have seen
numerous cases among their patients. "It has been my twenty-year

long experience," Willy Burgdorfer commented, however, "that once a physician loses a patient to spotted fever, he will not lose a second one, because death from spotted fever is an unnecessary loss of life."[39]

Burgdorfer had studied *Rickettsia rickettsii*, as well as numerous other organisms, since coming to the Rocky Mountain Laboratory in the 1950s from Switzerland. In the early 1980s his research on one longstanding mystery relating to Rocky Mountain spotted fever produced the spin-off solution to another mystery in an ancillary field, the discovery of the organism that caused Lyme disease. First identified in Old Lyme, Connecticut—hence its name—this disease caused a characteristic bull's-eye rash, followed by a variety of symptoms, including arthritis, heart complications, and neurological disorders. Investigators at Yale University, particularly Allan Steere, had discovered that Lyme disease responded to penicillin treatment, but the etiologic agent remained unidentified until Burgdorfer traveled to New York to search for ticks infected with *R. rickettsii* along the northeast coast.

Twenty-five to fifty cases of spotted fever occurred each year in this area, but *R. rickettsii* had never been isolated from local ticks. In 1979, Burgdorfer joined forces with Jorge L. Benach of the New York State Department of Health in a concerted effort to solve the puzzle. In areas where spotted fever had been contracted, Benach and Burgdorfer collected several thousand *Dermacentor variabilis* ticks—the common dog tick usually associated with the disease in the east. To test the ticks, Burgdorfer employed a "hemolymph" test he had developed in 1970 that allowed quick determination of the presence of rickettsiae. One leg of a tick was amputated and a drop of hemolymph from the wound placed on a microscopic slide. When stained by the Giménez method, rickettsiae were easily visible under the microscope. Positive specimens could then be subjected to fluorescent antibody studies to identify the particular rickettsial group to which the organisms belonged. This technique itself was a quantum leap from the older methods of injecting tick contents into guinea pigs and waiting to see whether they developed fever.[40]

Of the thousands of ticks tested, "not a single one was found to have *R. rickettsii*," Burgdorfer noted, although "about 15 percent of them were infected with a nonvirulent type [of rickettsia], *R. montana*." Thinking that perhaps they were investigating the wrong tick, Benach collected several hundred ticks of the species *Ixodes dammini*, which were usually parasites of deer but were more numerous in the area than the dog tick. He sent them to Burgdorfer, who examined them at the RML for rickettsiae. They, too, were all negative. "But in two ticks I found a microfilaria," Burgdorfer said in an interview, after which he smiled and noted, "Here comes the serendipity." Having found the earlier developmental stage of a similar microfilaria in *Ixodes* ticks in Switzerland during a sabbatical year in 1978, Burgdorfer began dissecting the two ticks very carefully, "tissue by tissue." He found no more microfilariae, but instead he found spirochetes. Burgdorfer knew that spirochetes had been considered as the possible cause of a European disease similar to Lyme disease, and he also knew that spirochetes were sensitive to penicillin, the drug that had been used successfully to treat Lyme disease victims. "I put two and two together and was convinced I had discovered the etiologic agent of Lyme disease." By 1982 serological and laboratory work had confirmed his hunch, and the organism was named in his honor, *Borrelia burgdorferi*.[41]

Reflecting the circuitous route by which scientific discovery often occurs, Burgdorfer's research had produced the answer to a problem totally unrelated to his initial work. The existence of virulent *R. rickettsii* in New York ticks, in fact, still has not been demonstrated. Other spotted fever mysteries long ignored, however, have yielded to intense study during the 1970s and 1980s. One line of research explained the phenomenon of reactivation, first noted in 1922 by Roscoe R. Spencer and Ralph R. Parker. At that time they experienced a scientific epiphany when they realized that the spotted fever organism was nonvirulent in flat ticks and virulent in engorged ticks. Spencer's experiments had revealed that either a blood meal or warming could produce a similar reactivation of virulence in *R. rickettsii*, but he was at a loss to explain the mechanism by which the process occurred. During the 1950s, Marianna R. Bovarnick and E. G. Allen demonstrated that metabolic changes produced by low temperatures affected the virulence of typhus rickettsiae. Winston H. Price and J. H. Gilford further characterized the reactivation phenomenon, showing that virulent *R. rickettsii* could be made avirulent by treatment with PABA. This process could be reversed, moreover, by incubation with particular coenzymes. In 1967, Emilio Weiss and his colleagues confirmed these findings and showed that *R. rickettsii* possessed metabolic requirements similar to *R. prowazekii*.[42]

In 1982, Stanley F. Hayes and Burgdorfer elucidated the specific physical characteristics that accompanied the metabolic changes of reactivation in *R. rickettsii*. Using the electron microscope, they described two structures in the organism that underwent profound alteration as it changed in virulence. The "microcapsular layer" was an outer structure of the organism, readily identified in electron microscopic examinations of engorged ticks. Around it was the "slime layer," which formed a "discrete electron-lucent zone" around the organism. In starved ticks "neither the microcapsular layer nor slime layer remains a discrete entity. Instead, they are shed and form stringy, shredded, and somewhat flocculent strands." Incubation at 37°C or feeding of starved infected ticks resulted in the restoration of these structures, and, as a corollary, the pathogenicity and virulence of the organism. Continuing study of the reactivation phenomenon may yield clues about the organism's pathogenic mechanism and about why it does so little damage to its tick host.[43]

In contrast to a satisfactory intellectual explanation for this mystery, the ecology of *Rickettsia rickettsii*—what Ralph R. Parker always called the disease's natural history—remains only partially understood. Research in this area has been based on a conceptual model articulated in the 1950s by a Soviet parasitologist, E. N. Pavlovsky. The geographic areas in which specific infections occurred, Pavlovsky suggested, were characterized by well-defined ecological peculiarities determined by topography, climate, vegetation, and other environmental factors. In such natural foci, the pathogens, their vectors, and vertebrate hosts formed a nidus, or biologically balanced ecological system. Only when humans unwittingly stumbled into this system did the pathogens become a hazard. J. R. Audy of the Institute for Medical Research in Kuala Lumpur, Malaya, colorfully summarized Pavlovsky's theory at a 1958 meeting of the Royal Society of Tropical Medicine and Hygiene at Manson House in London. "A man does not look for lion in a rain forest, nor for rhododendrons in a chalk-pit, because it is known that their preferred habitats are different from these." Pathogenic organisms similarly prefer different kinds of environments, and one principal difficulty in studying the biosystems of particular organisms, Audy maintained, was the human tendency to concentrate thought "on clinical disease in man, rather than on the pathogen in its natural environment." This has confused the picture greatly, "for the distribution of a pathogen is wider than that of disease caused by it and the latter cannot be understood without understanding the former as a whole." In an effort to enhance their understanding of biosystems inhabited by rickettsiae, Soviet and eastern bloc investigators have initiated an active program of field research. A rational method for controlling diseases based on environmental principles is the long-term goal of the work.[44]

Even before Pavlovsky gave voice to his theory, the peculiarities of several rickettsial diseases had already stimulated investigators in the United States to consider the natural histories of the organisms. The reason that scrub typhus attacked some troops and spared others

during World War II, for example, was explained by its natural occurrence in particular foci, the so-called islands of infection. Even older
was the enigma of why Rocky Mountain spotted fever had been limited
to the west side of the river in the Bitterroot Valley. All sorts of guesses
had been ventured, from the unwillingness of ground squirrels to cross
the river to analyses of the vegetation on each bank. In 1981, Willy
Burgdorfer, Stanley F. Hayes, and Anthony J. Mavros at the Rocky
Mountain Laboratory addressed the problem anew. Proceeding on the
initial hypothesis that genetic variations in *Dermacentor andersoni*
ticks on the east and west sides of the river might result in differences
of susceptibility to infection with *R. rickettsii*, they collected large
numbers of ticks from each area for study. Burgdorfer's hemolymph
test was used to identify east side ticks containing rickettsiae; larvae
from those female ticks showing none were allowed to engorge on
male guinea pigs. Surprisingly, although none of the guinea pigs developed fever, some of them showed low titers of antibodies to *R.
rickettsii* when tested a month later. "This suggested," the authors
noted in their paper, that some of the larvae were infected with "an
ovarially-acquired rickettsia" that was not detected by hemolymph
testing.[45]

Subsequent dissection confirmed their suspicions. In "large percentages" of the negative ticks—up to 80 percent of those from some east
side locations, a spotted fever group rickettsia, which was given the
name East side agent, was identified in specific tissues, especially the
ovaries. In one test, female ticks from the east side were fed on guinea
pigs infected with virulent *R. rickettsii* and allowed to lay their eggs.
Those females whose ovaries were heavily infected with the East side
agent showed no *R. rickettsii* in their ovaries, although it was present
in all other tissues. Their eggs, moreover, contained only the East side
agent—*R. rickettsii* had not been transmitted. This "interference phenomenon," by which the East side agent prevented the establishment
of virulent *R. rickettsii* in the ovaries of east side ticks offered one
explanation of why spotted fever was limited to the west side of the
river. "Indeed," wrote the investigators, "it may provide a logical
answer to the questions why in certain localities . . . virulent strains
of *R. rickettsii* are rare or have never been established."[46]

From the beginning of spotted fever investigations in 1902, when
the tick-borne nature of the disease was first postulated, investigators
had sought to understand and describe its maintenance in nature. Early
spotted fever investigations were strongly influenced by work on other
vector-borne diseases that had mammalian hosts thought to be their
natural reservoirs. Such an animal reservoir was assumed to exist for

Rocky Mountain spotted fever, and the earliest investigations had identified the Columbian ground squirrel and other small rodents as likely candidates. Once Howard Taylor Ricketts had demonstrated that the spotted fever organism could be transmitted through the eggs of the female tick to later generations, however, the tick itself was also viewed as a major disease reservoir.

In 1916, just after spotted fever had been identified in eastern Montana, Ralph R. Parker published the disturbing finding that immature stages of the spotted fever tick, *Dermacentor andersoni*, fed on rabbits, a potentially huge natural reservoir of the disease. Over the next three decades, Parker continued his research, assisted by several young entomologists who carried on the work after his death. They identified the rabbit tick *Haemaphysalis leporis-palustris*, which rarely bit humans, as a vector of one strain of *R. rickettsii*, and they carefully mapped the geographical locale of this tick and its major host, *Sylvilagus nuttallii*, more commonly known as Nuttall's cottontail.[47] For several decades entomologist William L. Jellison championed the theory that cottontails were probably the major reservoir of Rocky Mountain spotted fever in the United States. In 1980, however, he came out of retirement to join a younger generation of researchers in reopening the question. "The relationship in the U.S. between cottontail rabbits and several species of *Dermacentor* ticks, including the main vectors of the spotted fever agent, *R. rickettsii*, is recognized, and the close agreement in the distribution of cottontails to spotted fever cases in certain geographic areas cannot be disputed," the group reported. "However, our observations do not support the hypothesis that cottontail rabbits are the primary reservoirs of *Rickettsia rickettsii* in nature."[48]

Small rodents were also investigated as potential natural reservoirs of spotted fever. Early research by William Colby Rucker, Lunsford D. Fricks, and S. Burt Wolbach had indicated that the meadow "mouse"—or more precisely, a meadow vole—*Microtus modestus* was not susceptible to infection.[49] In 1934, however, Jellison demonstrated that these and other small rodents not only could be infected but also could transfer the infection to feeding nymphal ticks. Although this research suggested that rodents might play a role in the maintenance of the infection in nature, Jellison was not able to recover rickettsiae from animals in the wild. Twenty years later, however, Douglas J. Gould and Marie L. Miesse at the Walter Reed Army Medical Center confirmed Jellison's prediction. They recovered spotted fever group rickettsiae from the tissues of a meadow vole, *Microtus pennsylvanicus*, during a study in suburban Alexandria, Virginia. Their study did not indicate the actual prevalence of spotted fever among wild meadow voles, nor did it determine the role played by these mammals in the maintenance of spotted fever in nature. Additional research on small animal reservoirs and their tick vectors by Willy Burgdorfer and his colleagues during the 1960s pointed out the complexity of the problem, which will not easily be solved.[50]

In 1935, Ralph R. Parker had also raised the question of cycles in the occurrence of spotted fever, an observation that would prove prescient in the late 1960s when the disease began increasing in the United States for no identifiable reason. Parker's data on the yearly incidence of spotted fever in seven western states showed peaks of incidence in 1915, 1922, and 1929, which suggested a seven-year cycle. What caused this cycle, however, was not clear. Variations in the number of persons exposed, in tick abundance, and in the percentage of ticks carrying virulent organisms might all contribute to such a phenomenon. Parker also acknowledged that there were probably "even more fundamental" influences underlying these cycles. As two examples of this, he cited factors that benefited or harmed the hosts of each stage of the tick and meteorological conditions affecting the portions of the tick life cycle spent in estivation or hibernation. "The possible factors that affect the degree of virulence of the virus in ticks in nature, and which consequently determine whether it will cause frank or inapparent infections, are not understood. . . . That such factors are certainly involved, however, is shown by evidence" such as variations in wild ticks' ability to produce recognizable infections in laboratory animals some years and not in others.[51]

This line of research was continued after World War II as funds and interest permitted. In 1961, for example, a Virginia health officer, F. J. Spencer, published the results of data on the incidence of Rocky Mountain spotted fever and tularemia in Virginia between 1949 and 1958. His data indicated that 68.4 percent of the 588 cases of spotted fever occurred east of Virginia's western mountains. Within this eastern area, moreover, six counties in south-central Virginia reported 16.3 percent of the spotted fever cases and 25.7 percent of the tularemia cases. Spencer suggested that these figures represented Pavlovsky's concept of the nidality of disease and argued that they might indicate synergism between tularemia and spotted fever in this focal area.[52]

Another study, conducted by a group of investigators led by Verne F. Newhouse at the Centers for Disease Control, used sophisticated statistical analysis to examine ten geographic and sociologic variables in each of the 159 counties of Georgia in an attempt to determine how they were correlated with the occurrence of spotted fever. Through techniques known as principal-component analysis and cluster analysis, the group identified four geographically similar areas in Georgia that exhibited different incidences of spotted fever. The disease was low in the south and in the "upper north," moderate in the central region, and high in the "lower north." The most important variables, they found, were climate and geography—factors that annually enhanced or diminished tick populations. Of secondary but still major importance, they discovered, were the changes wrought during the fifteen-year period by humans on the environment. These changes included suburban development and the reclamation of wooded land for recreational purposes.[53]

Such recent ecological studies of spotted fever underscore the earliest observations about the disease, that it is a place disease, a disease of nature. Because of its generational transmission in ticks, Rocky Mountain spotted fever will probably never be eradicated. Unlike its close relative epidemic typhus, however, spotted fever does not represent a smoldering threat that could rapidly become a large-scale killer in time of war. A number of questions remain unanswered, and neither laboratory diagnosis nor prevention is ideally reliable. Nonetheless, Rocky Mountain spotted fever is curable and, in conjunction with public education programs, a manageable disease. The measures employed against spotted fever through the decades since it was first identified have reflected both the facility and the limitations of medical research during the twentieth century. As the number of martyrs to laboratory-acquired spotted fever suggests, however, this disease has been and remains a dangerous adversary. The history of Rocky Mountain spotted fever thus stands not only as a tribute to organized inquiry in the medical sciences but also as a reminder that, because humans and microorganisms share the earth's biosystem, vigilance against infectious diseases must continually be maintained.

Abbreviations

CC	Correspondence of Robert A. Cooley during his tenure as secretary of the Montana State Board of Entomology, 17 bound volumes, Montana State Archives, Helena
MSBE	Montana State Board of Entomology
MSBE, *First Biennial Report*	Montana State Board of Entomology, *First Biennial Report, 1913–1914* (Helena, 1915)
MSBE, *Second Biennial Report*	Montana State Board of Entomology, *Second Biennial Report, 1915–1916* (Helena, 1917)
MSBE, *Third Biennial Report*	Montana State Board of Entomology, *Third Biennial Report, 1917–1918* (Helena, 1919)
MSBE, *Fourth Biennial Report*	Montana State Board of Entomology, *Fourth Biennial Report, 1919–1920* (Helena, 1921)
MSBE, *Fifth Biennial Report*	Montana State Board of Entomology, *Fifth Biennial Report, 1922–1923* (Helena, 1924)
MSBE, *Seventh Biennial Report*	Montana State Board of Entomology, *Seventh Biennial Report, 1927–1928* (Great Falls [1929])
MSBE, *Eighth Biennial Report*	Montana State Board of Entomology, *Eighth Biennial Report, 1929–1930* (Great Falls [1931])
MSBE, *Ninth Biennial Report*	Montana State Board of Entomology, *Ninth Biennial Report, 1931–1932* (Helena [1933])
MSBH	Montana State Board of Health
MSBH Minutes	Minutes of the Montana State Board of Health, Montana State Archives, Helena

MSBH Records	Montana State Board of Health Records, Record Group 28, Montana State Archives, Helena
MSBH, *First Biennial Report*	Montana State Board of Health, *First Biennial Report of the Montana State Board of Health from Its Creation March 15, 1901 to November 30, 1902* (Helena, [1903])
MSBH, *Second Biennial Report*	Montana State Board of Health, *Second Biennial Report of the Montana State Board of Health from December 1, 1902 to November 30, 1904* (Helena, [1905])
MSBH, *Third Biennial Report*	Montana State Board of Health, *Third Biennial Report of the Montana State Board of Health from December 1, 1904 to November 30, 1906* (Helena, [1907])
MSBH, *Fourth Biennial Report*	Montana State Board of Health, *Fourth Biennial Report of the Montana State Board of Health and First Biennial Report of the State Registrar of Births and Deaths, 1907 and 1908* (Helena, [1909])
MSBH, *Tenth Biennial Report*	Montana State Board of Health, *Tenth Biennial Report of the Montana State Board of Health for the Years 1919–1920* (Helena, [1921])
NARA, Saint Louis	Federal Records Center, National Archives and Records Administration, Saint Louis, Missouri
NIAID	National Institute of Allergy and Infectious Diseases
NIAID files, NIH Historical Office	Vertical file of information on the history of Rocky Mountain spotted fever and on the National Institute of Allergy and Infectious Diseases, National Institutes of Health Historical Office, Bethesda, Maryland
NIH	National Institute(s) of Health
NLM	National Library of Medicine
PH-MHS, *Annual Report* (year)	U.S. Treasury Department, Public Health Service, *Annual Report of the Surgeon General of the United States Public Health and Marine Hospital*

	Service (Washington, D.C.: Government Printing Office, annual publication, 1902–12)
PHS Records	Records of the U.S. Public Health Service, Record Group 90, National Archives and Records Administration, Washington, D.C.
Ricketts Papers	Howard Taylor Ricketts Papers, Department of Special Collections, Joseph Regenstein Library, University of Chicago, Chicago
RML, *Annual Report* (year)	Rocky Mountain Laboratory, *Annual Report*, Rocky Mountain Laboratories, Hamilton, Montana
RML, Monthly Report, (month and year)	Monthly reports filed by the director of the Rocky Mountain Laboratory (or its earlier designations), Montana State Archives, Helena
RML Research Records	Research Records of the Rocky Mountain Laboratory, Records of the National Institutes of Health, Record Group 443, National Archives and Records Administration, Washington, D.C.
RML Scrapbook (period indicated)	Six Scrapbooks of the Rocky Mountain Laboratory, 1919–49, Rocky Mountain Laboratories, Hamilton, Montana
ZEA	Archives of the Department of Zoology and Entomology, Montana State University, Renne Library, Bozeman

Notes

Chapter One: A Twentieth-Century Disease of Nature

1. James W. Moulder, "The Rickettsias," in R. E. Buchanan and N. E. Gibbons, eds., *Bergey's Manual of Determinative Bacteriology*, 8th ed. (Baltimore: Williams & Wilkins Co., 1974), 882; S. Stanley Schneierson, *Atlas of Diagnostic Microbiology* (North Chicago: Abbott Laboratories, 1974), 4, 36.

2. Tsutsugamushi, or scrub typhus, was known in the Orient at least by the sixteenth century. Its history is discussed in chap. 6.

3. W. C. Rucker, "Rocky Mountain Spotted Fever," *Public Health Reports* 27 (1912):1471.

4. George T. Harrell, "Treatment of Rocky Mountain Spotted Fever with Antibiotics," *Annals of the New York Academy of Science* 55 (1952):1027–42.

5. William D. Tigertt, "A 1759 Spotted Fever Epidemic in North Carolina," *Journal of the History of Medicine and Allied Sciences* 42 (1987):296–304.

6. Mary A. Newcomb, *Four Years' Personal Experience in the War* (Chicago: H. S. Mills & Co., 1893). I am grateful to Fredrick Hambrecht for bringing this reference to my attention.

7. My discussion of the early history of typhus is based on Hans Zinsser, *Rats, Lice, and History* (Boston: Little, Brown & Co., 1935), and on John C. Snyder, "Typhus Fever Rickettsiae," in Frank L. Horsfall, Jr., and Igor Tamm, eds., *Viral and Rickettsial Infections of Man*, 4th ed. (Philadelphia: J. B. Lippincott Co., 1965), 1059–94.

8. Dale C. Smith, "The Rise and Fall of Typhomalarial Fever: II. Decline and Fall," *J. Hist. Med. Allied Sci.* 37 (1982):287–321.

9. See, for example, Erwin H. Ackerknecht, *Medicine in the Paris Hospital, 1794–1848* (Baltimore: Johns Hopkins Press, 1967); and Erna Lesky, *The Vienna Medical School in the Nineteenth Century* (Baltimore: Johns Hopkins University Press, 1976).

10. William Wood Gerhard, "On the Typhus Fever, Which Occurred at Philadelphia in the Spring and Summer of 1836," *American Journal of Medical Science* 19 (1837):289–92, 298–99, 302–3; Dale C. Smith, "Gerhard's Distinction between Typhoid and Typhus and Its Reception in America, 1833–1860," *Bulletin of the History of Medicine* 54 (1980):368–85.

11. Rudolf Virchow, "Report on the Typhus Epidemic in Upper Silesia," Eng. trans. in L. J. Rather, ed., *Rudolf Virchow: Collected Essays on Public Health and Epidemiology*, 2 vols. (Canton, Mass.: Science History Publications, 1985), 2:205–319.

12. See, for example, Claude Bernard, *An Introduction to Experimental Medicine*, trans. Henry C. Greene (New York: Macmillan Co., 1927); Rudolf Virchow, *Cellular Pathology*, trans. Frank Chance (Philadelphia: J. B. Lippincott Co., 1863); and Robert Hagelstein, "The History of the Microscope," *New York Microscopial Society Bulletin* 2 (1944):1–19.

Chapter Two: A Blight on the Bitterroot

1. Gretchen Jellison, Introduction, in Bitter Root Valley Historical Society, ed., *Bitterroot Trails*, 2 vols. (Darby, Mont.: Professional Impressions, 1982), 1:17. In recent years the words *Bitter* and *Root* have been combined officially. In the early years of the century, the two-word form was invariably used.

2. Samuel Lloyd Cappious, "A History of the Bitter Root Valley to 1914," M.A. thesis, University of Washington, 1939, 1–2. Curiously, Cappious never mentions spotted fever.

3. Peter Ronan, *History of the Flathead Indians* (Minneapolis: Ross & Haines, 1890); John Duffy, *The Healers: A History of American Medicine* (Urbana: University of Illinois Press, 1979), 2–4; idem, "Medicine and Medical Practices among Aboriginal American Indians," in Felix Marti-Ibañez, ed., *History of American Medicine: A Symposium* (New York: MD Publications, 1959), 15–33.

4. Duffy, "Medicine and Medical Practices"; Paul C. Phillips, *Medicine in the Making of Montana* (Missoula: Montana State University Press, 1962), 1; Ronan, *History of the Flathead Indians*, 13–14; Report of the investigation of Louis B. Wilson and William M. Chowning in MSBH, *First Biennial Report.*

5. Reuben G. Thwaites, ed., *The Journals of Lewis and Clark*, 8 vols. (New York, 1905; reprint, New York, Arno Press, 1969), 3:52–57, 5:246; Cappious, "History of the Bitter Root Valley," 6–10; Phyllis Twogood, Henry Grant, and Lena Bell, "History of Lewis and Clark Expedition in the Bitter Root Valley," in Bitter Root Valley Historical Society, ed., *Bitterroot Trails* 1:37–45; Phillips, *Medicine in the Making of Montana*, 20–31.

6. L. D. Fricks, "Rocky Mountain Spotted Fever," manuscript, file "S.F. History (Manuscript by Dr. Fricks on R.M.S.F.)," p. 2, RML Research Records.

7. Ibid., 2–3.

8. Monica G. Shannon, "Catholicity in the Bitter Root Valley," in "The Bitter Root Valley Illustrated," magazine suppl. to the *Western News*, May 1910, 35; Cappious, "History of the Bitter Root Valley," 54–61, 65–67; Ronan, *History of the Flathead Indians*, 22–33, 38–41; Phillips, *Medicine in the Making of Montana*, 34–40.

9. Cappious, "History of the Bitter Root Valley," 11–15, 16–17.

10. *Weekly Missoulian*, 28 May and 13 October, 1880, as cited in Robert N. Philip, "A Journalistic View of Western Montana, 1870–1910: Some Newspaper Items Relevant to the Development of the Bitter Root Valley and the Occurrence of Rocky Mountain Spotted Fever," manuscript, 1984, 1. Copies of this manuscript have been deposited in the Ravalli County Historical Museum and the library at the University of Montana.

11. "The World Famous Valley of the Bitter Root: Its Early History, Its Incomparable Resources and the Men Who Have Wrought Mightily in Its Development," in "The Bitter Root Valley Illustrated," magazine suppl. to the *Western News*, May 1910, 7; W. B. Harlan, "Pioneer Fruit Growers of the Bitter Root," in ibid., 10. *Missoula and Cedar Creek Pioneer*, 24 November 1870, and *Weekly Missoulian*, 20 April 1883, as quoted in Philip, "Journalistic View," 1, 27.

12. *Missoula Pioneer*, 9 December 1871, and *Pioneer*, 24 August 1872, as cited in Philip, "Journalistic View," 3; Ronan, *History of the Flathead Indians*, 58–62; *Western News*, 20 October 1891, as cited in Philip, "Journalistic View," 67.

13. See Philip, "Journalistic View," 18–68.

14. Ibid., 47, 61.

15. *Western News*, 8 April 1896, as cited in Philip, "Journalistic View," 85.

16. Philip, preface to "Journalistic View," n.p.

17. *Weekly Missoulian*, 22 August 1888, 23 and 30 October 1889, *Bitter Root Bugle*, 24 January, 5 June, 7 and 21 August, 4 and 11 September 1890, all as cited in Philip, "Journalistic View," 52, 55, 60.

18. Phillips, *Medicine in the Making of Montana*, 268–75.

19. *Weekly Missoulian*, 16 April 1880, as quoted in Phillips, *Medicine in the Making of Montana*, 289–90, n. 4.

20. Ibid., 278, 290, n. 7. There were twenty-seven reported smallpox cases in this epidemic.

21. The diphtheria epidemic was reported in the *Weekly Missoulian*, 6 March 1885, and the Indian deaths from apparent tuberculosis in the same paper, 24 July 1885. Both are cited in Philip, "Journalistic View," 36.

22. The figure for cases reported in the newspapers was tabulated from Philip, "Journalistic View," for each year. The official count was made by Wilson and Chowning and is given in their report. See MSBH, *First Biennial Report*, 32–41.

23. Wilson and Chowning's report, MSBH, *First Biennial Report*, 28, 30; Phillips, *Medicine in the Making of Montana*, 271.

24. Reports of two spotted fever deaths in 1882 are in the *Weekly Missoulian*, 10, 17, and 24 March 1882. On 6 July 1883 the paper reported one death from spotted fever. See Philip, "Journalistic View," 25, 29.

25. Phillips, *Medicine in the Making of Montana*, 164, 167–68.

26. Ibid., 278–81.

27. George Rosen, "The Bacteriological, Immunologic, and Chemotherapeutic Period, 1875–1950," *Bulletin of the New York Academy of Medicine*, second series, 40 (June 1964):487–93.

28. Erwin H. Ackerknecht, "Anticontagionism between 1821 and 1867," *Bull. Hist. Med.* 22 (1948):562–93.

29. Phillips, *Medicine in the Making of Montana*, 423, omits Minshall's practice in the Bitterroot. For more complete information on his career, see *Ravalli Republican*, 9 October 1895 and 23 March 1898, *Bitter Root Times*, 13 March 1896, *Western News*, 19 December 1906, all as cited in Philip, "Journalistic View," 83, 86, 96, 155.

30. *An Act to Increase the Efficiency and Change the Name of the United States Marine Hospital Service*, 1 July 1902, 32 *Stat. L.* 712.

31. MSBH, *First Biennial Report*, 4, 8. For biographical information on Longeway, see Phillips, *Medicine in the Making of Montana*, 356, 359.

32. The designations *black fever* and *blue disease* are noted in G. T. McCullough, "Spotted Fever," *Medical Sentinel* 10 (July 1902):225; "black typhus fever" is noted in several sources, including the *Bitter Root Times*, 24 June 1893, as cited in Philip, "Journalistic View," 75.

33. The diagnosis of "typhoid pneumonia and measles" was reported in the *Daily Missoulian*, 11 May 1896, as cited in Philip, "Journalistic View," 86; McCullough noted that "the new Standard dictionary" and "text books of authority" identified spotted fever as cerebrospinal meningitis or cerebrospinal fever, and *Journal of the American Medical Association* reported in

1902 an epidemic of spotted fever in Montana that was identified as cerebrospinal meningitis. See McCullough, "Spotted Fever," 225; "The 'Spotted Fever' Epidemic," *JAMA* 38 (1902):1313. Spotted fever was identified as a cognomen for typhus as well as for cerebrospinal meningitis in William Osler, *The Principles and Practice of Medicine* (New York: D. Appleton & Co., 1892), 39, 92.

34. McCullough stated that the disease was also known in Idaho and Alaska. See his "Spotted Fever," 225.

35. For biographical information on Wood see James F. Hammarsten, "The Contributions of Idaho Physicians to Knowledge of Rocky Mountain Spotted Fever," *Transactions of the American Clinical and Climatological Association* 94 (1982):28–29, 33–41.

36. Marshall W. Wood, "Spotted Fever as Reported from Idaho," U.S. War Department, *Report of the Surgeon General of the Army to the Secretary of War, 1896* (Washington, D.C.: Government Printing Office, 1896), 60.

37. On Wood's attack of spotted fever, see Edward E. Maxey, "Rocky Mountain Spotted Fever. A Summary of Progress," exerpts from speech given 3 August 1931, in Notebook "RMSF–Idaho–Early History," Notebooks of Ralph R. Parker (hereafter cited as R. R. Parker Notebooks, RML Research Records).

38. Wood, "Spotted Fever," 61, 63.

39. Edward E. Maxey, "Some Observations on the So-called Spotted Fever of Idaho," *Medical Sentinel* 7 (October 1899):433–38 (quotations from p. 434).

40. Ibid., 436. For additional information about the history of spotted fever in Idaho, see W. O. Spencer, "Mountain or Spotted Fever, as Seen in Idaho and Eastern Oregon," *Medical Sentinel* 15 (1907):532–37; "The Present Status of Rocky Mountain Spotted Fever in Idaho," in "Rocky Mountain Spotted Fever," Montana State Board of Health *Special Bulletin* no. 26 (1923):27–28; Notebook "RMSF–Idaho–Early History," R. R. Parker Notebooks, RML Research Records.

41. "Tick-borne Infections in Colorado," abstract in *JAMA* 94 (1930):1172; J. M. Braden, "Some Observations on Four Cases of Spotted Fever Occurring in Colorado," *Colorado Medicine* 3 (1906):213–19; Notebook, "RMSF–Colorado–Early History to 1929," R. R. Parker Notebooks, RML Research Records; Frederick D. Stricker, "The Prevalence and Distribution of Rocky Mountain Spotted Fever in Oregon," in "Rocky Mountain Spotted Fever," Montana State Board of Health *Special Bulletin* no. 26 (1923):18–20 (quotation from p. 18); Notebook "RMSF–Oregon–Early History to 1925," R. R. Parker Notebooks, RML Research Records.

42. Albert B. Tonkin, "Incidence of Rocky Mountain Spotted Fever in Wyoming," in "Rocky Mountain Spotted Fever," Montana State Board of Health *Special Bulletin* no. 26 (1923):23–27; Notebook "RMSF–Wyoming–Early History to 1926," R. R. Parker Notebooks, RML Research Records.

43. On Washington, see A. U. Simpson, "Rocky Mountain Tick Fever in the State of Washington," in "Rocky Mountain Spotted Fever," Montana State Board of Health *Special Bulletin* no. 26 (1923):20–23. On California, see F. L. Kelly, "Rocky Mountain Spotted Fever: Its Prevalence and Distribution in Modoc and Lassen counties, California: A Preliminary Report," *California State Journal of Medicine* 14 (1916):407–9; F. L. Kelly, "Rocky Mountain Spotted Fever in California," *Pub. Health Rep.* 31 (1916):2753–54; J. G.

Cumming, "Rocky Mountain Spotted Fever in California," *Journal of Infectious Diseases* 21 (1917):509–14; Notebook, "RMSF—California—Early History to 1929," R. R. Parker Notebooks, RML Research Records. On Utah and Nevada, see A. A. Robinson, "Rocky Mountain Spotted Fever, with Report of a Case," *Medical Record* 74 (1908):913–22; "RMSF—Utah—Early History to 1931," and "RMSF—Nevada—Early History to 1928," R. R. Parker Notebooks, RML Research Records.

44. *Daily Missoulian*, 5 May 1901, and *Western News*, 15 May 1901, as cited in Philip, "Journalistic View," 114.

45. Minutes of the MSBH, 9 May 1901, in MSBH, *First Biennial Report*, 9 10; *Western News*, 15 May 1901, and *Daily Missoulian*, 11 June 1901, as cited in Philip, "Journalistic View," 114–15.

46. *Daily Missoulian*, 11 June 1901, as cited in Philip, "Journalistic View," 115.

47. *Western News*, 17 April 1901, as cited in Philip, "Journalistic View," 115.

48. *Western News*, 22 May 1901, as cited in ibid. The physician was James William Howard.

49. Edward Burrows, letter to the editor of the *Western News*, 5 June 1901, clipping in RML Scrapbook "1919–1931"; also cited in Philip, "Journalistic View," 115.

50. Report of Louis B. Wilson and William M. Chowning in MSBH, *First Biennial Report*, 36.

Chapter Three: The Beginning of Scientific Investigations

1. Minutes of the meeting on 4 February 1902, of the MSBH in MSBH, *First Biennial Report*, 13; *Northwest Tribune*, 11 April 1902, as cited in Philip, "Journalistic View" (see chap. 2, n. 10), 124.

2. *Western News*, 30 April 1902, as cited in Philip, "Journalistic View," 121. Two local physicians presented clinical papers on spotted fever at the meeting of the Montana Medical Association in Anaconda on 23 May 1902. George T. McCullough's paper "Spotted Fever" was published in the *Medical Sentinel* (see chap. 2, n. 32). Russell Gwinn's paper was not published in a medical periodical.

3. *Daily Missoulian*, 2 May 1902, as cited in Philip, "Journalistic View," 121.

4. Esther Gaskins Price, *Fighting Spotted Fever in the Rockies* (Helena: Naegele Printing Co., 1948), 16–19, states that Strain suggested the significance of the tick to Longeway during a trip to the Bitterroot in 1901. No report of a 1901 visit appears in contemporary newspapers, but several obituaries of Strain repeat the story and give 1901 as the date. See "Dr. Earle Strain, Discoverer of Relationship between Wood Ticks, Spotted Fever, Dies," "Dr. Earle Strain Dies in Great Falls," and "Death Takes Expert on Spotted Fever," clippings dated 1953 in Scrapbook "1942–   ," RML Scrapbooks. The MSBH, *First Biennial Report*, 25, records Strain's 1902 visit to the valley. Other documentation of the 1902 visit is in *Daily Missoulian*, 6 May 1902, as cited in Philip, "Journalistic View," 121; Charles Wardell Stiles, "A Zoological Investigation into the Cause, Transmission, and Source of Rocky Mountain 'Spotted Fever,'" U.S. Hygienic Laboratory *Bulletin* no. 20 (1905), 17.

5. *Daily Missoulian*, 3, 6, 8, 9, and 10 May, *Western News*, 7, 14, 21 May 1902, as cited in Philip, "Journalistic View," 121–122.

6. For biographical information on Wilson see Samuel F. Haines and Clark W. Nelson's sketch of him in the *Dictionary of American Biography*, 20 vols., 6 supplements, (New York: Charles Scribner's Sons, 1932–80), suppl. 3 (1973):831–33 (hereafter cited as *DAB*). Wilson's papers, which are at the Mayo Clinic, unfortunately do not include manuscript materials relating to his spotted fever work.

7. Frank F. Wesbrook, Louis B. Wilson, and O. McDaniel, "Varieties of Bacillus Diphtheria," *Transactions of the Association of American Physicians* 15 (1900):198–223. For biographical information on Wesbrook see H. E. Robertson's sketch of him, *DAB* 20 (1936):3–4. For biographical information on Mallory, see Shields Warren's sketch of him, ibid., suppl. 3 (1973):502–3.

8. Biographical information on Chowning was kindly supplied by the Library and Information Management Section of the AMA. Because Chowning's license was revoked in 1936 following his conviction for "the crime of abortion," *JAMA* did not publish an obituary.

9. *Western News*, 21 May 1902, as cited in Philip, "Journalistic View," 122; Louis B. Wilson and William M. Chowning, "Studies in Pyroplasmosis Hominis ('Spotted Fever' or 'Tick Fever' of the Rocky Mountains)," *Journal of Infectious Diseases* 1 (1904):31–33; MSBH, *First Biennial Report*, 26–27.

10. MSBH, *First Biennial Report*, 26; Wilson and Chowning, "Studies in Pyroplasmosis Hominis," 41–42.

11. MSBH, *First Biennial Report*, 29; see also case records, ibid., 32–41.

12. Wilbur Catlin, a local civil engineer and draftsman, prepared the distribution maps for Wilson and Chowning. See *Western News*, 25 June 1902, as cited in Philip, "Journalistic View," 124. On the foci of spotted fever outside the Bitterroot, see Wilson and Chowning, "Studies in Pyroplasmosis Hominis," 34.

13. Percy M. Ashburn, "Piroplasmosis Hominis (?)—Spotted Fever of Montana," *Lancet-Clinic*, n.s. 54 (1905):481–94 (quotation from p. 492).

14. MSBH, *First Biennial Report*, 42–44.

15. Mortality figures computed by the author from Wilson and Chowning's tables, ibid., 32–41. Counts and computation by the author based on cases cited in Philip, "Journalistic View," 82–83, 86, 90–91, 95, 101–2, 107–8, 116–17, 124–25.

16. MSBH, *First Biennial Report*, 27; Wilson and Chowning, "Studies in Pyroplasmosis Hominis," 43–44.

17. Walter Reed, Victor C. Vaughn, and Edward O. Shakespeare, *Report on the Origin and Spread of Typhoid Fever in U.S. Military Camps during the Spanish War of 1898* (Washington, D.C.: Government Printing Office, 1904); M. A. Veeder, "Flies as Spreaders of Disease in Camps," *Medical Record*, 17 September 1898, 429–30; William B. Bean, *Walter Reed: A Biography* (Charlottesville: University Press of Virginia, 1982), 87–91; Edward F. Keuchel, "Chemicals and Meat: The Embalmed Beef Scandal of the Spanish-American War," *Bull. Hist. Med.* 48 (1974):249–64.

18. For surveys of scientific developments in parasitology, see William D. Foster, *A History of Parasitology* (Edinburgh: E. & S. Livingstone, 1965); Jean Théodoridès, "Les Grandes Etapes de la parasitologie," *Clio Medica* 1 (1966):129–45, 185–208. For a short survey of social and economic factors

in the professionalization of parasitology, see Michael Worboys, "The Emergence and Early Development of Parasitology," in Kenneth S. Warren and John Z. Bowers, eds., *Parasitology: A Global Perspective* (New York: Springer-Verlag, 1983), 1–18.

19. Patrick Manson, "On the Development of *Filaria sanguinis hominis*, and on the Mosquito Considered as a Nurse," *Journal of the Linnean Society* 14 (1878):304–11. This worm was later renamed *Wucheria bancrofti.*

20. L. O. Howard, "A Fifty Year Sketch History of Medical Entomology and Its Relation to Public Health," in Mazyck P. Ravenel, ed., *A Half Century of Public Health* (New York: American Public Health Association, 1921), 413; H. Harold Scott, *A History of Tropical Medicine*, 2 vols. (London: Edward Arnold, 1939), 2:1086–90.

21. Theobald Smith and F. L. Kilbourne, "Investigations into the Nature, Causation, and Prevention of Texas or Southern Cattle Fever," U.S. Department of Agriculture, Bureau of Animal Industry *Bulletin* no. 1 (1893); Tamara Miner Haygood, "Cows, Ticks, and Disease: A Medical Interpretation of the Southern Cattle Industry," *Journal of Southern History* 52 (1986):551–64.

22. Koch's postulates were articulated in his paper demonstrating the etiology of tuberculosis. He stated: "It was necessary to isolate the bacilli from the body, to grow them in pure culture until they were freed from any disease-product of the animal organism which might adhere to them; and, by administering the isolated bacilli to animals, to reproduce the same morbid condition which, as known, is obtained by inoculation with spontaneously developed tuberculous material." See Robert Koch, "Die Aetiologie der Tuberculose," *Berliner Klinische Wochenschrift* 19 (1882):221–30; hereafter cited as *Berl. klin. Wchnschr.* An English translation of this paper is in idem, *The Aetiology of Tuberculosis*, trans. Dr. and Mrs. Max Pinner (New York: National Tuberculosis Association, 1922) (quotation from p. 31). Lester S. King has pointed out that even for bacterial diseases, the postulates had to be understood as a method of elucidating a known disease process, not as a means of defining disease. See King, "Dr. Koch's Postulates," *J. Hist. Med. Allied Sci.* 7 (1952):350–61.

23. Sally Smith Hughes, *The Virus: A History of the Concept* (New York: Science History Publications, 1977), 12, 17–21. Evidence of the assumption that yellow fever was a protozoan disease may be seen in Herman B. Parker, George E. Beyer, and O. L. Pothier, "Report of Working Party No. 1, Yellow Fever Institute: A Study of the Etiology of Yellow Fever," U.S. Public Health and Marine Hospital Service *Yellow Fever Institute Bulletin* no. 13 (1903), esp. 28–32; Milton J. Rosenau, Herman B. Parker, Edward Francis, and George E. Beyer, "Report of Working Party No. 2, Yellow Fever Institute: Experimental Studies in Yellow Fever and Malaria at Vera Cruz, Mexico," in ibid. no. 14 (1905); Milton J. Rosenau and Joseph Goldberger, "Report of Working Party No. 3, Yellow Fever Institute: Attempts to Grow the Yellow Fever Parasite; the Hereditary Transmission of the Yellow Fever Parasite in the Mosquito," in ibid. no. 15 (1906); Joseph Goldberger, "Yellow Fever: Etiology, Symptoms, and Diagnosis," in ibid. no. 16 (1907), 8–9.

24. Hughes, *The Virus*, 61–73.

25. Victoria A. Harden, "Rocky Mountain Spotted Fever Research and the Development of the Insect Vector Theory, 1900–1930," *Bull. Hist. Med.* 59 (1985):451–52; George Henry Falkiner Nuttall, "On the Role of Insects, Arachnids, and Myriapods as Carriers in the Spread of Bacterial and Parasitic

Diseases of Man and Animals: A Critical and Historical Study," *Johns Hopkins Hospital Reports* 8 (1899):43–49, 71–75.

26. For examples of the association between ticks and blood poisoning, see *Bitter Root Times*, 12 June 1896, as cited in Philip, "Journalistic View," 86.

27. Wilson and Chowning, "Studies in Pyroplasmosis Hominis," 44–45. See also L. B. Wilson and W. M. Chowning, "The Hematozoon of the So-called 'Spotted Fever' of the Rocky Mountains," *Northwest Lancet* 22 (1902):440–42.

28. *Western News*, 11 June 1902, as cited in Philip, "Journalistic View," 123.

29. Wilson and Chowning, "Studies in Pyroplasmosis Hominis," 47–48.

30. MSBH, *First Biennial Report*, 82.

31. J. O. Cobb, "The So-called 'Spotted Fever' of the Rocky Mountains— A New Disease in the Bitter Root Valley, Mont.," *Pub. Health Rep.* 17 (1902):1869. In 1902 the ground squirrel was known as *Spermophilus columbianus*.

32. MSBH, *First Biennial Report*, 83.

33. Charles Wardell Stiles, "Zoological Pitfalls for the Pathologist," *Proceedings of the New York Pathological Society*, 1905, 16.

34. *Northwest Tribune*, 4 July 1902, as cited in Philip, "Journalistic View," 123.

35. *Sundry Civil Appropriations Act*, 3 March 1901, 31 *Stat. L.* 1137. On the history of federal medical research policy, see Victoria A. Harden, *Inventing the NIH: Federal Biomedical Research Policy, 1887–1937* (Baltimore: Johns Hopkins University Press, 1986), chs. 1–2; Cobb, "The So-called 'Spotted Fever,' " 1868.

36. For biographical information on Cobb see his personnel file, Record Group 090–78, Accession no. 0001, Agency Box no. OF, Records Center Location no. FU#134867 through FU#134992, box # 22, NARA, Saint Louis; Cobb, "The So-Called 'Spotted Fever,' " 1868, 1870; Wilson and Chowning, "The So-called 'Spotted Fever' of the Rocky Mountains: A Preliminary Report to the Montana State Board of Health," *JAMA* 39 (1902):131– 36.

37. MSBH, *First Biennial Report*, 13.

38. *Ravalli Republican*, 24 April 1903, and *Daily Missoulian*, 16 April 1903, as cited in Philip, "Journalistic View," 130.

39. For biographical information on Anderson, see Ralph C. Williams, *The United States Public Health Service, 1798–1950* (Washington, D.C.: Commissioned Officers Association, 1951), 251–52; Paul F. Clark, *Pioneer Microbiologists of America* (Madison: University of Wisconsin Press, 1961), 211; Anderson's personnel file, Record Group 090–78, Accession no. 0001, Agency Box no. OF, Records Center Location no. FU#134867 through FU#134992, Box # 3, NARA, Saint Louis.

40. John F. Anderson, "Spotted Fever (Tick Fever) of the Rocky Mountains: A New Disease," U.S. Hygienic Laboratory *Bulletin* no. 14 (1903): 7, 10, 21 (quotation from p. 10); Wilson and Chowning, "Studies in Pyroplasmosis Hominis," 32; *Daily Missoulian*, 21 May 1903, as cited in Philip, "Journalistic View," 130.

41. See Anderson, "Spotted Fever." This report also appeared in MSBH, *Second Biennial Report*, 123–58; and in summary form with the same title,

"Spotted Fever (Tick Fever) of the Rocky Mountains: A New Disease," in *American Medicine* 6 (1903):506–8.

42. Stiles, "Zoological Investigation," 25; see also Stiles's discussion of the infectivity of *Piroplasma* in idem, "Zoological Pitfalls," 18.

43. Ashburn, "Piroplasmosis Hominis (?)," 492.

44. *Western News*, 6 May 1903, as cited in Philip, "Journalistic View," 129.

45. *Western News*, 20 April 1904, as cited in Philip, "Journalistic View," 136.

46. *Stevensville Register*, 18 May 1904, and *Ravalli Republican*, 29 April 1904, as cited in Philip, "Journalistic View," 137.

47. *Northwest Tribune*, 6 May 1904, as cited in Philip, "Journalistic View," 137.

48. *Western News*, 6 May 1903, as cited in Philip, "Journalistic View," 129.

49. *Western News*, 20 May 1903, and *Ravalli Republican*, 17 June 1904, as cited in Philip, "Journalistic View," 129, 138.

50. Elsie McCormick, "Death in a Hard Shell," *Saturday Evening Post*, 15 November 1941, 24ff. (quotation from p. 47); advertisement in the *Daily Missoulian*, 20 June 1902, as cited in Philip, "Journalistic View," 125.

51. *Stevensville Register*, 15 June 1904, as cited in Philip, "Journalistic View," 138. For a survey of the history of quackery and patent medicines before the passage of the 1906 Pure Food and Drugs Act, see James Harvey Young, *The Toadstool Millionaires: A Social History of Patent Medicines in America before Federal Regulation* (Princeton, N.J.: Princeton University Press, 1961); idem, *Pure Food: Securing the Federal Food and Drug Act of 1906* (Princeton, N.J.: Princeton University Press, 1989).

52. Anderson, "Spotted Fever," 40; MSBH, *Second Biennial Report*, 156; Anderson, summary version of "Spotted Fever," *American Medicine* 6 (1903): 508.

53. See, for example, an instance reported in the *Daily Missoulian*, 21 April and 24 May 1903, as cited in Philip, "Journalistic View," 132.

54. MSBH, *Second Biennial Report*, 6–7.

55. For biographical information on Tuttle, see his obituary in *Montana Record Herald* (Helena), 9 July 1942.

56. During his first three months in office, Tuttle reinstated a three-week quarantine for measles, threatened county and local state health officers with lawsuits if they failed to report births, deaths, and infectious diseases, and initiated publication of the *Montana Health Bulletin*. See MSBH, *Second Biennial Report*, 8–13.

57. Ibid., 9, 44–45.

58. There are many biographical articles on Stiles, including James H. Cassedy's sketch of him, *DAB*, suppl. 3 (1903):737–39; and an autobiographical article, "Early History, in Part Esoteric, of the Hookworm (Uncinariasis) Campaign in Our Southern U.S.," *Journal of Parasitology* 25 (1939):283–308. For accounts of Stiles's work with hookworm, see Stiles, "Early History"; James H. Cassedy, "The 'Germ of Laziness' in the South, 1900–1915: Charles Wardell Stiles and the Progressive Paradox," *Bull. Hist. Med.* 45 (1971):159–69; John Ettling, *The Germ of Laziness: Rockefeller Philanthropy and Public Policy in the New South* (Cambridge, Mass.: Harvard University Press, 1981).

59. Stiles, "Zoological Investigation," 10.
60. Charles Wardell Stiles, "Insects as Disseminators of Disease," *Virginia Medical Semi-Monthly* 6 (1901):53–58 (quotation from p. 54). Stiles's italics.
61. Stiles, "Zoological Investigation," 11; PH-MHS, *Annual Report, 1904,* 362.
62. Stiles, "Zoological Pitfalls," 11–12.
63. Stiles, "Zoological Investigation," 7, 19; PH-MHS, *Annual Report, 1904,* 362–63.
64. Charles F. Craig, "The Relation of the So-called Piroplasma Hominis and Certain Degenerative Changes in the Erythrocytes," *American Medicine* 8 (1904):1016. For biographical information on Craig, who from 1918 to 1920 served as curator of the Army Medical Museum, see Robert S. Henry, *The Armed Forces Institute of Pathology: Its First Century, 1862–1962* (Washington, D.C.: Office of the Surgeon General of the Army, 1964), 189; "Charles F. Craig," in *American Men of Science,* 5th ed., ed. J. McKeen Cattell and Jacques Cattell (New York: Science Press, 1933), 239. In a personal communication to the author, 16 February 1988, Robert N. Philip suggested that Wilson and Chowning's observations could have been affected if their patients' blood were infected with Colorado tick fever virus, also present in the Bitterroot, although unknown at that time.
65. Stiles, "Zoological Investigation," 29–30.
66. Ibid., 8, 49, 65.
67. Ibid., 20. Ashburn likewise believed that if no protozoan organism were found in the blood, "the tick and gopher hypothesis would seem to die of inanition, as it was merely a hypothesis advanced to account for the protozoon infection." See Ashburn, "Piroplasmosis Hominis (?)," 491. The spelling of the Latin words *protozoan* and *protozoon* changes according to the word's grammatical use in the sentence.
68. Stiles, "Zoological Investigation," 10.
69. Ibid., 44; Ashburn, "Piroplasmosis Hominis (?)," 483–85.
70. Stiles, "Zoological Investigation," 23.
71. Ibid., 32, 35.
72. PH-MHS, *Annual Report,* 1904, 363. Stiles's summary report also appeared in MSBH, *Second Biennial Report,* 160–62 (quotation from p. 162).
73. Price, *Fighting Spotted Fever,* 34–36.
74. Cassedy, " 'Germ of Laziness,' " 161; James H. Cassedy, "Applied Microscopy and American Pork Diplomacy: Charles Wardell Stiles in Germany, 1898–1899," *Isis* 62 (1971):5–20.
75. Stiles, "Zoological Pitfalls," 20.
76. Stiles noted the lack of any such experiment, ibid., 15.
77. Rankin's death was reported in the *Daily Missoulian,* 4 May 1904. His and other cases of spotted fever in 1904 are cited in Philip, "Journalistic View," 137–38.
78. Percy M. Ashburn, "A Suggestion as to the Treatment of the 'Spotted Fever' of Montana," *Lancet-Clinic,* n.s. 54 (1905):579–84 (quotation from p. 579).
79. On hydrotherapy see Marshall Scott Legan, "Hydropathy in America: A Nineteenth Century Panacea," *Bull. Hist. Med.* 45 (1971):267–80; John Harvey Kellogg, *Rational Hydrotherapy: A Manual of the Physiological and Therapeutic Effects of Hydriatic Procedures, and the Technique of Their Ap-*

plication in the Treatment of Disease, 2d ed. (Philadelphia: F. A. Davis Co., 1903); Simon Baruch, *Principles and Practice of Hydrotherapy* (London: Bailliere, Tindall & Co., 1900). Osler's recommendation is in *Principles and Practice of Medicine*, 43.

80. Ashburn, "Suggestion as to the Treatment," 583, 581; Robert N. Philip, personal communication to the author, 16 February 1988.

81. "Spotted Fever," *JAMA* 44 (1905):1686.

Chapter Four: Dr. Ricketts's Discoveries

1. See, for example, references to such changes in *Western News*, 3 July 1907, 1 July 1908, and 27 July and 9 September 1910, and *Ravalli Republican*, 26 March 1909, all cited in Philip, "Journalistic View" (see chap. 2, n. 10), 158–59, 165, 176, 180.

2. MSBH, *Second Biennial Report*, 66, 58, 67–68.

3. Robert William Hadlow, "The Big Ditch and the McIntosh Red: Early Boosterism in Montana's Bitter Root Valley," *Pacific Northwest Forum* 8 (Fall 1983):2–13; *Western News*, 30 October 1907, as cited in Philip, "Journalistic View," 157.

4. Philip identified the following cases and deaths from spotted fever in this period—1904: 14 cases, 9 deaths; 1905: 10 cases, 8 deaths; 1906: 14 cases, 11 deaths; 1907, 6 cases, 6 deaths; 1908: 10 cases, 4 deaths; 1909, 10 cases, 8 deaths; 1910: 8 cases, 8 deaths. See "Journalistic View," 137–38, 146–47, 154–55, 161, 167–68, 176, 180. His figures for 1909 include four fatal cases in Northern Pacific Railroad workers that were never reported in the press. On the creation of the Montana Bureau of Vital Statistics and registration of births and deaths, see *Daily Missoulian*, 30 May 1907, as cited in Philip, "Journalistic View," 156.

5. Wyman to the Secretary of the Treasury, 19 April 1905, file 1266, box 119, Central File, 1897–1923, PHS Records. For biographical information on Francis see *American Men of Science*, 5th ed. (see chap. 3, n. 64), 378; Williams, *United States Public Health Service* (see chap. 3, n. 39), 190–92; and Clark, *Pioneer Microbiologists* (see chap. 3, n. 39), 62, 296–97.

6. *Daily Missoulian*, 11 June 1905, as cited in Philip, "Journalistic View," 146. Francis's investigation was mentioned in the 1905 and 1906 annual reports of the Service, but no report of substance was ever published. See PHMHS, *Annual Report*, 1905, 211; and 1906, 219.

7. Stiles, "Zoological Pitfalls" (see chap. 3, n. 33). The observer was S. Burt Wolbach, whose comment was published in "Studies on Rocky Mountain Spotted Fever," *Journal of Medical Research* 41 (1919):1–197 (quotation from p. 9).

8. Chowning to Ricketts, 15 March 1906; and Ricketts to Chowning, 17 March 1905 (letter misdated; should be 1906), box 8, folder 9, Ricketts Papers.

9. Chowning to Ricketts, 15 March 1906, box 8, folder 9, Ricketts Papers; Lucien P. McCalla, "Direct Transmission from Man to Man of the Rocky Mountain Spotted (Tick) Fever," *Medical Sentinel* 16 (1908):87–88. For biographical information on McCalla see Hammarsten, "Contributions of Idaho Physicians" (see chap. 2, n. 35), 31–33.

10. Howard Taylor Ricketts, *Infection, Immunity, and Serum Therapy* (Chicago: American Medical Association, 1906). For biographical information on

Ricketts, see Pierce C. Mullen's sketch of him in Charles Coulston Gillispie, ed., *Dictionary of Scientific Biography*, 16 vols. (New York: Charles Scribner's Sons, 1970–80), 11 (1975):442–43; William K. Beatty and Virginia L. Beatty, "Howard Taylor Ricketts—Imaginative Investigator," *Proceedings of the Institute of Medicine of Chicago* 34 (1981):46–48; Ludvig Hektoen's memorial address on Ricketts, in Howard T. Ricketts, *Contributions to Medical Science by Howard Taylor Ricketts, 1870–1910* (Chicago: University of Chicago Press, 1911), 3–7; H. Gideon Wells's sketch of him, *DAB* (see chap. 3, n. 6), suppl. 1 (1944), 628–29; Clark, *Pioneer Microbiologists*, 285–91; obituary, *JAMA* 54 (1910):1640. No book-length biography of Ricketts has yet been written. On Ricketts's study with Henry B. Ward, see Edwin F. Hirsch, "The Insect Vector as Transmitter of Disease," *Proceedings of the Institute of Medicine of Chicago* 27 (1969):294. On medical education during this period, see the classic report of Abraham Flexner, *Medical Education in the United States and Canada* (New York: Carnegie Foundation, 1910). An excellent recent study is Kenneth M. Ludmerer, *Learning to Heal: The Development of American Medical Education* (New York: Basic Books, 1985).

11. Spottswood to Ricketts, 10 April 1906; and Ricketts to Tuttle, 29 June 1906, box 8, folder 9, Ricketts Papers; Ricketts's report in MSBH, *Third Biennial Report*, 22–23; William M. Chowning, "Rocky Mountain Spotted Fever: Preliminary Reports," *Journal of the Minnesota State Medical Association and the Northwest Lancet* 27 (1907):101.

12. Williams, *United States Public Health Service*, 261–62; "Science Takes Doctors' Lives: Voluntarily They Assume Risks in Studying Various Forms of Disease," *Boston Herald*, 17 July 1910, clipping in "1909–1911 Scrapbook," box 3, U.S. Public Health Service Scrapbooks, Manuscripts Collection, NLM; PH-MHS, *Annual Report*, 1905, 216–17. Some of the hookworm control methods developed by King, Ashford, and Gutierrez were later adapted by the Rockefeller Hookworm Commission for use in the southern United States.

13. There are virtually no primary records available regarding King's work on spotted fever. His comments on Ricketts were made to a newspaper reporter shortly after Ricketts died of typhus. See "Science Takes Doctors' Lives," cited above.

14. My discussion of these methods follows Paul Clark's summary in *Pioneer Microbiologists*, 96–98.

15. Ricketts to Tuttle, 29 June 1906, box 8, folder 9, Ricketts Papers; MSBH, *Third Biennial Report*, 23–24, 26; Howard Taylor Ricketts, "The Study of 'Rocky Mountain Spotted Fever' (Tick Fever?) by Means of Animal Inoculations," *JAMA* 47 (1906):33. Rabbits were later proven to be susceptible to spotted fever, but they never displayed so marked a reaction as did guinea pigs. See Liborio Gomez, "Rocky Mountain Spotted Fever in the Rabbit," *J. Inf. Dis.* 6 (1909):383–86.

16. *Daily Missoulian*, 15 and 24 May 1906, as cited in Philip, "Journalistic View," 153; MSBH, *Third Biennial Report*, 34.

17. MSBH, *Third Biennial Report*, 24–28; Ricketts to Tuttle, 29 June 1906, box 8, folder 9, Ricketts Papers; Ricketts, "Study of 'Rocky Mountain Spotted Fever' (Tick Fever?) by means of Animal Inoculations," 33–36.

18. A newspaper account stated that "it is feared" Etta Bradley "cannot recover." She did recover, however, and lived in the Bitterroot until her death in 1980. See *Daily Missoulian*, 13 June 1906, as cited in Philip, "Journalistic

View," 155; William L. Jellison, "Jellison Recalls Bradley Contribution," *Ravalli Republic*, 19 November 1980, 9. Robert N. Philip, in a personal communication to the author, 16 February 1988, noted that in 1962, fifty-six years after her illness, Etta Bradley McKinney's blood still produced a complement fixation titer of 1:8.

19. Ricketts to Tuttle, 29 June 1906, box 8, folder 9, Ricketts Papers; MSBH, *Third Biennial Report*, 25–26; Ricketts, "Study of 'Rocky Mountain Spotted Fever' (Tick Fever?) by Means of Animal Inoculations," 34.

20. R. R. Parker, "Certain Phases of the Problem of Rocky Mountain Spotted Fever: A Summary of Present Information," *Archives of Pathology* 15 (1933):398–429 (first demonstration of tick transmission of human disease in United States noted on p. 400); Walter W. King, "Experimental Transmission of Rocky Mountain Spotted Fever by Means of the Tick," *Pub. Health Rep.* 21 (1906):863–64; Ricketts, "The Transmission of Rocky Mountain Spotted Fever by the Bite of the Wood Tick (*Dermacentor occidentalis*)," *JAMA* 47 (1906):358.

21. Ricketts, "Transmission of Rocky Mountain Spotted Fever," 358. The question of scientific priority has always been a sensitive issue. Rolla E. Dyer, himself a distinguished rickettsial investigator and director of the NIH, inserted a handwritten note on King's article—in the copy now held in the NIH library—to reemphasize King's priority to later readers. Dated 12 May 1931, it reads: "W. W. King returned to Hy. Lab. from Montana June 29, 1906. Ricketts fed his first ticks on an infected pig June 19, 1906. Placed them on non-infected pig on June 23, 1906. This pig developed fever June 27, 1906. Therefore the experiments of King and Ricketts must have run concurrently. King certainly started his experiment before Ricketts's experiment was positive. King's publication precedes Ricketts. Therefore, the priority belongs to King—although Ricketts may have first suggested the experiment."

22. Ricketts to Tuttle, 25 June 1906, box 8, folder 9, Ricketts Papers.

23. For example, in 1908, Ricketts refused the request of a Dr. Smith for ticks infected with spotted fever. "It doesn't sound generous," he wrote, but explained that he had reached this position "as a result of some unpleasant experiences which I want to avoid in the future." See Ricketts to Maria B. Maver, 18 June 1908, box 8, folder 11, Ricketts Papers. Walter W. King also noted that Ricketts was "a little given to reticence about results he had obtained until ready to make them public." See "Science Takes Doctors' Lives."

24. "The Transmission of Rocky Mountain Spotted Fever by Ticks," *JAMA* 47 (1906):366.

25. MSBH, *Third Biennial Report*, 34–35; "State Association Meeting," *JAMA* 46 (1906):1704.

26. "The Value of the People of Montana," in MSBH, *Third Biennial Report*, 12–20 (quotations from pp. 18–20); "Investigation of the Cause and Means of Prevention of Rocky Mountain Spotted Fever Carried on During 1907 and 1908 by Dr. Howard Taylor Ricketts of the University of Chicago," in MSBH, *Fourth Biennial Report*, 78.

27. Ricketts to Tuttle, 29 June 1906, box 8, folder 9, Ricketts Papers; MSBH, *Third Biennial Report*, 29.

28. See newspaper requests for citizens to collect ticks for both King and Ricketts in *Western News*, 29 November and 19 December 1906, and *Stevensville Register*, 8 August and 26 December 1906, as cited in Philip, "Journalistic View," 153–54.

29. T. W. Goodspeed to Ricketts, 21 March 1907, box 4, folder 15, Ricketts Papers. Goodspeed was secretary of the University of Chicago Board of Trustees. In a personal communication to the author, 16 February 1988, Robert N. Philip commented on the four nymphal ticks "taken from horses" that Ricketts used for his early experiments: "Very likely these were *D. albipictus* (the elk winter tick), which at that time had not yet been distinguished from '*D. occidentalis*' [actually *D. andersoni*]. *D. albipictus* is a one-host tick, active in the winter time. *D. andersoni* nymphs are seldom active in the winter, and seldom found on large animals. Because it is strictly a one-host tick, *D. albipictus* was never considered to be important in the transmission cycle and hence, to my knowledge, was never tested for its experimental transmission potential by Ralph R. Parker. My father [Cornelius B. Philip] raised this question some years ago." See C. B. Philip and G. M. Kohls, "Elk, Winter Ticks, and Rocky Mountain Spotted Fever: A Query," *Pub. Health Rep.* 66 (1952):1672–75.

30. Ricketts to Hektoen, 4 June 1907, box 8, folder 10, Ricketts papers; Howard Taylor Ricketts, "Observations on the Virus and Means of Transmission of Rocky Mountain Spotted Fever," *J. Inf. Dis.* 4 (1907):141–53.

31. Ricketts to Tuttle, 19 April 1907, box 8, folder 10, Ricketts Papers; Tuttle to Ricketts, 3 May 1907, in Howard Taylor Ricketts, Scrapbook, 39, prepared by his family and deposited in selected libraries. The NLM has a copy. Holden's death on 22 April was reported in the *Western News*, 23 April 1907, as cited in Philip, "Journalistic View," 161.

32. William M. Chowning, "Studies in Rocky Mountain Spotted Fever," *J. Minn. Med. Assn. & Northwest Lancet* 28 (1908):45–49. Chowning included eighteen microphotographs from case studies in this paper, but because of the diversity of the organisms, he did not claim that any particular one caused spotted fever.

33. Ricketts to [Hektoen], n.d., box 8, folder 10, Ricketts Papers. The first page of this letter is missing, but from the context it is clearly addressed to Hektoen.

34. Ricketts to Hektoen, 4 June 1907, box 8, folder 10, Ricketts Papers.

35. King's detachment from the Hygienic Laboratory and detail to San Francisco are noted in the Hygienic Laboratory Register, 30 July and 22 August 1907, U.S. Hygienic Laboratory Registers, 1901–23, Manuscripts Collection, NLM (hereafter cited as Hygienic Laboratory Registers, NLM); his later positions are noted in "Science Takes Doctors' Lives"; PH-MHS, *Annual Report*, 1911, 272.

36. Howard Taylor Ricketts, "A Micro-Organism Which Apparently Has a Specific Relationship to Rocky Mountain Spotted Fever: A Preliminary Report," *JAMA* 52 (1909):379–80. Ricketts also discussed these findings in the Wesley M. Carpenter Lecture at the New York Academy of Medicine. See idem, "Some Aspects of Rocky Mountain Spotted Fever as Shown by Recent Investigations," in idem, *Contributions to Medical Science*, 373–408.

37. Howard Taylor Ricketts, "Spotted Fever Report No. 1: General Report of an Investigation of Rocky Mountain Spotted Fever, Carried on during 1906 and 1907," in MSBH, *Fourth Biennial Report*, 109; idem, "A Summary of Investigations of the Nature and Means of Transmission of Rocky Mountain Spotted Fever," *Transactions of the Chicago Pathological Society* 7 (1907):73–82.

38. Ricketts to Tuttle, 24 June 1909, folder 1, "Rocky Mountain Spotted Fever, 1908–1911," box 1, "General Correspondence," MSBH Records. See also Ricketts, "The Role of the Wood-tick (*Dermacentor occidentalis*) in Rocky Mountain Spotted Fever, and the Susceptibility of Local Animals to This Disease: A Preliminary Report," *JAMA* 49 (1907):24–27; idem, "Further Experiments with the Wood-Tick in Relation to Rocky Mountain Spotted Fever," *JAMA* 49 (1907): 1278–81.

39. Maria B. Maver, "Transmission of Spotted Fever by Other Than Montana and Idaho Ticks," *J. Inf. Dis.* 8 (1911):322–26; idem, "Transmission of Spotted Fever by the Tick in Nature," ibid., 327–29. See also correspondence about these experiments in box 8, folder 12, Ricketts Papers. The common dog tick is known as *Dermacentor variabilis* (Say), the "lone star" tick as *Amblyomma americanum* (Linnaeus), and the Utah rabbit tick as *Dermacentor parumapertus*.

40. Ricketts, "Spotted Fever Report No. 1," 99–100.

41. Ibid., 100–105.

42. Ibid., 120; Ricketts to Tuttle, 23 November 1908, folder 1, "Rocky Mountain Spotted Fever, 1908–1911," box 1, "General Correspondence," MSBH Records.

43. Ricketts, "Spotted Fever Report No. 1," 121–24.

44. Ricketts to Tuttle, 8 January 1908; and Morgan to Ricketts, n.d. but late January 1908, from context, folder 1, "Rocky Mountain Spotted Fever, 1908–1911," box 1, "General Correspondence," MSBH Records; Ricketts, "Spotted Fever Report No. 1," 124.

45. Ricketts, "Spotted Fever Report No. 1," 129–30; Ricketts to Tuttle, 19 January 1908, folder 1, "Rocky Mountain Spotted Fever, 1908–1911," box 1, "General Correspondence," MSBH Records. Montana State College is now called Montana State University.

46. Ricketts to Tuttle, 14 January 1908, folder 1, "Rocky Mountain Spotted Fever, 1908–1911," box 1, "General Correspondence," MSBH Records.

47. Ricketts, "Spotted Fever Report No. 1," 126.

48. Ibid., 126–27.

49. Quotation from ibid., 127; Josiah J. Moore, "Time Relationships of the Wood-Tick in the Transmission of Rocky Mountain Spotted Fever," *J. Inf. Dis.* 8 (1911):339–47.

50. *Western News*, 19 June 1907, as cited in Philip, "Journalistic View," 161; "Investors Flock to the Bitter Root Valley: Exhibition Takes Chicago by Storm!" *Western News*, 13 November 1907, and, on cherries, *Western News*, 5 August 1908, both cited in Philip, "Journalistic View," 157, 164; Tuttle to Ricketts, 23 October 1909; and Ricketts to Tuttle, 9 November 1909, folder 1, "Rocky Mountain Spotted Fever, 1908–1911," box 1, "General Correspondence," MSBH Records.

51. Ricketts to Hektoen, 4 June 1907, box 8, folder 10, Ricketts Papers. For a more complete discussion of these techniques, see George Clark and Frederick H. Kasten, *History of Staining*, 3d ed. (Baltimore: Williams & Wilkins, 1983), esp. 113–17. For a complete statement of Koch's postulates, see chap. 3, n. 22.

52. W. A. Hooker, "A Review of the Present Knowledge of the Role of Ticks in the Transmission of Disease," *Journal of Economic Entomology* 1 (1908):65–76, esp. charts on pp. 68, 69, 74; Rennie W. Doane, *Insects and*

Disease: A Popular Account of the Way in Which Insects May Spread or Cause Some of Our Common Diseases (New York: Henry Holt, 1910), 32.

53. Ricketts, "A Micro-Organism," 379, 380. In this original article, Ricketts gave the dilutions as "up to 1 to 160." This was in error; the actual dilutions were up to 1 to 320. See Ricketts, letter of correction to the editor, *JAMA* 52 (1909): 491.

54. Ricketts, "Some Aspects of Rocky Mountain Spotted Fever as Shown by Recent Investigations," 397–98.

55. Idem, "A Micro-Organism," 380.

56. Ricketts to Tuttle, 25 January 1909, folder 1, "Rocky Mountain Spotted Fever, 1908–1911," box 1, "General Correspondence," MSBH Records; Novy to Ricketts, 6 April 1909; and Chowning to Ricketts, 13 July 1909, box 8, folder 12, Ricketts Papers.

57. Ricketts to Tuttle, 17 March 1909; and Ricketts to Tuttle, 24 June 1909, folder 1, "Rocky Mountain Spotted Fever, 1908–1911," box 1, "General Correspondence," MSBH Records; McCampbell to Ricketts, 22 November 1909, box 8, folder 12, Ricketts Papers.

58. Ricketts to Hektoen, 4 June 1907, box 8, folder 10, Ricketts Papers; Howard Taylor Ricketts and Liborio Gomez, "Studies on Immunity in Rocky Mountain Spotted Fever: First Communication," *J. Inf. Dis.* 5 (1908):221–44 (quotations from p. 235).

59. Ricketts and Gomez, "Studies on Immunity," 224, 236.

60. Ibid., 228–30, 236–42.

61. Ricketts to Tuttle, 17 March 1909; and Ricketts to Tuttle, 24 June 1909, folder 1, "Rocky Mountain Spotted Fever, 1908–1911," box 1, "General Correspondence," MSBH Records.

62. McCampbell to Ricketts, 8 August 1909; Ricketts to Hektoen, 23 December 1909; and Ricketts to S. A. Matthews, 8 October 1909, box 8, folder 12, Ricketts Papers.

63. Ricketts to Hektoen, 4 June 1907, box 8, folder 10, Ricketts Papers.

64. Ricketts and Gomez, "Studies on Immunity," 230–32; Howard Taylor Ricketts, "Spotted Fever Report No. 2: A Report of Investigations Carried on during the Winter of 1907–8 and the Spring and Summer of 1908," in MSBH, *Fourth Biennial Report*, 138–42; Ricketts to Tuttle, 21 March 1908, folder 1, "Rocky Mountain Spotted Fever, 1908–1911," box 1, "General Correspondence," MSBH Records.

65. These cases are discussed in Ricketts, "Spotted Fever Report No. 2," 144–49 (quotation from p. 146).

66. All three recovered cases are identifiable in local press accounts. One paper attributed to the serum the recovery of a case that Ricketts himself never recorded. For all these cases see Philip, "Journalistic View," 167–68.

67. Ricketts to Tuttle, 29 March 1909; and Ricketts to Tuttle, 24 June 1909, folder 1, "Rocky Mountain Spotted Fever, 1908–1911," box 1, "General Correspondence," MSBH Records. The serum sent in 1909 reportedly saved the life of Mrs. Harry H. Townsend, whose grateful husband wrote a letter of appreciation to their perceived benefactor. See *Stevensville Register*, 17 June 1909, as cited in Philip, "Journalistic View," 176; Harry H. Townsend to Ricketts, 31 March 1910, box 8, folder 13, Ricketts Papers.

68. Tuttle to Ricketts, 25 February 1908, folder 1, "Rocky Mountain Spotted Fever, 1908–1911," box 1, "General Correspondence," MSBH Records;

MSBH Minutes, special session, 19 February 1908; Ricketts to Tuttle, 22 October 1908; and [Ricketts and Tuttle], unsigned letter, to E. E. Maxey, 24 October 1908, folder 1, "Rocky Mountain Spotted Fever, 1908–1911," box 1, "General Correspondence," MSBH Records.

69. Tuttle to Ricketts, 5 March 1909; and Ricketts to Tuttle, 17 March 1909, folder 1, "Rocky Mountain Spotted Fever, 1908–1911," box 1, "General Correspondence," MSBH Records. The bill passed the legislature on 4 March.

70. MSBH Minutes, 1 April 1909; Tuttle to Cooley, 22 March 1909, folder 1, "Rocky Mountain Spotted Fever, 1908–1911," box 1, "General Correspondence," MSBH Records.

71. Romney to Tuttle, 25 April 1909; President, Montana Medical Association, to Board of Education, 4 June 1909; and Ricketts to Tuttle, 24 June 1909, folder 1, "Rocky Mountain Spotted Fever, 1908–1911," box 1, "General Correspondence," MSBH Records; *Daily Missoulian*, 14 May 1909, as cited in Philip, "Journalistic View," 176.

72. MSBH Minutes, 1 April 1909. See also correspondence in box 8, folder 12, Ricketts Papers, regarding Ricketts's attempt to discuss this with the state board of examiners when the members of that body went to Chicago in late April 1909.

73. See correspondence in box 4, folder 15, Ricketts Papers, about Ricketts's offers of positions. Ricketts received the gold medal for an exhibit on spotted fever research prepared by his assistant Maria B. Maver. See Ricketts to Maver, 18 June 1908, box 8, folder 11, Ricketts Papers.

74. Preliminary negotiations and financial arrangements for the typhus investigations are documented in box 8, folder 12, and box 4, folder 15, Ricketts Papers; quotation from Ricketts to H. G. Wells, 12 February 1910, box 8, folder 13, Ricketts Papers. On Ricketts's decision to go to Mexico, see also Russell M. Wilder, "The Rickettsial Diseases: Discovery and Conquest," *Arch. Pathol.* 49 (1950):479–89.

75. Charles Nicolle, C. Comte, and E. Conseil, "Transmission expérimentale du typhus exanthématique par le pou du corps," *Comptes Rendus de l'Academie des Sciences* 149 (1909):486–89 (hereafter cited as *Compt. Rend. Acad. d. Sc.*); Wilder, "Rickettsial Diseases," 483–84; John F. Anderson and Joseph Goldberger, "On the Relation of Rocky Mountain Spotted Fever to the Typhus Fever of Mexico: A Preliminary Note," *Pub. Health Rep.* 24 (1909):1861–62; Goldberger to Ricketts, 8 March 1910, Ricketts, Scrapbook, 109; Howard Taylor Ricketts and Russell M. Wilder, "The Etiology of the Typhus Fever (Tabardillo) of Mexico City: A Further Preliminary Report," *JAMA* 54 (1910):1373–75. The entire series of Ricketts's and Wilder's papers on typhus are in Ricketts, *Contributions to Medical Science*, 451–500.

76. Ricketts to Tuttle, 13 February 1910; Ricketts to Tuttle, 12 March 1910; Tuttle to Ricketts, 18 March 1910; and Ricketts to Moore, 14 April 1910, box 8, folder 13, Ricketts Papers.

77. Ricketts to Moore, 14 April 1910; Moore to Ricketts, 13 April 1910; and Ricketts to H. G. Wells, 12 February 1910, box 8, folder 13, Ricketts Papers.

78. Wilder to Tuttle, 25 April 1910, folder 1, "Rocky Mountain Spotted Fever, 1908–1911," box 1, "General Correspondence," MSBH Records. See references to Ricketts's illness in box 8, folder 12, Ricketts Papers. *Daily Missoulian*, 5 May 1910, as cited in Philip, "Journalistic View," 179.

79. Tuttle to Moore, telegram, 4 May 1910; and Wilder to Tuttle, 25 April 1910, folder 1, "Rocky Mountain Spotted Fever, 1908–1911," box 1, "General Correspondence," MSBH Records; Ricketts to Judson, 23 April 1909, box 4, folder 15, Ricketts Papers.

80. P. G. Heinemann and Josiah J. Moore, for example, attempted to develop a more concentrated form of Ricketts's antiserum. The few human trials of its efficacy, however, were inconclusive. See Heinemann and Moore, "The Production and Concentration of a Serum for Rocky Mountain Spotted Fever: Preliminary Note," *JAMA* 57 (1911):198; idem, "Experimental Therapy of Rocky Mountain Spotted Fever: The Preventive and Curative Action of a Serum for Spotted Fever, and the Inefficiency of Sodium Cacodylate as a Curative Agent for This Disease in Guinea Pigs," *J. Inf. Dis.* 10 (1912):294–304. Other work by Ricketts's students and colleagues, published in Ricketts, *Contributions to Medical Science,* will be discussed and cited in later chapters.

81. See correspondence regarding this in box 8, folder 13, Ricketts Papers.

Chapter Five: Tick Eradication Efforts, 1911–1920

1. Cornelius B. Philip and Lloyd E. Rozeboom, "Medico-Veterinary Entomology: A Generation of Progress," in Ray F. Smith, Thomas E. Mittler, and Carroll N. Smith, eds., *History of Entomology* (Palo Alto, Calif.: Annual Reviews, 1973), 333; R. Hoeppli, *Parasites and Parasitic Infections in Early Medicine and Science* (Singapore: University of Malaya Press, 1959), 187–88.

2. Taxonomic systematics are discussed in most textbooks of zoology. My discussion follows that in William B. Herms, *Medical Entomology: With Special Reference to the Health and Well-Being of Man and Animals* (New York: Macmillan, 1939), 29–31, 422–23; and Wolbach's review of the spotted fever tick in his "Studies on Rocky Mountain Spotted Fever" (see chap. 4, n. 7), 46–48. The word *Dermacentor* is derived from the Greek *dermis,* "skin," and *kentor,* "stinger," "pricker," or "goader."

3. Report of Louis B. Wilson and William M. Chowning in MSBH, *First Biennial Report,* 27.

4. Wilson and Chowning, "Studies in Pyroplasmosis Hominis" (see chap. 3, n. 9), 51–52.

5. Stiles, "Zoological Investigation" (see chap. 3, n. 4), 7; King, "Experimental Transmission" (see chap. 4, n. 20), 863; Ricketts, "Role of the Wood-Tick" (see chap. 4, n. 38), 24.

6. Nathan Banks, "A Revision of the Ixodoidea, or Ticks, of the United States," Technical Services, Bureau of Entomology, U.S. Department of Agriculture *Bulletin* no. 15 (1908). The species name *venustus* means "lovely," "charming," or "beautiful."

7. Charles Wardell Stiles, "The Common Tick (*Dermacentor andersoni*) of the Bitter Root Valley," *Pub. Health Rep.* 23 (1908):949; idem, "The Taxonomic Value of the Microscopic Structure of the Stigmal Plates in the Tick Genus Dermacentor," U.S. Hygienic Laboratory *Bulletin* no. 62 (August 1910), 72 pp. and 43 plates; idem, "The Correct Name of the Rocky Mountain Spotted Fever Tick," *JAMA* 55 (1910):1909–10; Nathan Banks, letter to the editor, JAMA 55 (1910): 1574–75.

8. See, for example, MSBE, *First Biennial Report,* 12, 28.

9. "Opinion 78: Case of Dermacentor andersoni vs. Dermacentor venustus," in "Opinions Rendered by the International Commission on Zoological Nomenclature: Opinions 78 to 81," *Smithsonian Miscellaneous Collections* 73, no. 2 (1924):1–14 (quotation from pp. 13–14). The effect of this ruling, however, made *D. venustus* a valid "senior synonym" for *D. andersoni* if the names were applied to a single species. In 1976 an RML entomologist, James E. Keirans, with the support of many of his colleagues, successfully applied to the International Commission on Zoological Nomenclature to have the name *D. venustus* suppressed entirely, so that the name *D. andersoni* alone is now the official name for the Rocky Mountain wood tick. See James E. Keirans, "*Dermacentor venustus* Marx MS. in Neumann, 1897: Proposed Suppression under the Plenary Powers so as to Conserve *Dermacentor andersoni* Stiles, 1908 (Acarina: Ixodidae). Z.N.(S.) 260," *Bulletin of Zoological Nomenclature* 32 (1976):261–64. I am grateful to Dr. Keirans for providing me with a copy of this paper.

10. As late as 1928, for example, L. O. Howard, chief of the U.S. Bureau of Entomology, told delegates to an international congress of entomologists that zoologists, because of their conservatism, had consistently "slighted" entomology. See "Age of Insects, Not Man, Says Dr. L. O. Howard Opening Entomology Congress Here," *Journal-News* (Ithaca, N.Y.), 13 August 1928, clipping in RML Scrapbook "1919–1931."

11. On early entomological research see Gustavus A. Weber, *The Bureau of Entomology: Its History, Activities, and Organization*, Institute for Government Research, Service Monographs of the United States Government no. 60 (Washington, D.C.: Brookings Institution, 1930), 1–13. On insect threats in 1876 see James Harvey Young, "Harper's Weekly on Health in America, 1876," *J. Hist. Med. Allied Sci.* 41 (1986):156–74, esp. 162.

12. Robert H. Wiebe, *The Search for Order, 1877–1920* (New York: Hill & Wang, 1967); William B. Herms, "Medical Entomology, Its Scope and Methods," *J. Econ. Entomol.* 2 (1909):265–68.

13. It has been argued, for example, that veterinarian Fred L. Kilbourne was slighted in the allocation of credit for the Texas cattle fever tick transmission experiments because his physician-supervisor, Theobald Smith, claimed first-author privilege on their classic report. See J. F. Smithcors, "Discovery of the Arthropod Vector of Disease," *Modern Veterinary Practice* 62 (1981):371–74.

14. Tuttle to Wyman, 2 March 1911; and Thomas B. McClintic, "Memorandum Relative to Investigations of Rocky Mountain Spotted Fever," 5 July 1911, file 1266, box 119, Central File, 1897–1923, PHS Records; PH-MHS, *Annual Report*, 1911, 40–42.

15. Biographical information on McClintic is taken from his personnel file, Record Group 090–78, Accession no. 0001, Agency Box no. OF, Records Center Location no. FU#134867 through FU#134992, box # 77, NARA, Saint Louis (hereafter cited as McClintic personnel file, NARA, Saint Louis); Blue to F. M. Wilmot, 25 November 1912, in ibid.; McClintic, "Memorandum Relative to Investigations."

16. McClintic to Wyman, 5 July 1911, file 1266, box 119, Central File, 1897–1923, PHS Records.

17. McClintic to Wyman, 7 July 1911, file 1266, box 119, Central File, 1897–1923, PHS Records.

18. For biographical information on Cooley see his curriculum vitae, file "Zoology and Entomology Bibliography," Archives Department, Renne Library, Montana State University, Bozeman; obituary by Glen M. Kohls, *J. Econ. Entomol.* 62 (1969):972. For a history of the development of entomology as a graduate program at Massachusetts Agricultural College, see *Entomology and Zoology at the Massachusetts Agricultural College* (Amherst, Mass.: Massachusetts Agricultural College, 1911) (esp. Warren E. Hinds's article by the same title), 15–27. This institution later became the University of Massachusetts.

19. Robert A. Cooley, "Notes on Spotted Fever," manuscript, 1953, in RML Scrapbook "1942–   "; idem, "Preliminary Report on the Wood Tick, *Dermacentor sp.*," Montana Agricultural Experiment Station *Bulletin* no. 75 (1909):95–104. Ricketts to Tuttle, 9 November 1908, folder 1, "Rocky Mountain Spotted Fever, 1908–1911," box 1, "General Correspondence," MSBH Records; Cooley to Tuttle, 16 November 1908, vol. "W. F. Cogswell, A. H. McCray, T. D. Tuttle," CC.

20. The results of the tick survey were published in F. C. Bishopp, "The Distribution of the Rocky Mountain Spotted Fever Tick," U.S. Bureau of Entomology *Circular* no. 136 (1911); W. D. Hunter and F. C. Bishopp, "The Rocky Mountain Spotted Fever Tick, with Special Reference to the Problem of Its Control in the Bitter Root Valley in Montana," U.S. Bureau of Entomology *Bulletin* no. 105 (1911). On the history of the Bureau of Biological Survey, see Jenks Cameron, *The Bureau of Biological Survey: Its History, Activities, and Organization*, Institute for Government Research Service Monographs of the United States Government no. 54 (Baltimore: Johns Hopkins Press, 1929).

21. Cooley, "Notes on Spotted Fever," 2–3. Price relates the anecdote in more detail in *Fighting Spotted Fever* (see chap. 3, n. 4), 74–76. Birdseye succeeded in publishing as first author of one paper and as junior author of another, but King did not. His work, although acknowledged, appeared in 1911 under the authorship of Cooley and representatives of the Bureau of Entomology. See citations in n. 22, 24, and 27 below. King wrote to Cooley about Bishopp's claiming of first-author status in King to Cooley, 23 December 1912, vol. "W. V. King," CC.

22. Robert A. Cooley, "Tick Control in Relation to the Rocky Mountain Spotted Fever: A Report of Cooperative Investigations Conducted by the Bureau of Entomology and the Montana Experiment Station," Montana Agricultural College Experiment Station *Bulletin* no. 85 (1911):18–19.

23. Ibid., 20. Although the men noted that they used a "woolen" cloth, flannel was soon adopted to flag ticks because it is much lighter and easier to handle. Game Warden J. L. DeHart reminded Cooley in 1914 about "the wanton slaughter of game in 1910 by Mr. Birdseye's party." See DeHart to Cooley, 7 August 1914, vol. "Montana State Officials," CC.

24. Cooley, "Tick Control," 20–27; Cooley to W. E. McMurry, 17 January 1911, vol. "Montana State Officials," CC; W. H. Henshaw and Clarence Birdseye, "The Mammals of the Bitter Root Valley, Montana and Their Relation to Spotted Fever," U.S. Bureau of Biological Survey *Bulletin* no. 82 (1911).

25. See correspondence regarding this in vol. "W. F. Cogswell, A. H. McCray, T. D. Tuttle," CC.

26. Cooley to Norris, 13 October 1910; and Cooley to McMurry, 17 January 1911, vol. "Montana State Officials"; Cooley to H. T. Fernald, 4 May 1911, vol. "Professors at Various Universities"; and Cooley to W. D. Hunter, 23 May 1911, vol. "W. F. Cogswell, A. H. McCray, T. D. Tuttle," CC (quotation from Cooley to McMurry).

27. Cooley, "Notes on Spotted Fever," 3; Clarence Birdseye, "Some Common Mammals of Western Montana in Relation to Agriculture and Spotted Fever," U.S. Department of Agriculture *Farmer's Bulletin* no. 484 (1912).

28. Cooley, "Notes on Spotted Fever," 4. According to the entomologists' version of this larger controversy, Tuttle later made outrageous and false charges about the dangerous conditions under which this experiment was conducted. See Cooley to King, 13 May 1912, vol. "W. V. King," CC; King to Cooley, 3 May 1912, file 1266, box 119, Central File, 1897–1923, PHS Records.

29. Cooley, "Tick Control," 27–28; Thomas D. Tuttle, untitled statement opposing Cooley's independent work, n.d., folder 1, "Rocky Mountain Spotted Fever, 1908–1911," box 1, "General Correspondence," MSBH Records.

30. MSBH Minutes, 5 June 1911.

31. Thomas D. Tuttle, untitled statement opposing Cooley's independent work (see n. 29 above); MSBH Minutes, 24 July 1911.

32. King to Cooley, 3 May 1912; and Cooley to King, 13 May 1912, vol. "W. V. King," CC; MSBH Minutes, 6 June 1911; Montana State Archives. Howard to Cooley, 29 May 1911, vol. "W. F. Cogswell, A. H. McCray, T. D. Tuttle," CC.

33. Thomas B. McClintic, "Investigations of and Tick Eradication in Rocky Mountain Spotted Fever: A Report of Work Done on Spotted Fever in Cooperation with the State Board of Health of Montana," *Pub. Health Rep.* 27 (1912):732–60.

34. Ibid., 734.

35. Ibid., 735; H. W. Graybill, "Methods of Exterminating the Texas Fever Ticks," U.S. Department of Agriculture *Farmer's Bulletin* no. 378 (1909). After the Florence vat was dynamited in 1913, it was replaced by a galvanized iron vat.

36. McClintic, "Investigations and Tick Eradication," 735–36.

37. Ibid., 736–38.

38. Ibid., 733–34; Harden, *Inventing the NIH* (see chap. 3, n. 35), 27–39; Manfred Waserman, "The Quest for a National Health Department in the Progressive Era," *Bull. Hist. Med.* 49 (1975):353–80; George Rosen, "The Committee of One Hundred on National Health and the Campaign for a National Health Department, 1906–1912," *American Journal of Public Health* 62 (1972):261–63.

39. Entry dated 21 November 1911, Hygienic Laboratory Registers, NLM; Harden, *Inventing the NIH*, 38–39; *An Act to Change the Name of the Public Health and Marine Hospital Service, to Increase the Pay of Officers of Said Service, and for Other Purposes*, 14 August 1912, 37 *Stat. L.* 309.

40. Various secondary sources contain conflicting accounts of McClintic's marriage and death from spotted fever. My account is based largely on a letter seeking a pension for McClintic's widow and initialed by Service administrators who knew McClintic personally: Andrew Mellon to Harold Knutson, 5 February 1930, McClintic personnel file, NARA, Saint Louis.

41. McClintic, "Investigations and Tick Eradication," 746–47; L. D. Fricks, ed., "Rocky Mountain Spotted Fever: Some Investigations Made During 1912 by Passed Asst. Surg. T. B. McClintic," *Pub. Health Rep.* 29 (1914):1008–20.

42. Fricks, ed., "Rocky Mountain Spotted Fever: McClintic," 1012, 1019–20; McClintic, "Investigations and Tick Eradication," 744–46. Experiments with coyotes and domestic cats gave inconclusive results.

43. McClintic, "Investigations and Tick Eradication," 740–42; Fricks, ed., "Rocky Mountain Spotted Fever: McClintic," 1012–19.

44. Fricks, ed., "Rocky Mountain Spotted Fever: McClintic," 1009–12.

45. Andrew Mellon to Harold Knutson, 5 February 1930, McClintic personnel file, NARA, Saint Louis; "Specialist Dies on Day of Arrival at Washington," *Northwest Tribune*, 16 August 1912; "Dr. McClintic Dies after Long Journey," *Western News*, 16 August 1912; "Spotted Fever," *Western News*, 3 September 1912.

46. For biographical information on Fricks see Williams, *United States Public Health Service* (see chap. 3, n. 39), 195, 296, 302, 545, 559; Fricks's personnel file, Record Group 090–78, Accession no. 0001, Agency Box no. OF, Records Center Location no. FU#134867 through FU#134992, box # 41, NARA, Saint Louis; "Takes Up Study of the Deadly Spotted Fever Bearing Tick: Passed Assistant Surgeon L. D. Fricks Designated to Resume Work of Dr. McClintic, Who Caught Malady While Investigating It, and Died," clipping, n.d., RML Scrapbook "1919–1931."

47. Price, *Fighting Spotted Fever*, 96–97; MSBE, *First Biennial Report*, 6; *An Act to Create the State Board of Entomology. To Define its Powers and Duties and Appropriate Money Therefor*, cited in MSBE, *First Biennial Report*, 5.

48. Tuttle obituary in *Montana Record Herald* (Helena), 9 July 1942. During World War I, Tuttle served as director of medical administration at the cantonments of Fort Lewis and Bremerton, Washington; later he held a post at the U.S. Veterans Hospital at Saint Paul, Minnesota. He died on 24 June 1942 at age seventy-three from heart disease.

49. Tuttle to W. C. Rucker, 23 September 1913, file 1266, box 119, Central File, 1897–1923, PHS Records. For biographical information on Cogswell see John S. Anderson, "A Strange Disease in a Beautiful Land," *Treasure State Health*, Fall 1976, 13–16; obituary in *JAMA* 161 (1956):1494.

50. MSBH Minutes, 16 December 1912; Price, *Fighting Spotted Fever*, 96–97.

51. Price, *Fighting Spotted Fever*, 98–103; Hunter to Cooley, 31 March 1913, folder 2, "Rocky Mountain Spotted Fever, 1912–1919," box 1, "General Correspondence," MSBH Records.

52. W. V. King, "Work of Bureau of Entomology against Spotted Fever Tick in Co-operation with Board," in MSBE, *First Biennial Report*, 18; Fricks to Montana State Board of Entomology, 14 May 1915, vol. "Montana State Officials," CC; "Start War on Wood Tick," *Northwest Tribune*, 18 April 1913.

53. Robert A. Cooley, "Communication from the State Entomologist to the State Board of Entomology," n.d., folder E1, "Rocky Mountain Spotted Fever—Research and Control (R. A. Cooley), 1909–1916," box 10, ZEA.

54. Fricks to Blue, 15 September 1913; and Howard to Blue, 20 August 1913, file 1266, box 119, Central File, 1897–1923, PHS Records.

55. Blue to Howard; and memorandum for the Secretary, signed Rupert Blue, 29 September 1913, file 1266, box 119, Central File, 1897–1923, PHS Records.

56. Unsigned letter to Fricks, 16 September 1913, file 1266, box 119, Central File, 1897–1923, PHS Records. The writer appears to have been Surgeon General Rupert Blue.

57. L. D. Fricks, "Rocky Mountain Spotted Fever: A Report of Its Investigation and of Work in Tick Eradication for Its Control During 1913," *Pub. Health Rep.* 29 (1914):449–61 (strength of dipping solutions is discussed on p. 452); Price, *Fighting Spotted Fever*, 107.

58. Price, *Fighting Spotted Fever*, 107–9. On the official ban against compensation from state funds, see Butler to Cooley, 22 July 1915, vol. "Montana State Officials"; also letters regarding compensation in vol. "Numerous Persons in the Bitterroot Valley," CC.

59. Known as the "Laboratory Dip," the improved formula had been worked out by a South African researcher and included arsenite of soda, soft soap, kerosene, and water. See King, "Work of Bureau of Entomology," 20.

60. These incidents are briefly covered in Price, *Fighting Spotted Fever*, 111–13. They received scant mention in the press and in official archival correspondence. See, for example, "Dipping Vats Destroyed," *Northwest Tribune*, 20 June 1913, which reported that John Dunbar had been charged with destroying the vat on the James Dunbar ranch northwest of Hamilton. Prosecution of Dunbar is mentioned only briefly in D. M. Kelly to Cooley, 12 September 1913, vol. "Montana State Officials"; and destruction of the Florence vat is mentioned but not described in Cooley to J. D. Taylor, 24 June 1913, vol. "Numerous Persons in the Bitterroot Valley," CC. There is no discussion of either incident in the files of the National Archives or in any official publications. Robert N. Philip, however, in a personal communication to the author, 16 February 1988, illuminated the incident of the dynamiting of the Florence vat. His information was based on an interview he conducted on 20 February 1986, with Carl Wemple, who had survived spotted fever after a prolonged illness. The boys' father, Philip stated, denied having had anything to do with the dynamiting.

61. Cooley to King, 1 August 1913, vol. "W. V. King"; and C. H. Stevens to Cooley, 3 August 1913, vol. "Montana State Officials," CC; King, "Work of Bureau of Entomology," 17–18.

62. Fricks, "Rocky Mountain Spotted Fever: A Report, 1913," 455; King, "Work of the Bureau of Entomology," 23.

63. King, "Work of the Bureau of Entomology," 19–23; Fricks, "Rocky Mountain Spotted Fever: A Report, 1913," 451.

64. L. D. Fricks, "Rocky Mountain Spotted (or Tick) Fever: Sheep Grazing as a Possible Means of Controlling the Wood Tick (Dermacentor andersoni) in the Bitter Root Valley," *Pub. Health Rep.* 28 (1913):1647–53 (quotation from p. 1649); King to Cooley, 6 November 1915; and Cooley to King, 19 November 1915, vol. "W. V. King," CC.

65. Fricks, "Rocky Mountain Spotted Fever: A Report, 1913," 454.

66. Idem, "Rocky Mountain Spotted (or Tick) Fever: Sheep Grazing," 1647–49, 1653; idem, "Rocky Mountain Spotted Fever: A Report, 1913," 455.

67. Idem, "Rocky Mountain Spotted Fever: A Report, 1913," 456; idem, "Rocky Mountain Spotted (or Tick) Fever: Sheep Grazing," 1653.

68. W. V. King, "Report on the Investigation and Control of the Rocky Mountain Spotted Fever Tick in Montana During 1915–1916," in MSBE, *Second Biennial Report*, 23; King to Cooley, 6 November 1915, vol. "W. V. King," CC.

69. "Bitter Root Sheep Come to the Rescue," *Western News*, 14 April 1914; "Sheep Death on Ticks, Experiments Prove," ibid., 8 May 1914.

70. Smith and Kilbourne, "Investigations into Texas or Southern Cattle Fever" (see chap. 3, n. 21).

71. Fricks, "Rocky Mountain Spotted Fever: A Report, 1913," 452–53.

72. Cooley to R. R. Parker, 24 May 1915, vol. "R. R. Parker, 1913–1917," CC.

73. Tabulation of spotted fever cases in Montana by county, 1915, n.d., vol. "W. F. Cogswell, A. H. McCray, T. D. Tuttle," CC; Robert A. Cooley, "Control of the Rocky Mountain Spotted Fever Tick in Montana," in MSBE, *Second Biennial Report*, 6; "Report 18 Cases of Spotted Fever," *Western News*, 18 May 1915.

74. R. R. Spencer, "The Fleas, the Ticks, Spotted Fever, and Me," *Saturday Review* 46 (2 November 1963):48. Spencer's background will be discussed in detail in chap. 7.

75. For biographical information on Parker see Victor H. Haas, "Ralph R. Parker: 1888–1949," *Science* 111 (1950):56–57; *American Men of Science*, 5th ed. (see chap. 3, n. 64), 857; *Who's Who in America: A Biographical Dictionary of Notable Living Men and Women*, 1938–39 (Chicago: Marquis-Who's Who, 1939), 1935; "Ralph R. Parker," in Jeanette Barry, comp., *Notable Contributions to Medical Research by Public Health Service Scientists: A Bibliography to 1940* (Washington, D.C.: Government Printing Office, 1960), 63–65.

76. Cooley to Fernald, 10 March 1914; and Fernald to Cooley, 17 March 1914, vol. "Professors at Various Universities," CC; MSBE, *First Biennial Report*, 32–34; R. R. Parker and R. W. Wells, "Some Facts of Importance Concerning the Rocky Mountain Spotted Fever Tick (Dermacentor venustus Banks) in Eastern Montana," in MSBE, *Second Biennial Report*, 45–56; R. R. Parker, "Second Report on Investigations of the Rocky Mountain Spotted Fever Tick in Eastern Montana," in MSBE, *Third Biennial Report*, 41–54. During his 1917 work, Parker was assisted by young Harold C. Urey, who in 1934 won a Nobel prize in chemistry.

77. "Regulations of the Montana State Board of Entomology," in MSBE, *Second Biennial Report*, 11; Fricks to Montana State Board of Entomology, 8 November 1916, vol. "Montana State Officials"; Cooley to King, 16 December 1916; and King to Cooley, 26 and 31 December 1916, vol. "W. V. King," CC; Fricks to Blue, 4 December 1916, file 1266, box 119, Central File, 1897–1923, PHS Records.

78. Fricks to Cooley, 1 February 1917, folder 2, "Rocky Mountain Spotted Fever, 1912–1919," box 1, "General Correspondence," MSBH Records.

79. Malburn to Stewart, 12 December 1916; Cogswell to Malburn, 27 December 1916; and McAdoo to Cogswell, 10 January 1917, folder 2, "Rocky Mountain Spotted Fever, 1912–1919," box 1, "General Correspondence," MSBH Records.

80. Fricks to Blue, 9 April 1917; Blue to Fricks, 24 April 1917; Blue to Cogswell, 24 April 1917; and "Tick Quarantine in Valley Lifted by State

Board," clipping from *Daily Missoulian*, n.d., file 1266, box 119, Central File, 1897–1923, PHS Records; "Tick Quarantine Is Lifted along the West Side," *Western News*, 12 April 1917.

81. Cooley to Rankin, 17 July 1917; and Secretary of Agriculture David F. Houston to Rankin, 12 September 1917, vol. "Montana State Officials," CC.

82. Cooley to S. Burt Wolbach, 26 February 1918, vol. "Professors at Various Universities," CC. On Parker's work at Harvard and an illness he suffered during this period, see his correspondence with Cooley from August through November 1917, vol. "R. R. Parker, 1913–1917"; and Parker to Cooley, 12 and 30 March 1918, vol. "R. R. Parker, 1918–1919," CC.

83. Parker to Cooley, 25 April 1918, vol. "R. R. Parker, 1918–1919," CC; "Controlling the Tick," *Western News*, 6 March 1919; Robert A. Cooley, "Control Methods in Use," in MSBE, *Third Biennial Report*, 6; R. R. Parker, "Report of Tick Control Operations in the Bitter Root Valley during the Season of 1918, Facts in Connection Therewith; Recommendations for the Further Prosecution of the Work," in MSBE, *Third Biennial Report*, 25–40; R. R. Parker, "Report of Tick Control Operations in the Bitter Root Valley during the Seasons of 1919 and 1920," in MSBE, *Fourth Biennial Report*, 18–44.

84. Parker to Cooley, 27 January 1919; and correspondence in April 1919 between Parker and Cooley on stock owners' opposition to grazing restrictions, vol. "R. R. Parker, 1918–1919," CC; Robert A. Cooley, "Results," in MSBE, *Third Biennial Report*, 10–11, 17.

85. Robert A. Cooley, introductory remarks in MSBE, *Fourth Biennial Report*, 5; idem, in *Fifth Biennial Report*, 4; Price, *Fighting Spotted Fever*, 169. The Montana State Board of Entomology did not publish a report to cover the year 1921.

86. Robert A. Cooley, letter of transmittal, in MSBE, *Fourth Biennial Report*, 4. The possible extermination of the mountain goat was first proposed in Cooley, "Control Methods," 7. See also idem, "The Goat Question," press release, 18 September 1923, folder E4, "Rocky Mountain Spotted Fever and General and Miscellaneous Health Services, 1925–1946," box 10, ZEA; "The Mountain Goat or the Taxpayers Goat," *Northwest Tribune*, 12 October 1923, clipping in RML Scrapbook "1919–1931."

87. Cogswell to Surgeon General Cumming, telegram, 22 June 1921, cited in Price, *Fighting Spotted Fever*, 169; "Spotted Fever Causes 2 Deaths," *Western News*, 9 June 1921; "Tyler Worden of Missoula Dies," *Western News*, 16 June 1921. I am grateful to Robert N. Philip for information about the epidemiology of the 1921 cases.

Chapter Six: A Wholly New Type of Microorganism

1. For a statement of Koch's postulates, see chap. 3, n. 22; see also Victoria A. Harden, "Koch's Postulates and the Etiology of Rickettsial Diseases," *J. Hist. Med. Allied Sci.* 42 (1987):277–95.

2. E. R. LeCount, "A Contribution to the Pathological Anatomy of Rocky Mountain Spotted Fever," *J. Inf. Dis.* 8 (1911):421–26 (quotations from pp. 422, 423, 424).

3. On Councilman and Mallory see Esmond R. Long, *A History of American Pathology* (Springfield, Ill.: Charles C. Thomas, 1962), 153–55. For biographical information on Wolbach see Charles A. Janeway, "S. Burt Wolbach, 1880–

1954," *Trans. Assn. Am. Physicians* 67 (1954):30–35; Shields Warren, "Simeon Burt Wolbach, 3rd July 1880–19th March 1954," *Journal of Pathology and Bacteriology* 68 (1954):656–57; Sidney Farber and Charlotte L. Maddock, "S. Burt Wolbach, M.D., 1880–1954," *A.M.A. Archives of Pathology* 59 (1955):624–30; "S. Burt Wolbach," in Esmond R. Long, *History of the American Society for Experimental Pathology* (Bethesda, Md.: American Society for Experimental Pathology, 1972), 89–90; "Dr. S. B. Wolbach, Pathologist, Dies," *New York Times*, 20 March 1954; Jeffrey D. Hubbard, "S. Burt Wolbach, M.D., 1880–1954," *Pediatric Pathology* 7 (1987):507–14. I am grateful to Dr. Hubbard for providing me with a preprint of his paper.

4. Wolbach, "Studies on Rocky Mountain Spotted Fever," 55, as cited in chap. 4, n. 7.

5. For biographical information on Noguchi see Isabel R. Plesset, *Noguchi and His Patrons* (Rutherford, N.J.: Fairleigh Dickinson University Press, 1980); Gustav Eckstein, *Noguchi* (New York: Harper, 1931); Paul Franklin Clark, "Hideyo Noguchi, 1876–1928," *Bull. Hist. Med.* 33 (1959):18–19. My discussion of Noguchi's early spotted fever work follows Plesset, *Noguchi*, 166–73.

6. Hideyo Noguchi, *Snake Venoms: An Investigation of Venomous Snakes with Special Reference to the Phenomena of Their Venoms* (Washington, D.C.: Carnegie Institution of Washington, 1909); idem, "A Method for the Pure Cultivation of Pathogenic Treponema Pallidum (*Spirocheta pallida*)," *Journal of Experimental Medicine* 14 (1911):99–108; Plesset, *Noguchi*, 166; Noguchi to Fricks, 15 February 1916, file "S. F. History (Correspondence with Noguchi, 1916)," RML Research Records. Tsutsugamushi is discussed in more detail later in this chapter.

7. L. D. Fricks, "Rocky Mountain Spotted Fever: A Report of Laboratory Investigations of the Virus," *Pub. Health Rep.* 31 (1916):516–21, reprinted in MSBE, *Second Biennial Report*, 28–34 (quotations from the latter, p. 33).

8. Wolbach to Cogswell, 21 February 1916, folder 2, "Rocky Mountain Spotted Fever, 1912–1919," box 1, "General Correspondence," MSBH Records; Wolbach to Cooley, 21 February and 21 April 1916; Cooley to Wolbach, telegram, 1 March, and letter, 8 June 1916, vol. "Professors at Various Universities"; and Cogswell to Wolbach, 29 April 1916, vol. "W. F. Cogswell, A. H. McCray, T. D. Tuttle," CC.

9. "I hastened into print," Wolbach confided in a letter to Fricks, "because of Noguchi's competition." See Wolbach to Fricks, 21 April 1916, file "S. F. History (Correspondence with Wolbach—1916)," RML Research Records.

10. Wolbach to Cooley, 14 November 1916, vol. "Professors at Various Universities," CC.

11. S. Burt Wolbach, "The Etiology of Rocky Mountain Spotted Fever (A Preliminary Report)," *J. Med. Res.* 34 (1916):121–25 (quotations from pp. 122–23), reprinted in MSBE, *Second Biennial Report*, 35–44; idem, "The Etiology of Rocky Mountain Spotted Fever: Occurrence of the Parasite in the Tick (Second Preliminary Report)," *J. Med. Res.* 35 (1916):147–50.

12. Plesset, *Noguchi*, 170–71; Noguchi to Fricks, 16 October 1916, file "S. F. History (Correspondence with Noguchi—1916)," RML Research Records.

13. Wolbach to Cooley, 13 May 1918, vol. "Professors at Various Universities," CC.

14. McCoy to Fricks, 1 May and 12 June 1916, file "S. F. History (Correspondence, McCoy and Fricks—General—1916)," RML Research Records.

15. Wolbach to Cooley, 13 December 1916, vol. "Professors at Various Universities," CC.

16. S. Burt Wolbach, "The Etiology and Pathology of Rocky Mountain Spotted Fever: The Occurrence of the Parasite and the Pathology of the Disease in Man; Additional Notes on the Parasite (Third Preliminary Report)," *J. Med. Res.* 37 (1918):499–508 (quotation from p. 501).

17. Ibid.; Wolbach to Chairmen of the State Boards of Entomology and Health, 18 January 1918, vol. "Professors at Various Universities," CC (quotation from the letter).

18. Wolbach to Cooley, 20 February 1918, vol. "Professors at Various Universities," CC.

19. Parker to Cooley, 4 June 1918, vol. "R. R. Parker, 1918–1919"; and Wolbach to Cooley, 2 November 1918, vol. "Professors at Various Universities," CC.

20. My discussion of Molinscek's illness is based on his hospital report, folder "Molinscek," box 20, Record Group no. 210.3, Rockefeller University Archives, New York; and on Plesset's discussion of the accident in *Noguchi*, 173.

21. The records on Molinscek's death also provide an interesting view of legal and societal attitudes toward institutional responsibility for the families of people who died from laboratory-acquired infections. Under the New York labor laws in force at the time of Molinscek's death, the Rockefeller Institute had no legal responsibility to provide financial remuneration to his wife and daughter, both named Mary. As the institute's attorney advised its officials, however, there was a "moral obligation" to do so, and failure to provide something might precipitate "attacks from persons hostile to the Institute." Consequently, the board of trustees settled a pension on Molinscek's family that was more liberal than prevailing Workmen's Compensation requirements for deaths covered by the law. See copies of the final financial arrangement approved by members of the Executive Committee of the Board of Scientific Directors of the Rockefeller Institute dated 29 June 1918, folder "Molinscek," box 20, Record Group no. 210.3, Rockefeller University Archives, New York.

22. Wolbach, "Studies on Rocky Mountain Spotted Fever," 83, 87 (see chap. 4, n. 7).

23. Ibid., 84.

24. E. V. Cowdry, "The Distribution of Rickettsia in the Tissues of Insects and Arachnids," *J. Exp. Med.* 37 (1923):431–56 (quotation from pp. 431–32). The first major work on the laboratory regulation of acidity levels, or pH, was William Mansfield Clark, *The Determination of Hydrogen Ions: An Elementary Treatise on the Hydrogen Electrode, Indicators, and Supplementary Methods, with an Indexed Bibliography on Applications* (Baltimore: Williams & Wilkins Co., 1920).

25. Fricks consistently denied that the two organisms were the same. When the Montana State Board of Entomology published the two reports side by side, Fricks complained. "I wish to disclaim any connection with the bacillus first reported by Prof. Wolbach, and at the same time remind the Board that the small, double granules or protozoan bodies" were "first described by me."

See Fricks to the Montana State Board of Entomology, 29 March 1917, vol. "Montana State Officials," CC.

26. Harry Plotz, "The Etiology of Typhus Fever (and of Brill's Disease)," *JAMA* 62 (1914):1556; Henrique da Rocha Lima, "Beobachtungen bei Fleck-typhusläusen," *Archiv für Schiffs- und Tropen-Hygiene* 21 (1916):17–31; Henrique da Rocha Lima, "Zur Aetiologie des Fleckfiebers," *Berl. klin. Wchnschr.* 53 (1916):567–72, Eng. trans. in Nicholas Hahon, ed., *Selected Papers on the Pathogenic Rickettsiae* (Cambridge, Mass.: Harvard University Press, 1968), 74–78 (quotation from pp. 76–77). Da Rocha Lima's articles on typhus are also reproduced in Henrique da Rocha Lima, *Estudos sôbre o Tifo Exantemático*, comp. Edgard de Cerqueira Falcão, with commentary by Otto G. Bier (São Paulo, Brazil, 1966).

27. Wolbach, "Studies on Rocky Mountain Spotted Fever," 87–88.

28. A. Conor and A. Bruch, "Une Fièvre éruptive observée en Tunisie," *Bulletin de la Société de Pathologie Exotique et de Ses Filiales* 3 (1910):492–96 (hereafter cited as *Bull. Soc. Path. Exotique*), Eng. trans. in Hahon, ed., *Selected Papers*, 47–52 (quotations from pp. 47–48).

29. Nathan E. Brill, "A Study of 17 Cases of a Disease Clinically Resembling Typhoid Fever, but without the Widal Reaction," *New York Medical Journal* 67 (1898):48–54, 77–82; idem, "An Acute Infectious Disease of Unknown Origin: A Clinical Study Based on 221 Cases," *Am. J. Med. Sci.* 139 (1910):484–502.

30. José F. Sant'Anna, "On a Disease in Man Following Tick Bites and Occurring in Lourenço Marques," *Parasitology* 4 (1911):87–88.

31. George H. F. Nuttall, "On Symptoms Following Tick-Bites in Man," *Parasitology* 4 (1911):89–93.

32. J. G. McNaught, "Paratyphoid Fevers in South Africa," *Journal of the Royal Army Medical Corps* 16 (1911):505–14.

33. J. W. D. Megaw, "A Case of Fever Resembling Brill's Disease," *Indian Medical Gazette* 52 (1917):15–18 (quotation from p. 18..

34. Oliver Smithson, "Mossman Fever," *Journal of Tropical Medicine and Hygiene* 13 (1910):351–52. A review of reports from the Federated Malay States is in William Fletcher, "Typhus-Like Fevers of Unknown Etiology, with Special Reference to the Malay States," *Proceedings of the Royal Society of Medicine* 23 (1930):1021–27 (discussion, pp. 1027–30).

35. My discussion follows Francis G. Blake, Kenneth F. Maxcy, J. F. Sadusk, G. M. Kohls, and E. J. Bell, "Studies on Tsutsugamushi Disease (Scrub Typhus, Mite-Borne Typhus) in New Guinea and Adjacent Islands: Epidemiology, Clinical Observations, and Etiology in the Dobadura Area," *American Journal of Hygiene* 41 (1945):243–72; J. R. Audy, *Red Mites and Typhus* (London: Athlone Press, 1968); and Rinya Kawamura, "Studies on Tsutsugamushi Dis-ease," College of Medicine of the University of Cincinnati *Medical Bulletin* 4 (1926), special nos. 1, 2.

36. Percy M. Ashburn and Charles F. Craig, "Comparative Study of Tsut-sugamushi Disease and Spotted or Tick Fever of Montana," *Boston Medical and Surgical Journal* 159 (1908):749–61.

37. The three initial papers describing trench fever were H. Töpfer, "Zur Aetiologie des 'Febris Wolhynica,'" *Berl. klin. Wchnschr.* 53 (1916):323; idem, "Der Fleckfiebererreger in der Laus," *Deutsche Medizinische Wochenschrift* 42 (1916):1251–54 (hereafter cited as *Deutsche med. Wchnschr.*); and idem,

"Zur Ursache und Übertragung des Wolhynischen Fiebers," *Muenchener Medizinische Wochenschrift* 63 (1916):1495–96. For reviews of trench fever research written shortly after World War I, see David Bruce, "Trench Fever: Final Report of the War Office Trench Fever Investigation Committee," *Journal of Hygiene* 20 (1921):258–88; American Red Cross Medical Research Committee, *Trench Fever: Report of Commission, Medical Research Committee, American Red Cross,* by Richard P. Strong (Oxford: Oxford University Press, 1918); H. F. Swift, "Trench Fever," *Archives of Internal Medicine* 26 (1920):76–98.

38. "Typhus Fever and Plague in Central Europe," *JAMA* 99 (1932):1369.

39. The report of their work is in League of Red Cross Societies, Typhus Research Commission to Poland, *The Etiology and Pathology of Typhus,* by S. Burt Wolbach, John L. Todd, and Francis W. Palfrey (Cambridge, Mass.: League of Red Cross Societies, Harvard University Press, 1922) (hereafter cited as Wolbach, Todd, and Palfrey, *Etiology and Pathology of Typhus*).

40. Parker to Cooley, 14 October 1919; and Parker to Wolbach, 2 December 1919, vol. "R. R. Parker, 1918–1919," CC. Parker's illness is referred to variously as influenza and pneumonia; it may well have been a combination. See vol. "R. R. Parker, 1920," CC.

41. Wolbach to Cooley, 26 August 1920, vol. "Professors at Various Universities," CC. On Bacot see J. C. G. Ledingham, "In Memoriam: Arthur W. Bacot, F. E. S.," *British Journal of Experimental Pathology* 3 (1922):117–24.

42. Wolbach, Todd, and Palfrey, *Etiology and Pathology of Typhus,* 3.

43. Wolbach, "Studies on Rocky Mountain Spotted Fever," 183; Wolbach, Todd, and Palfrey, *Etiology and Pathology of Typhus,* 202.

44. Wolbach, Todd, and Palfrey, *Etiology and Pathology of Typhus,* 123–24. One point of disagreement about the definition of Rickettsia-bodies concerned human pathogenicity. Wolbach maintained that only pathogenic organisms should be classified as Rickettsia-bodies. Edmund V. Cowdry of the Rockefeller Institute, in contrast, argued that this was not a necessary criterion. For Cowdry's view see E. V. Cowdry, "Rickettsiae and Disease," *Archives of Pathology and Laboratory Medicine* 2 (1926):59–90.

45. Report of Berlin correspondent, *JAMA* 76 (1921):1780; D. Montfallet, "A Protozoon in Relation to Typhus," *Revista Médica de Chile* 48 (1920):718, as abstracted in ibid., 900.

46. This work was mentioned and rebutted in Peter K. Olitsky, "Definition of Experimental Typhus in Guinea-Pigs," ibid. 78 (1922):571–74.

47. H. M. Woodcock, " 'Rickettsia'-Bodies as a Result of Cell-Digestion or Lysis," *J. Royal Army Med. Corps* 40 (1923):81–97, 241–69; idem, "On the Modes of Production of 'Rickettsia'-Bodies in the Louse," ibid. 42 (1924):121–31, 175–86 (quotation from p. 186); Leo Loewe, Saul Ritter, and George Baehr, "Cultivation of Rickettsia-Like Bodies in Typhus Fever," *JAMA* 77 (1921):1967–69.

48. Edmund Weil and Arthur Felix, "Zur serologischen Diagnose des Fleckfiebers," *Wiener klinische Wochenschrift* 29 (1916):33–35, Eng. trans. in Hahon, ed., *Selected Papers,* 79–86.

49. My description follows Hahon's comments in preface to Weil and Felix's article, in Hahon, ed., *Selected Papers,* 79.

50. W. J. Wilson, "Serologic Test in Typhus," *Lancet* 1 (1922):222; Fletcher, "Typhus-Like Fevers," 1024.

51. Report of Berlin correspondent, *JAMA* 76 (1921):1780; B. Fejgin, "Au sujet du sérum de Kuczynski et d'une variation du Protéus X19 obtenue à partir de Rikettsia provazeki," *Comptes Rendus des Séances de la Société de Biologie et de Ses Filiales* 95 (1926):1208–10 (hereafter cited as *Compt. rend. Soc. de biol.*); L. Anigstein and R. Amzel, "Recherches sur l'étiologie du typhus exanthématique. Le typhus exanthématique chez les cobazes infectés par les cultures du germe," *Comt. rend. Soc. de biol.* 96 (1927):1502; M. H. Kuczynski and Elisabeth Brandt, "Neue ätiologische und pathogenetische Untersuchungen in der 'Rickettsiengruppe,'" *Krankheitsforschung* 3 (1926):26–74; Kuczynski and Brandt, *Die Erreger des Fleck- und Felsenfiebers, Biologische und Pathogenetische Studien* (Berlin: Julius Springer, 1927); abstract of M. Ruiz Castaneda and S. Zia, "Antigenic Relationship of Proteus X19 to Typhus Rickettsiae," in *Arch. Pathol.* 16 (1933):419. Elisabeth Brandt's death was noted in Richard Otto, "Fleckfieber und Amerikanisches Felsengebirgsfieber," *Centralblatt für Bakteriologie, Parasitenkunde, und Infektionskrankheiten* 106 (1928):279–91. Theodore E. Woodward, who knew Felix, communicated to me that Felix never gave up his conviction that the etiological agent of typhus was a variant of *B. proteus*.

52. Frederick Breinl, "Betrachtungen, über die Immunität bei einigen Erkrankungen mit ultravisiblem Erreger," *Deutsche med. Wchnschr.* 51 (1925):264; Rudolf Weigl, "Der Gegenwärtige Stand der Rickettsiaforschung," *Klinische Wochenschrift* 3 (1924):1590–94, 1636–41; abstract of I. W. Hach, "Experimental Typhus. IV. Filterability of Virus of Typhus," in *Arch. Pathol. Lab. Med.* 3 (1927):318; abstract of P. Hauduroy, "Etiology of Typhus," in "Recent Research on Typhus," *JAMA* 85 (1925):1844; E. V. Cowdry, "Rickettsiae and Disease," *Arch. Pathol. Lab. Med.* 2 (1926):59–90 (reference to Trench Fever Commission on p. 63).

53. S. B. Wolbach and M. J. Schlesinger, "The Cultivation of the Microorganisms of Rocky Mountain Spotted Fever (*Dermacentroxenus rickettsi*) and of Typhus (*Rickettsia prowazeki*) in Tissue Plasma Cultures," *J. Med. Res.* 44 (1923):231–56; P. K. Olitsky and J. E. McCartney, "Experimental Studies on the Etiology of Typhus Fever. V. Survival of the Virus in Collodion Sacs Implanted Intra-Abdominally in Guinea Pigs," *J. Exp. Med.* 38 (1928):691; Clara Nigg and Karl Landsteiner, "Studies on Cultivation of Typhus Fever Rickettsia in Presence of Live Tissue," *J. Exp. Med.* 55 (1932):563–76.

54. S. Burt Wolbach, "The Rickettsiae and Their Relationship to Disease," *JAMA* 84 (1925):723–28 (quotations from pp. 723, 728).

55. Quoted in Hughes, *The Virus* (see chap. 3, n. 23), 86.

56. W. G. MacCullum, "A Survey of Our Present Knowledge of Filterable Viruses," *Arch. Pathol. Lab. Med.* 1 (1926):487–88 (quotations from p. 488). An excellent view of the development of virology is offered in Saul Benison, *Tom Rivers: Reflections on a Life in Medicine and Science* (Cambridge: MIT Press, 1967); on this early period see esp. chaps. 3–6. Rivers's views on the state of knowledge regarding virus diseases were similar to those of MacCullum; see excerpts from a paper on the subject given by Rivers at a symposium sponsored by the Society of American Bacteriologists in Benison, *Tom Rivers*, 110–11; the entire text is in T. M. Rivers, "Filterable Viruses: A Critical Review," *Arch. Pathol. Lab. Med.* 3 (1927):525–28.

57. "Dwarf Bacteria and Pigmy Protozoa," *JAMA* 94 (1930):795–96.

58. Wendell M. Stanley, "Isolation of a Crystalline Protein Possessing the Properties of Tobacco-Mosaic Virus," *Science* 81 (1935):644–45; Lily E. Kay,

"W. M. Stanley's Crystallization of the Tobacco Mosaic Virus, 1930–1940," *Isis* 77 (1986):450–72.

59. Earlier definitions of "life" turned on the ability of organisms to metabolize and to reproduce themselves independently. Viruses cannot perform these functions alone but must take over the genetic machinery of a functioning cell. Sally Smith Hughes observed, "With regard to the nature of viruses, biochemical findings appeared to support the idea that viruses are very large molecules, a refinement of the nonmicrobial concept of the virus. Yet it was also true that the ability of viruses to multiply and to infect were properties traditionally associated with the living state. Hence they possessed both animate and inanimate characteristics." See Hughes, *The Virus*, 89–92.

60. *Virus and Rickettsial Diseases, with Especial Consideration of Their Public Health Significance*, Proceedings of a symposium, Harvard School of Public Health, 12–17 June 1939 (Cambridge, Mass.: Harvard University Press, 1940).

61. S. Burt Wolbach, "The Rickettsial Diseases: A General Survey," ibid., 797–801. Wolbach also noted that heartwater disease of sheep, goats, and cattle was the single rickettsial infection known to infect animals. Its etiological agent was known as *R. ruminantium*, and its vector was the tick *Amblyomma hebraeum*.

62. Emile Brumpt, *Précis de Parasitologie* (Paris: Masson et Cie., 1927), 883; Henry Pinkerton, "Criteria for the Accurate Classification of the Rickettsial Diseases (Rickettsioses) and of Their Etiological Agents," *Parasitology* 28 (1936):172–89 (quotation from pp. 185–86); C. B. Philip, "Nomenclature of the Pathogenic Rickettsiae," *Am. J. Hyg.* 37 (1943):301–9; Philip, "Family Rickettsiaceae Pinkerton," in *Bergey's Manual of Determinative Bacteriology*, 7th ed. (Baltimore: Williams & Wilkins, 1957), 934–57. On the evolution of rickettsial nomenclature, see also Ida A. Bengtson, "Family Rickettsiaceae Pinkerton," in *Bergey's Manual of Determinative Bacteriology*, 6th ed. (Baltimore: Williams & Wilkins, 1948), 1083–99; Philip, "Nomenclature of the Rickettsiaceae Pathogenic to Vertebrates," *Ann. New York Acad. Sci.* 56 (1953):484–94.

Chapter Seven: The Spencer-Parker Vaccine

1. On land prices see F. J. Clifford to Surgeon General, 26 November 1920; and Surgeon General to Clifford, 7 December 1920, folder 3, "Rocky Mountain Spotted Fever, 1920–1926," box 1, "General Correspondence," MSBH Records. On tourism, see Cooley to James C. Evenden, 3 May 1922, folder E2, "Tick Control—General Correspondence, 1918–1928," box 10, ZEA; Cogswell to Fricks, 27 March 1922, file "S. F. History (Correspondence, Spencer and Fricks with Others—1916–1925)," RML Research Records.

2. Charles H. Roberts to Cogswell, 20 July 1921, folder 3, "Rocky Mountain Spotted Fever, 1920–1926," box 1, "General Correspondence," MSBH Records.

3. Report of Hygienic Laboratory, in MSBH, *Tenth Biennial Report*, 5; Price, *Fighting Spotted Fever* (see chap. 3, n. 4), 162.

4. Cogswell to Surgeon General Cumming, and Cogswell to Henry L. Meyers, telegrams, 22 June 1921, vol. "W. F. Cogswell, A. H. McCray, T. D. Tuttle," CC; "U.S. Launches New Fight on Spotted Fever," *Montana Record-Herald* (Helena), 18 July 1921, and "Spotted Fever Aid Is Urged," *Montana*

Record-Herald, 21 July 1921; "Would Ask U.S. to Help Fever Fight," *Independent* (Helena), 22 July 1921, clippings in file 1266, box 120, Central File, 1897–1923, PHS Records.

5. Parran to Cumming, 25 July 1921, folder 3, "Rocky Mountain Spotted Fever, 1920–1926," box 1, "General Correspondence," MSBH Records.

6. Cogswell to Parran, 26 August 1921; and Eliot Wadsworth to Cogswell, telegram, 31 August 1921, folder 3, "Rocky Mountain Spotted Fever, 1920–1926," box 1, "General Correspondence," MSBH Records.

7. Fricks to Surgeon General, 24 February 1922, vol. "Montana State Officials," CC.

8. J. W. Kerr to R. R. Spencer, 4 March 1922, folder E9, "Bitter Root Field Station, Correspondence, 1922–1927," box 10, ZEA. For biographical information on Spencer see Spencer, "The Fleas, the Ticks, Spotted Fever, and Me" cited in chap. 5, n. 74 (quotation from p. 47); R. R. Spencer oral history interview by Harlan Phillips, in George Rosen, "Transcripts of Oral History Project, 1962–1964," NLM (hereafter cited as Spencer oral history); Michael B. Shimkin, "Historical Note: Roscoe Roy Spencer (1888–1982)," *Journal of the National Cancer Institute* 72 (1984):969–71; "Roscoe R. Spencer," in Barry, *Notable Contributions* (see chap. 5, n. 75), 79–81; "Roscoe R. Spencer," *Pittsburgh Medical Bulletin* 39 (1948):397; Williams, *United States Public Health Service* (see chap. 3, n. 39), 195–99.

9. Fricks to Cogswell, 22 March 1922; and Cogswell to Fricks, 27 March 1922, file "S. F. History (Correspondence, Spencer and Fricks with Others—1916–1925)," RML Research Records.

10. Spencer to J. W. Schereschewsky, 16 March 1922; and Parker to Cooley, 23 May 1923, folder E9, "Bitter Root Field Station, Correspondence, 1922–1927," box 10, ZEA.

11. Fricks to J. W. Schereschewsky, 23 November 1923, file "S. F. History (Correspondence, Spencer and Fricks with Others—1916–1925)," RML Research Records. There was much correspondence about this issue during 1923 between Parker and Cooley. See folder E9, "Bitter Root Field Station, Correspondence, 1922–1927," box 10, ZEA.

12. Spencer to Surgeon General, 10 April and 5 June 1922, file 1266, box 119, Central File, 1897–1923, PHS Records.

13. Spencer to Surgeon General, 5 June 1922, file 1266, box 119, Central File, 1897–1923, PHS Records. This work was published as R. R. Spencer and R. R. Parker, "Rocky Mountain Spotted Fever: Infectivity of Fasting and Recently Fed Ticks," *Pub. Health Rep.* 38 (1923):333–39. It was reprinted as a part of a collection of Spencer and Parker's spotted fever papers in "Studies on Rocky Mountain Spotted Fever," U.S. Hygienic Laboratory *Bulletin* no. 154 (1930), 1–7.

14. Spencer to Surgeon General, 5 June 1922; and 10 April 1922, file 1266, box 119, Central File, 1897–1923, PHS Records.

15. Spencer to Fricks, 15 June 1922, file "S. F. History (Correspondence, Spencer and Fricks with Others—1916–1925)," RML Research Records.

16. "A Hero of the Bitter Root Valley"; and "Research Worker Dies of Virulence He Is Combatting," *Daily Missoulian,* 1 July 1922, clippings in folder E3, "Rocky Mountain Spotted Fever Fatalities, 1922–1928," box 10, ZEA; Price, *Fighting Spotted Fever* (see chap. 3, n. 4), 179–81.

17. Spencer to Surgeon General, 13 April 1923; and Spencer to A. M. Stimson, 14 May 1923, file 1266, box 119, Central File, 1897–1923, PHS Records; R. R. Spencer, "Experimental Studies on the Virus of Rocky Mountain Spotted Fever," in "Rocky Mountain Spotted Fever," Montana State Board of Health *Special Bulletin* no. 26 (1923):40–44; R. R. Spencer and R. R. Parker, "Rocky Mountain Spotted Fever: Viability of the Virus in Animal Tissues," *Pub. Health Rep.* 39 (1924):55–57.

18. Spencer to Surgeon General, 13 April 1923; untitled memo, apparently to the surgeon general from G. W. McCoy, 7 May 1923; and Cumming to Spencer, 10 May 1923, file 1266, box 119, Central File, 1897–1923, PHS Records.

19. Hideyo Noguchi, "Immunity Studies of Rocky Mountain Spotted Fever. I. Usefulness of Immune Serum in Suppressing an Impending Infection," *J. Exp. Med.* 37 (1923):383–94 (quotations from pp. 383, 394).

20. Parker to Cooley, 18 November 1922, vol. "R. R. Parker, 1921–1925," CC; Noguchi to Cogswell, 30 December 1922, folder 3, "Rocky Mountain Spotted Fever, 1920–1926," box 1, "General Correspondence," MSBH Records.

21. Hideyo Noguchi, "Immunity Studies of Rocky Mountain Spotted Fever. II. Prophylactic Inoculation in Animals," *J. Exp. Med.* 38 (1923):605–26 (quotation from p. 625); idem, "Prophylactic Inoculation against Rocky Mountain Spotted Fever," in "Rocky Mountain Spotted Fever," Montana State Board of Health *Special Bulletin* no. 26 (1923):44–47.

22. Foreword, in "Rocky Mountain Spotted Fever," Montana State Board of Health *Special Bulletin* no. 26 (1923):3.

23. "Dr. H. Noguchi Is Enthusiastic Man," 6 April 1923, clipping marked "either *Daily Missoulian* or *Missoula Sentinel*"; and "Spotted Fever Heroes: Noguchi's Countrymen Submit to His Serum," *Missoula Sentinel*, 12 April 1923, clippings in RML Scrapbook "1919–1931"; "A Death Gamble: Martyrs to Risk Lives to Aid Science," press release in folder 3, "Rocky Mountain Spotted Fever, 1920–1926," box 1, "General Correspondence," MSBH Records.

24. Spencer oral history, 59–62; "Annual Report on Rocky Mountain Spotted Fever Investigations," [1923], file 1266, box 119, Central File, 1897–1923, PHS Records.

25. Parker to Cooley, 12 July 1923, vol. "R. R. Parker, 1921–1925," CC.

26. Michky lived in the schoolhouse laboratory in order to be available twenty-four hours a day. See job description on untitled personnel list, 1921, file 1266, box 119, Central File, 1897–1923, PHS Records.

27. Cogswell to Noguchi, 7 September 1923; Spencer to Noguchi, 20 September 1923; and Noguchi to Spencer, 27 September 1923, folder 3, "Rocky Mountain Spotted Fever, 1920–1926," box 1, "General Correspondence," MSBH Records; Spencer to Surgeon General, 15 August 1923; and "Spotted Fever Vaccine Fails to Protect Boy," *Anaconda Standard*, 13 August 1923, clipping in file 1266, box 119, Central File, 1897–1923, PHS Records.

28. Parker to Cooley, 28 February 1925, vol. "R. R. Parker, 1921–1925," CC. For Noguchi's later work on spotted fever, see Hideyo Noguchi, "Cultivation of *Rickettsia*-Like Microorganisms from the Rocky Mountain Spotted Fever Tick, *Dermacentor andersoni*," *J. Exp. Med.* 43 (1926):515–32; Hideyo

Noguchi, "A Filter-Passing Virus Obtained from *Dermacentor andersoni*," *J. Exp. Med.* 44 (1926):1–10. On the yellow fever research that led to Noguchi's death, see Plesset, *Noguchi* (see chap. 6, n. 5), chaps. 21–22; and Claude E. Dolman, "Hideyo Noguchi (1876–1928): His Final Effort," *Clio Medica* 12 (1977):131–45.

29. R. R. Spencer and R. R. Parker, "Rocky Mountain Spotted Fever: Experimental Studies on Tick Virus," *Pub. Health Rep.* 39 (1924):3027–40; idem, "Rocky Mountain Spotted Fever: Nonfiltrability of Tick and Blood Virus," ibid., 3251–55; R. R. Parker and R. R. Spencer, "A Study of the Relationship between the Presence of Rickettsialike Organisms in Tick Smears and the Infectiveness of the Same Ticks," ibid., 41 (1926):461–69; idem, "Certain Characteristics of Blood Virus," ibid., 1817–22.

30. Frederick Breinl, "Studies on Typhus Virus in the Louse," *J. Inf. Dis.* 34 (1924):1–12, abstracted in *JAMA* 82 (1924):497–98. Spencer's accounts of his work in developing the vaccine are in Spencer to Esther Gaskins Price Ingraham, 10 October 1945, folder E5, "Rocky Mountain Spotted Fever History—Correspondence, 1942–1947," box 10, ZEA; Spencer oral history, 85–87; Spencer, "The Fleas, the Ticks, Spotted Fever, and Me."

31. Spencer and Parker, "Rocky Mountain Spotted Fever: Experimental Studies on Tick Virus," 21–22. There was some debate at first about whether the phenol killed or attenuated the organisms, for prevailing opinion argued that only attenuated organisms conferred immunity. Guinea pig studies convinced Spencer that the organism was indeed killed, and he observed, "We are inclined to believe that the killed as well as the live virus of Rocky Mountain spotted fever can immunize." See R. R. Spencer and R. R. Parker, "Improved Method of Manufacture of the Vaccine and a Study of Its Properties," in idem, "Studies on Rocky Mountain Spotted Fever," 68–69.

32. Price, *Fighting Spotted Fever*, 195–96. Earl W. Malone, who became chief vaccine maker, also wanted to take the experimental vaccine, but Spencer cautioned him to wait until it was clear how the vaccine affected one person. See Spencer to W. L. Jellison, 9 May 1966, NIAID files, NIH Historical Office.

33. G. W. McCoy, "A Plague-Like Disease in Rodents," *Public Health Bulletin* no. 43 (1911):53–71; G. W. McCoy and C. W. Chapin, "Further Observations on a Plague-Like Disease of Rodents with a Preliminary Note on the Causative Agent, *Bacterium tularense*," *J. Inf. Dis.* 10 (1912):61–72; G. W. McCoy and C. W. Chapin, "*Bacterium tularense*, the Cause of a Plague-Like Disease of Rodents," *Public Health Bulletin* no. 53 (1912):17–23; Edward Francis, "Deer-Fly Fever, or Pahvant Valley Plague: A Disease of Man of Hitherto Unknown Etiology," *Pub. Health Rep.* 34 (1919):2061–62; "Tularemia Francis 1921: A New Disease of Man," U.S. Hygienic Laboratory *Bulletin* no. 130 (1922), 87 pp.; Edward Francis, "Tularemia," *JAMA* 84 (1925):1243–50; Parker to Cooley, 24 August 1924, vol. "R. R. Parker, 1921–1925," CC; Price, *Fighting Spotted Fever*, 194–97.

34. Untitled personnel list, 1921, file 1266, box 119. Central File, 1897–1923, PHS Records; "Tick Worker Succumbs; Spotted Fever Is Fatal," *Daily Missoulian*, 30 October 1924, clipping in notebook "RMSF Laboratory Infections—Book I," R. R. Parker Notebooks, RML Research Records.

35. "Tick Worker Succumbs," *Daily Missoulian*, 30 October 1924; Spencer, "The Fleas, the Ticks, Spotted Fever, and Me," 49.

36. Noguchi, cited in Spencer to Surgeon General, 28 March 1925, file 0425–32, "Spotted Fever—Hamilton, Montana," box 158, "Domestic Stations, Hamilton, Montana," PHS Records; R. R. Spencer and R. R. Parker, "Rocky Mountain Spotted Fever: Vaccination of Monkeys and Man," *Pub. Health Rep.* 40 (1925):2159–67; reprinted in idem, "Studies on Rocky Mountain Spotted Fever," 28–36.

37. Cooley to Parker, 24 May 1926, vol. "R. R. Parker, 1926–1931," CC; R. R. Spencer and R. R. Parker, "Rocky Mountain Spotted Fever: Vaccination of Monkeys and Man," in idem, "Studies on Rocky Mountain Spotted Fever," 31–32.

38. Spencer and Parker, "Rocky Mountain Spotted Fever. Vaccination of Monkeys and Man," 34–35.

39. Spencer to Surgeon General, 28 March 1925, file 0425–32, "Spotted Fever—Hamilton, Montana," box 158, "Domestic Stations, Hamilton, Montana," PHS Records; Parker's cover letter to Surgeon General, 9 April 1926 in RML, Monthly Report, March 1926. On Spencer's illness see Parker to Cooley, 16 March 1926, vol. "R. R. Parker, 1926–1931," CC.

40. R. R. Spencer and R. R. Parker, "Results of Four Years' Human Vaccination," in idem, "Studies on Rocky Mountain Spotted Fever," 72–103, esp. 89–95; [Parker] to Cooley, 7 July 1926, folder 3, "Rocky Mountain Spotted Fever, 1920–1926," box 1, "General Correspondence," MSBH Records.

41. Spencer and Parker, "Results of Four Years' Human Vaccination," 75–78; Parker to Surgeon General, telegram, 18 August 1926, file 0425–183, "Spotted Fever, Hamilton, Montana," box 158, "Domestic Stations—Hamilton, Montana," PHS Records; Parker to Surgeon General, 31 August 1926, folder 3, "Rocky Mountain Spotted Fever, 1920–1926," box 1, "General Correspondence," MSBH Records; Parker to Surgeon General, 30 September 1926, RML Monthly Report, August and September 1926 (quotations from this report).

42. Spencer and Parker, "Results of Four Years' Human Vaccination," 81–89.

43. R. R. Parker, "Rocky Mountain Spotted Fever: Results of Ten Years' Prophylactic Vaccination," *J. Inf. Dis.* 57 (1935):78–93; idem, "Rocky Mountain Spotted Fever: Results of Fifteen Years' Prophylactic Vaccination," *American Journal of Tropical Medicine* 21 (1941):369–83.

44. The various methods tried are documented in RML, Monthly Reports; RML, *Annual Reports*; Earl W. Malone, "Methods of Rearing *Dermacentor andersoni* for the Manufacture of Rocky Mountain Spotted Fever Vaccine"; Earl W. Malone, "Preparation of Rocky Mountain Spotted Fever Tick-Tissue Vaccine," unpublished technical reports, RML; R. R. Spencer and R. R. Parker, "Improved Method of Manufacture of the Vaccine and a Study of Its Properties," in idem, "Studies on Rocky Mountain Spotted Fever," 63–72. My description of the vaccine-making process is based on these documents and on Price, *Fighting Spotted Fever*, 213–21.

45. As the quantity of vaccine increased over the years, it became necessary to arrange for on-site sterility testing. In 1934 technician Max T. McKee was sent to Bethesda to learn the techniques, and funds were allocated for a special room with incubators necessary for the process at the Spotted Fever Laboratory in Montana. See RML, Monthly Report, November 1934, 3; RML, *Annual Report*, 1935, 3–4.

46. This article was reprinted as one chapter in Paul de Kruif, *Men against Death* (New York: Harcourt, Brace & Co., 1932), 119–45.

47. The quotations were noted as objectionable passages in "An Outside View of Bitter Root Valley," *Ravalli Republican*, 31 March 1927, clipping in RML Scrapbook "1919–1931."

48. Ibid.; "Bitter Root Valley Is Up in Arms," *Northwest Tribune*, 3 March 1927, clipping in RML Scrapbook "1919–1931"; Knight to Leavitt, 28 February 1929, file 0243–183, "Hamilton, Montana, Chamber of Commerce," box 44, "Montana Cities and Counties," State Boards of Health, 1924–1935; and Cumming to Parker, 9 March 1929, file 0425–183, "Hamilton, Montana," box 158. "Domestic Stations, Hamilton, Montana," PHS Records.

49. Cogswell to Pearl I. Smith, n.d.; and F. J. O'Donnell to Cogswell, 15 and 16 April (two letters), 1926, folder 3, "Rocky Mountain Spotted Fever, 1920–1926," box 1, "General Correspondence," MSBH Records.

50. Parker to Cooley, 9 August 1926, vol. "R. R. Parker, 1926–1931," CC.

51. Parker to Cooley, 18 May 1925; and Parker to Cooley, 29 January 1926, vol. "R. R. Parker, 1926–1931," CC; Cooley to Cogswell, 14 July 1927, folder 4, "Rocky Mountain Spotted Fever, 1927–1929," box 1, "General Correspondence," MSBH Records.

52. Cooley to Kenneth Ross, 24 April 1925; and Parker to Cooley, 14 May 1926, folder 3, "Rocky Mountain Spotted Fever, 1920–1926," box 1, "General Correspondence," MSBH Records; Cooley's correspondence with Albert B. Tonkin, former Wyoming state health officer, vol. "R. R. Parker, 1926–1931," CC.

53. Cooley to W. J. Butler and Cogswell, 12 February 1926, vol. "W. F. Cogswell, A. H. McCray, T. D. Tuttle," CC.

54. Wolbach to McCoy, 19 October 1926, vol. "R. R. Parker, 1926–1931," CC; Cogswell to Spencer, 5 November 1926; and Cumming to Cogswell, 16 November 1926, file 0425–32, "Montana—Spotted Fever—Hamilton," box 158, "Domestic Stations—Hamilton, Montana," PHS Records.

55. Cooley to Wolbach, 24 January 1927, vol. "Professors at Various Universities," CC; Spencer to Cooley, 16 March 1927; and Cooley to Spencer, 5 April 1927, folder E7, "U.S. Public Health Service, Correspondence 1927," box 10, ZEA; George L. Knight to Scott Leavitt, 28 February 1929, file 0243–183, "Hamilton, Montana, Chamber of Commerce," box 44, "Montana Cities and Counties," State Boards of Health, 1924–1935, PHS Records.

56. Louis Nelson, Harry G. Bullock, Ralph B. Robinson, William S. Schraedl, and James A. Shields to Cogswell, 7 April 1927, folder 12, "1912, 1927–29, Rocky Mountain Laboratory," box 1, "General Correspondence and Subject Files, 1908–1949," MSBH Records.

57. The other plaintiffs were identified as G. A. Gordon, a physician; F. M. Hagens, an engineer for the Bitter Root Irrigation District; Ben Ogg, a pharmacist; Bert C. Lee, a dentist; and Judge J. M. Self—all residents of Pine Grove. See F. J. O'Donnell to Cogswell, 4 April 1927, folder 4, "Rocky Mountain Spotted Fever, 1927–1929," box 1, "General Correspondence," MSBH Records.

58. Cooley to Cogswell, 2 April 1927; and H. C. Groff to Cogswell, 14 April 1927, folder 12, "1912, 1927–29, Rocky Mountain Laboratory," box 1, "General Correspondence and Subject Files, 1908–1949," MSBH Records.

59. "Work on Laboratory Began Here Yesterday," *Western News*, 16 June 1927; "Tick Laboratory Hearing July 27," ibid., 14 July 1927; "Pine Grove Folk Go to Court in Effort to Rid Lab from Midst," ibid., 30 June 1927; "Laboratory Will Be Build [*sic*] in Pine Grove as Result of Judge's Decision," ibid., 11 August 1927. Quotations from plaintiffs' testimony were taken from the transcript of a portion of the proceedings in RML Research Records. Cogswell's testimony was cited in the *JAMA* coverage of the case, "Citizens Fear Experimental Spotted Fever Ticks," *JAMA* 89 (1927):530. On final negotiations with the Waddells, see Parker to Cooley, 17 June 1927, folder E7, "U.S. Public Health Service, Correspondence 1927," box 10, ZEA.

60. Description in attachment to request for bids to construct laboratory, Standard Form no. 33, "Standard Government Short Form Contract," 5 December 1927, vol. "W. F. Cogswell, A. H. McCray, T. D. Tuttle," CC.

61. Cooley to Cogswell and Butler, 19 April 1930, vol. "W. F. Cogswell, A. H. McCray, T. D. Tuttle," CC.

62. Ibid.

63. There are numerous accounts of Kerlee's illness and death. Mine is drawn primarily from F. J. O'Donnell to Cogswell, 23 February 1928, folder 4, "Rocky Mountain Spotted Fever, 1927–1929," box 1, "General Correspondence," MSBH Records; Spencer to Surgeon General, 14 February 1928, RML, Monthly Report, February 1928; Montana State Board of Health Special Spotted [Tick] Fever Report on LeRoy Kerlee, notebook "R.M.S.F.—Laboratory Infections—Book I," R. R. Parker Notebooks, RML Research Records; "Health Secretary Explains Conditions Accounting for Death from Spotted Fever," 21 February 1928, clipping in RML Scrapbook "1919–1931." Brian Thrailkill, a student associate of Kerlee's in the schoolhouse laboratory, stated in an interview with Robert N. Philip, 3 August 1983, that Kerlee probably acquired his illness from washing contaminated glassware. Kerlee's family were longtime residents of the Bitterroot Valley. His aunt, Bessie K. Monroe, wrote a column for the *Ravalli Republic* until her death in 1987. See B. K. Monroe, "The Kerlees of Darby," in Bitter Root Historical Society, ed., *Bitterroot Trails* (see chap. 2, n. 1), 2:290–99.

64. Montana State Board of Health Special Spotted [Tick] Fever Report on LeRoy Kerlee, notebook "R.M.S.F.—Laboratory Infections—Book I," R. R. Parker Notebooks, RML Research Records.

65. "Health Secretary Explains" (see n. 63 above); Spencer to Surgeon General, 14 February 1928, RML, Monthly Report, February 1928.

66. Parker to Cooley, 26 February 1928, vol. "R. R. Parker, 1926–1931," CC; Spencer oral history, 98.

67. In the published account of this speech, however, Spencer was mentioned several times as being a colleague in the work. See R. R. Parker, "Rocky Mountain Spotted Fever," in MSBE, *Seventh Biennial Report*, 39–62.

68. Spencer oral history, 97–98.

69. Spencer's popular articles include "The Fleas, the Ticks, Spotted Fever, and Me," and "Rocky Mountain Spotted Fever: A Remarkable American Malady and Its Insect Vector," *Hygeia* 4 (1926):461–63.

70. Fricks to Surgeon General, 13 August 1929; Cumming to Fricks, 24 September 1929; and A. M. Stimson to "Dr. Pierce," memorandum, 20 September 1929, file 1850-95, "Rocky Mountain Spotted Fever Laboratory,"

box 158, "Domestic Stations, Hamilton, Montana," PHS Records. Parker's industrious habits eventually received favorable comment from Fricks himself. See Fricks to Surgeon General, 19 August 1930, file 1850–95, "Rocky Mountain Spotted Fever Laboratory," box 158, "Domestic Stations, Hamilton, Montana," PHS Records. Gordon E. Davis, who had just completed his D.Sc. degree in bacteriology at Johns Hopkins University and had spent time in Nigeria working with the Rockefeller Yellow Fever Commission, joined the laboratory as bacteriologist in October 1930. See RML, Monthly Report, October 1930.

71. McCoy to Surgeon General, 11 April 1928, file 1850,"Hamilton, Montana," box 158, "Domestic Stations, Hamilton, Montana," PHS Records.

Chapter Eight: Spotted Fever outside the Rockies

1. Abstract of C. R. LaBier, "Rocky Mountain Spotted Fever in Indiana," *JAMA* 86 (1926):150.

2. John F. Anderson and Joseph Goldberger, "The Relation of So-called Brill's Disease to Typhus Fever," *Pub. Health Rep.* 27 (1912):149–60. The identification of Brill's disease and its use as a catchall diagnostic category were discussed in chap. 6.

3. Kenneth F. Maxcy, "An Epidemiological Study of Endemic Typhus (Brill's Disease) in the Southeastern United States with Special Reference to Its Mode of Transmission," *Pub. Health Rep.* 41 (1926):2967–95. For biographical information on Maxcy, see K. F. Meyer, "Presentation of Sedgwick Memorial Award to Dr. Maxcy for 1952," *Am. J. Pub. Health* 42 (1952):1618–21; Barry, *Notable Contributions* (see chap. 5, n. 75), 52–54. Maxcy's study was apparently generated by questions raised when he presented a paper on "dengue fever with a rash" at a Hygienic Laboratory review of staff research. Joseph Goldberger suggested that the symptoms sounded suspiciously like typhus fever. Maxcy thus held back a pending publication until he could do additional research, which confirmed the senior typhus investigator's view. As a result, Maxcy's publication contained not a description of atypical dengue fever but an authoritative study of endemic typhus. See Rolla Eugene Dyer, oral history interview by Harlan Phillips, 13 November 1962, p. 9, in George Rosen, Transcripts of Oral History Project, 1962–64, NLM (hereafter cited as Dyer oral history).

4. R. D. Glasser, "Case of Typhus-Like Fever Following Tick Bite," *Virginia Medical Monthly* 56 (1930):670–71.

5. *Washington Post* article cited in "Outbreak of Typhus Fever," *JAMA* 95 (1930):53; "Spread of Typhus Fever," *JAMA* 95 (1930):207; "Conference on Typhus Fever," *JAMA* 95 (1930):349; Robert Hickman Riley and Charles H. Halliday, *Typhus, Spotted Fever in Maryland* (Baltimore: Maryland State Department of Health, 1932).

6. For biographical information on Dyer see Dyer oral history; Abel Wolman, "Sedgwick Memorial Medal to Dr. Dyer for 1950," *Am. J. Pub. Health* 40 (1950):1584–87; "Rolla Dyer Retires," *JAMA* 144 (1950):248; and Barry, *Notable Contributions*, 19–22.

7. Harden, *Inventing the NIH* (see chap. 3, n. 35), 50–159.

8. Dyer oral history, 10; L. F. Badger, R. E. Dyer, and A. Rumreich, "An Infection of the Rocky Mountain Spotted Fever Type: Identification in the Eastern Part of the United States," *Pub. Health Rep.* 46 (1931):463–70.

9. A. Rumreich, R. E. Dyer, and L. F. Badger, "The Typhus-Rocky Mountain Spotted Fever Group: An Epidemiological and Clinical Study in the Eastern and Southeastern States," *Pub. Health Rep.* 46 (1931):470–80 (quotations from pp. 470, 478); "Is Rocky Mountain Fever Present in the Eastern United States?" *JAMA* 96 (1931):1146–47 (quotation from p. 1147).

10. Rumreich, Dyer, and Badger, "Typhus-Rocky Mountain Spotted Fever Group: Eastern and Southeastern States," 479; R. E. Dyer, L. F. Badger, and A. Rumreich, "Rocky Mountain Spotted Fever (Eastern Type): Transmission by the American Dog Tick (*Dermacentor variabilis*)," *Pub. Health Rep.* 46 (1931):1403–13; L. F. Badger, "Rocky Mountain Spotted Fever (Eastern Type): Virus Recovered from the Dog Tick *Dermacentor variabilis* Found in Nature," *Pub. Health Rep.* 47 (1932):2365–69.

11. Herman Mooser, M. Ruiz Castaneda, and Hans Zinsser, "Rats as Carriers of Mexican Typhus Fever," *JAMA* 97 (1931):231–32; R. E. Dyer, A. Rumreich, and L. F. Badger, "The Typhus-Rocky Mountain Spotted Fever Group in the United States," ibid., 589–94 (discussion, pp. 594–95).

12. Ibid., 594.

13. For a review of the status of typhus research in 1932, see R. E. Dyer, L. F. Badger, E. T. Ceder, and W. G. Workman, "Endemic Typhus Fever of the United States: History, Epidemiology, and Mode of Transmission," *JAMA* 99 (1932):795–801. I am grateful to Kimberly Pelis for copies of her two untitled seminar papers, February and May 1988, Institute of the History of Medicine, Johns Hopkins University School of Medicine, Baltimore, Maryland, which stimulated my thinking about the changing definition of tabardillo.

14. M. H. Neill, "Experimental Typhus Fever in Guinea Pigs," *Pub. Health Rep.* 32 (1917):1105–8; Herman Mooser, "Reaction of Guinea-Pigs to Mexican Typhus (Tabardillo): Preliminary Note on Bacteriologic Observations," *JAMA* 91 (1928):19–20; Herman Mooser, "Experiments Relating to the Pathology and the Etiology of Mexican Typhus (Tabardillo)," *J. Inf. Dis.* 43 (1928):241–72.

15. Herman Mooser, "Essai sur l'histoire naturelle du typhus exanthématique," *Archives de l'Institut Pasteur de Tunis* 21 (1932):1–19. In honor of Mooser's contribution to the knowledge of this disease, Brazilian investigator José Lemos Monteiro suggested that the rickettsiae of endemic typhus be called *Rickettsia mooseri*. See José Lemos Monteiro, "Estudos Sobre o Typho Exantematico de São Paulo," *Memorias do Instituto Butantan* 6 (1931):1–135 (hereafter cited as *Mem. Inst. Butantan*). The name of the organism was later changed to *Rickettsia typhi*.

16. Hans Zinsser, "Varieties of Typhus Virus and the Epidemiology of the American Form of European Typhus Fever (Brill's Disease)," *Am. J. Hyg.* 20 (1934):513–32; E. S. Murray, G. Baehr, G. Schwartzman, R. A. Mandelbaum, N. Rosenthal, J. C. Doane, L. B. Weiss, S. Cohen, and J. C. Snyder, "Brill's Disease. I. Clinical and Laboratory Diagnosis," *JAMA* 142 (1950):1059–66; E. S. Murray and J. C. Snyder, "Brill's Disease. II. Etiology," *Am. J. Hyg.* 53 (1951):22–32; John C. Snyder, "Typhus Fever Rickettsiae," in Horsfall and Tamm, eds., *Viral and Rickettsial Infections of Man*, 4th ed. (see chap. 1, n. 7), 1078–87.

17. William Fletcher, "Typhus-Like Fevers of Unknown Ætiology, with Special Reference to the Malay States," *Proc. R. Soc. Med.* 23 (1930):1021–27 (discussion, pp. 1027–30; quotation from p. 1029). Fletcher noted the following local names for the typhus-like diseases: Rocky Mountain spotted

fever, endemic typhus, and Brill's disease in the United States; tick-typhus in India; urban tropical typhus, or shop typhus, and rural tropical typhus, or scrub typhus, in the Malay States; tropical typhus in Java and Sumatra; sporadic typhus in French Indochina; endemic typhus and Mossman fever in Australia; *fièvre boutonneuse* in North Africa; twelve-day fever in Nigeria; Brill's disease in South Africa; typhus-like fever in Kenya and Southern Rhodesia; *fièvre exanthématique* and *typhus endémique bénin* in the south of France; and *febbre eruttiva* in Italy.

18. J. W. D. Megaw, "A Typhus-Like Fever in India, Possibly Transmitted by Ticks," *Indian Med. Gaz.* 56 (1921):361; idem, "Typhus Group of Fevers," ibid. 59 (1924):169–73; idem, "Indian Tick Typhus," ibid. 60 (1925):58–61.

19. Fletcher, "Typhus-Like Fevers of Unknown Ætiology," 1023.

20. Ibid.; Charles Nicolle, "Unité ou pluralité des typhus exanthématiques," *Bull. Soc. Path. Exot.* 26 (1933):316–40; Charles Nicolle, "Unité ou pluralité des typhus exanthématiques (A propos de la discussion de mon rapport à la séance du 9 février)," *Bull. Soc. Path. Exot.* 26 (1933):375–76.

21. "Small Epidemic of Mild Typhus," abstract in *JAMA* 89 (1927):705; "Exanthematic Typhus and Typhoid Infection with Exanthem" and "Epidemics of Infectious Exanthems of Indeterminate Nature," abstracts in ibid. 90 (1928):424; "Epidemic in Marseilles Due to Ticks," ibid. 95 (1930):1846; Emile Brumpt, "Longévité du virus de la fièvre boutonneuse (*R. conori*, n. sp.) chez la tique, *Rhipicephalus sanguineus*," *Compt. rend. Soc. de biol.* 110 (1932):1199–1202. Later taxonomic convention called for doubling the final *i*, hence this organism is known at present as *R. conorii*.

22. Accounts of Brumpt's illness are in "Case of Rocky Mountain Spotted Fever in Paris," *JAMA* 100 (1933):1190; RML, Monthly Report, March 1933; "Single Injection of Spotted Fever Serum Saves French Doctor," *Helena* [Montana] *Record*, 15 April 1933, clipping in RML Scrapbook "1932–1940." *JAMA* reported that at the Hôpital Pasteur, Brumpt received three doses of typhus serum, flown in from convalescents at the Pasteur Institute in Casablanca and at the hygienic institute in Warsaw. French parasitologist Jean Théodoridès provided a slightly different version of Brumpt's therapy, told to him by a relative of Charles Nicolle. In this account, Nicolle advised Brumpt to be treated at the Hôpital Pasteur, where Brumpt was cured by inoculation from his roommate, Paul Giroud, who was convalescing from a grave typhus infection. I am grateful to Dr. Théodoridès for providing me with a preprint of the chapter on rickettsial diseases from his forthcoming book.

23. "Case of Rocky Mountain Spotted Fever in Paris," 1190; RML, Monthly Report, March 1933.

24. L. F. Badger, "Rocky Mountain Spotted Fever and Boutonneuse Fever: A Study of Their Immunological Relationship," *Pub. Health Rep.* 48 (1933):507–11; Gordon E. Davis and R. R. Parker, "Comparative Experiments on Spotted Fever and Boutonneuse Fever (I)," ibid. 49 (1934):423–28.

25. "A New Type of Typhus Fever," *JAMA* 96 (1931):1968; "Typhus Epidemics in 1932," ibid. 100 (1933):1266; Robin L. Anderson, "Public Health and Public Healthiness, São Paulo, Brazil, 1876–1893," *J. Hist. Med. Allied Sci.* 41 (1986):293–307; George Browne, "Government Immigration in Imperial Brazil, 1822–1870," Ph.D. dissertation, Catholic University, 1972; Michael Hall, "The Origins of Mass Immigration in Brazil, 1871–1914," Ph.D. dissertation, Columbia University, 1969.

26. Ronald Hilton, in *The Scientific Institutions of Latin America, with Special Reference to Their Organization and Information Facilities* (Stanford: California Institute of International Studies, 1970), 564.

27. "Experiments with Virus of Exanthematic Typhus," *JAMA* 97 (1931):262–63. "Experiments with Virus of Typhus Fever," ibid., 1480 (quotation this article); Emmanuel Dias and Amilcar Vianna Martins, "Spotted Fever in Brazil: A Summary," *Am. J. Trop. Med.* 19 (1939):103–8. See also José de Toledo Piza, *Typho exantematico de São Paulo* (São Paulo, Brazil: Sociedade Impressora Paulista, 1932); J. Lemos Monteiro, "Estudos sôbre o typho exantematico de São Paulo," *Mem. Inst. Butantan* 6 (1931):5–13; J. Lemos Monteiro, F. Fonseca, and A. Prado, "Pesquisas epidemiologicas sôbre o typho exantemático de São Paulo," *Mem. Inst. Butantan* 6 (1931):139; J. Lemos Montiero, "Tentativos de transmissao experimentale do 'typho exantemático' de São Paulo por percevejos (*Cimex lenticularis*)," *Mem. Inst. Butantan* 9 (1935):1; J. Lemos Monteiro and F. Fonseca, "Typho exantemático de São Paulo. XII. Sôbre un virus isolado de ratos da zona urbana da cidade e suas relacoes com o do typho exantemático de São Paulo," *Brasil Médico* 59 (1932):137 (hereafter cited as *Brasil Med.*); J. Travassos, "Studies on Rickettsial Diseases in Brazil," in Carolyn Whitlock, ed., *Proceedings of the Fourth International Congresses on Tropical Medicine and Malaria, Washington, D.C., May 10–18, 1948* (Washington, D.C.: Government Printing Office, 1948), 414–21 (discussion, pp. 421–25).

28. R. R. Parker and Gordon E. Davis, "Protective Value of Convalescent Sera of Sao Paulo Exanthematic Typhus against Virus of Rocky Mountain Spotted Fever," *Pub. Health Rep.* 48 (1933):501–7; R. E. Dyer, "Relationship between Rocky Mountain Spotted Fever and 'Exanthematic Typhus of Sao Paulo,'" ibid., 521–22; R. R. Parker and Gordon E. Davis, "Further Studies on the Relationship of the Viruses of Rocky Mountain Spotted Fever and Sao Paulo Exanthematic Typhus," ibid., 839–43; Gordon E. Davis and R. R. Parker, "Additional Studies on the Relationship of the Viruses of Rocky Mountain Spotted Fever and Sao Paulo Exanthematic Typhus," ibid., 1006–11.

29. RML, Monthly Report, January 1934, 2–3; RML, *Annual Report*, 1934, 2; "Tick Fever Serum Sent to Tropics," n.d., n.p., clipping in RML Scrapbook "1932–1940."

30. RML, Monthly Report, February 1936, 8–9; list of spotted fever deaths from laboratory infections, "RMSF—Laboratory Infections—Book 1," R. R. Parker Notebooks, RML Research Records; RML, Monthly Reports, April 1937, 6; and May 1937, 12; "Brazil Doctors Leave Hamilton," *Daily Missoulian*, 19 May 1937; and "News Bits of Montanans," paper and date not cited, clippings in RML Scrapbook 2, "1932–1940"; Travassos, "Studies on Rickettsial Diseases in Brazil," 418–19.

31. L. Patiño-Camargo, A. Afanador, and J. H. Paul, "A Spotted Fever in Tobia, Colombia: Preliminary Report," *Am. J. Trop. Med.* 17 (1937):639–53.

32. Luis Patiño-Camargo, "Neuvas observaciones sobre un tercer foco de fiebre petequial (maculosa) en el hemisferio americano," *Boletin de la Oficina Sanitaria Panamerica* 20 (1941):1112–23 (hereafter cited as *Bol. Offic. San. Panam.*); RML, *Annual Report*, 1941, 1. Calderón Cuervo's death in 1942 is noted in Aristides A. Moll, *Aesculapius in Latin America* (Philadelphia: W. B. Saunders Co., 1944), 463; R. R. Parker, "RMSF—Laboratory Infections—Book 1," R. R. Parker Notebooks, RML Research Records.

33. RML, Monthly Report, December 1941, 8.

34. Badger, Dyer, and Rumreich, "An Infection," 466; Dyer, Badger, and Rumreich, "Rocky Mountain Spotted Fever: Transmission," 1403.

35. Parker to G. W. McCoy, 21 July 1931, RML, Monthly Report, July 1931.

36. Ibid.

37. For biographical information on Lillie, see Frederick H. Kasten, "Ralph Dougall Lillie," in Clark and Kasten, *History of Staining* (see chap. 4, n. 51), 1–34; G. G. Glenner, "Ralph D. Lillie: Pioneer in Three Specialties," *Journal of Histochemistry and Cytochemistry* 16 (1968):3–16; J. D. Longley, "Ralph Dougall Lillie, 1896–1979," *J. Histochem. Cytochem.* 28 (1980):291–96; Frederick H. Kasten, "Ralph D. Lillie," *Stain Technology* 55 (1980):201–15; S. S. Spicer, "A Tribute to Dr. Ralph Dougall Lillie (1896–1979)," *Histochemical Journal* 12 (1980):495–98; "Ralph Dougall Lillie," in *American Men and Women of Science*, 14th ed., ed. Jacques Cattell Press, *Physical and Biological Sciences*, vol. 4 (New York: R. R. Bowker, 1979), 2991.

38. Ralph D. Lillie, "Pathology of the Eastern Type of Rocky Mountain Spotted Fever," *Pub. Health Rep.* 46 (1931):2840–59 (quotations from p. 2858).

39. P. N. Harris, "Histological Study of a Case of the Eastern Type of Rocky Mountain Spotted Fever," *American Journal of Pathology* 7 (1933):91–104. M. C. Pincoffs and C. C. Shaw, "The Eastern Type of Rocky Mountain Spotted Fever: Report of a Case with Demonstration of Rickettsiae," *Medical Clinics of North America* 16 (1933):1097–1114; Ralph D. Lillie, "Histologic Reaction to the Virus of Rocky Mountain Spotted Fever in Chick Embryos," *Pub. Health Rep.* 50 (1935):1498–1501; Ralph D. Lillie and R. E. Dyer, "Brain Reaction in Guinea Pigs Infected with Endemic Typhus, Epidemic (European) Typhus and Rocky Mountain Spotted Fever, Eastern and Western Types," *Pub. Health Rep.* 51 (1936):1293–1307.

40. E. R. Maillard and E. L. Hazen, "Rocky Mountain Spotted Fever in New York State Outside of New York City," *Am. J. Pub. Health* 25 (1935):1012–17; Norman H. Topping and R. E. Dyer, "A Highly Virulent Strain of Rocky Mountain Spotted Fever Virus Isolated in the Eastern United States," *Pub. Health Rep.* 55 (1940):728–31; George D. Brigham and James Watt, "Highly Virulent Strains of Rocky Mountain Spotted Fever Virus Isolated from Ticks (*D. variabilis*) in Georgia," *Pub. Health Rep.* 55 (1940):2125–26; George D. Brigham and James Watt, "Additional Highly Virulent Strains of Rocky Mountain Spotted Fever Virus Isolated in Georgia," *Pub. Health Rep.* 57 (1942):1342–44; Norman H. Topping, "A Strain of Rocky Mountain Spotted Fever Virus of Low Virulence Isolated in the Western United States," *Pub. Health Rep.* 56 (1941):2041–43; Norman H. Topping, "Rocky Mountain Spotted Fever: A Note on Some Aspects of Its Epidemiology," *Pub. Health Rep.* 56 (1941):1699–1703; Norman H. Topping, "The Epidemiology of Rocky Mountain Spotted Fever," *New York State Journal of Medicine* 47 (1947):1585–87.

41. Eugene P. Campbell and Walter H. Ketchum, "Rocky Mountain Spotted Fever: An Analysis of Seven Cases, Including One Laboratory Infection," *New England Journal of Medicine* 223 (1940):540–43 (quotation from p. 540); Alfred L. Florman and Joseph Hafkenschiel, "The Eastern Variety of Rocky Mountain Spotted Fever: The Experience on the Adult Medical Service of The

Johns Hopkins Hospital, Including the Report of a Fatal Case Showing Thrombocytopenia," *Bulletin of the Johns Hopkins Hospital* 66 (1940):123–33 (quotations from p. 132).

42. Ralph D. Lillie, "Pathology of Rocky Mountain Spotted Fever. I. The Pathology of Rocky Mountain Spotted Fever. II. The Pathologic Histology of Rocky Mountain Spotted Fever in the Rhesus Monkey *Macaca mulatta*," U.S. National Institute of Health *Bulletin* no. 177 (1941), 53 pp. (quotations from pp. 1, 27).

43. "Epidemic in Marseilles Due to Ticks," *JAMA* 95 (1930):1846; R. A. Cooley, "Preliminary Report on the Tick Parasite, *Ixodiphagus caucurtei* du Buysson," in MSBE, *Seventh Biennial Report*, 17–31.

44. C. P. Clausen, "Parasites and Predators," *Yearbook of Agriculture* (Washington, D.C.: Government Printing Office, 1952), 380–88; idem, "Biological Control of Insect Pests in the Continental United States," U.S. Department of Agriculture *Technical Bulletin* no. 1139 (1956), 151 pp.; Marshall Hertig and David Smiley, Jr., "The Problem of Controlling Wood Ticks on Martha's Vineyard," *Vineyard Gazette* (Martha's Vineyard, Mass.), 15 January 1937, clipping in RML Scrapbook "1935–1941"; Harvey L. Sweetman, *The Principles of Biological Control: Interrelation of Hosts and Pests and Utilization in Regulation of Animal and Plant Populations* (Dubuque, Iowa: William C. Brown Co., 1958), 157.

45. Cooley to Wolbach, 4 February 1928; and J. R. Parker to Wolbach, 17 October 1928, vol. "Professors at Various Universities," CC. Several other volumes of the Cooley Correspondence also document Cooley's experiments with tick parasites. For published material see Cooley, "Tick Parasites—Executive Report," in MSBE, *Seventh Biennial Report*, 10–16; Fred A. Morton, "Quantity Production of Tick Parasites," MSBE, *Seventh Biennial Report*, 32–35; J. R. Parker and W. J. Butler, "Tick Parasite Liberation in Montana During 1928," MSBE, *Seventh Biennial Report*, 35–38.

46. Application and correspondence, vol. "Tick Parasite Work—Africa, 1928–1932," CC; Price, *Fighting Spotted Fever* (see chap. 3, n. 4), 208–11.

47. RML, Monthly Report, May–June 1933.

48. Ibid.; RML, *Annual Report*, 1933, 11–13.

49. RML, Monthly Reports, January 1934, 6–8; February 1935, 8–9; RML, *Annual Report*, 1934, 3.

50. F. J. O'Donnell, "Control Work: Rocky Mountain Spotted Fever Control Districts, Bitter Root Valley, for the Biennium Ending December 31, 1932," in MSBE, *Ninth Biennial Report*, 7; RML, Monthly Reports, May 1935, 6, 13–15; July 1935, 13–14; September 1935, 5; January 1936, 7; April 1936, 4–5; RML, *Annual Report*, 1936, 13.

51. Occasionally the press in other western states took politicians to task over the situation. One author reminded Idaho readers that although spotted fever had been "one of Idaho's most serious problems," the financial burden of battling the disease had been borne by Montana alone. "Thus Idaho governors" had been "spared the awkwardness of asking their legislatures for a few dollars to control a dread disease in this state." See H. H. Miller, "Battling a Dread Disease—Rocky Mountain Spotted Fever," *Idaho Sunday Statesman* (Boise), 5 April 1936, clipping in RML Scrapbook "1935–41."

52. "Proposal to Surrender the Board's Research Work to the United States Government," in MSBE, *Eighth Biennial Report*, 13–14.

53. "Rocky Mountain Spotted Fever Committee Report," n.d., folder 11, "Rocky Mountain Spotted Fever Committee, 1930," box 1, "General Correspondence," MSBH Records; Hardy A. Kemp and C. M. Gribsby, "The Occurrence and Identification of an Infection of the Rocky Mountain Spotted Fever Type in Texas," *Texas State Medical Journal* 27 (1931):395–98. For the text of the resolution, see "Proposal to Surrender," 14–15.

54. U.S. Congress, Senate, *A Bill Authorizing the Purchase of the State Laboratory at Hamilton, Montana, Constructed for the Prevention, Eradication, and Cure of Spotted Fever*, S. 5959, 71st Cong., 3d sess., 26 January (calendar day 30 January) 1931. Senator Walsh's speech, the discussion, and inserted letters are in U.S. Congress, Senate, *Congressional Record*, 71st Cong., 3d sess., 30 January 1930, 3634–38. The identical bill was introduced by Congressman Scott Leavitt, 6 February 1931, into the House of Representatives as H.R. 16915. Copies of both bills and of correspondence about the bill circulated in the U.S. Public Health Service are in file 1960–62, "Hamilton—Spotted Fever," box 159, "Domestic Stations," PHS Records.

55. U.S. Congress, Senate, *Congressional Record*, 71st Cong., 3d sess., 30 January 1930, 3638.

56. Correspondence and other records in file 1960–62, "Hamilton— Spotted Fever," box 159, "Domestic Stations," PHS Records; Price, *Fighting Spotted Fever*, 223–27; Harden, *Inventing the NIH*, 140–59; "Rocky Mountain Spotted Fever Committee Report," n.p.

57. Parker to Surgeon General, telegram, 25 February 1931; and Thompson to Parker, 3 March 1931, file 1960–62, "Hamilton—Spotted Fever," box 159, "Domestic Stations," PHS Records; "Rocky Mountain Spotted Fever Committee Report," n.p.

58. The original draft erroneously authorized the Surgeon General of the U.S. Public Health Service to purchase the laboratory. This was revised, and the secretary of the Treasury was designated as the appropriate official. The second change was an addition stipulating that the laboratory would be administered and maintained as a part of the U.S. Public Health Service. See U.S. Congress, S. Rept. 1660 to Accompany S. 5959, 71st Cong., 3d sess., 17 February 1931.

59. U.S. Congress, Senate, *Congressional Record*, 71st Cong., 3d sess., 20 February 1931, 5575–76; *An Act Authorizing the Purchase of the State Laboratory at Hamilton, Montana, Constructed for the Prevention, Eradication, and Cure of Spotted Fever*, 2 March 1931, 46 *Stat. L.* 319; *Second Deficiency Act, Fiscal Year 1931*, 4 March 1931, 46 *Stat. L.* 522.

60. Spencer to Parker, 20 March 1932, file "Senior Surgeon R. R. Spencer," RML Director's Office files, Hamilton, Montana (hereafter cited as RML Director's Files).

61. Budget projections and correspondence in file "Federal Government Reorganization—Recommendations of 1933," General Correspondence, Thomas Parran Papers, University Archives, University of Pittsburgh, Pittsburgh (hereafter cited as Parran Papers); "Possible Cut in Funds for War Against Fever Menaces Hamilton Work," *Daily Missoulian*, 28 May 1933; "Dangerous Economy," *Daily Missoulian*, 29 May 1933; "Spotted Fever Research Fund May Be Slashed," *Bozeman* [Mont.] *Chronicle*, 28 May 1933; "Wood-Tick Fund May Be Reduced," *Billings* [Mont.] *Gazette*, 29 May 1933, clippings in RML Scrapbook "1932–1940."

62. Cumming to Ballantine, 17 April 1933, file "Federal Government Reorganization—Recommendations of 1933," General Correspondence, Parran Papers.

63. "No Let-Up in Fight against Tick Fever," *Cheyenne* [Wyo.] *Tribune*, 4 June 1933; "U.S. Will Continue Fight on Tick Fever," *Denver* [Colo.] *Morning Post*, 3 June 1933, clippings in RML Scrapbook "1932–1940."

64. Spencer to Parker, 5 July 1932, file "Senior Surgeon R. R. Spencer," RML Director's Files; Dedication, *Fernald Club Yearbook*, University of Massachusetts, no. 19, January 1950, 2, NIAID files, NIH Historical Office; RML, Monthly Report, January–February 1933, 8–9. In 1931, Parker also suffered the loss of his wife Adah Nicolet Parker, who had assisted him in his early career despite physical handicaps. They had two children. In 1932 Parker remarried, to Vivian Kaa, daughter of a prominent Hamilton surgeon.

65. RML, *Annual Reports*, 1934, 1; and 1936, 6–7.

66. RML, *Annual Report*, 1933, 15–16; RML, Monthly Report, May 1934, 2.

67. R. R. Parker, "Tick-Borne Diseases of Man in Montana and Methods of Prevention," Montana State Department of Health *Special Bulletin* no. 47 (1933), 12 pp.; RML, Monthly Report, March 1926, 9; Parker to Surgeon General, 17 July 1931, letter bound with RML Monthly Reports.

68. RML, Monthly Reports, August 1935, 9–10; and March 1936, 3; RML, *Annual Report*, 1936, 8–10; G. E. Davis and H. R. Cox, "A Filter-Passing Infectious Agent Isolated from Ticks: I. Isolation from *Dermacentor andersoni*, Reactions in Animals, and Filtration Experiments," *Pub. Health Rep.* 53 (1938):2259–67; H. R. Cox, "Studies of a Filter-Passing Agent Isolated from Ticks. V. Further Attempts to Cultivate in Cell-Free Media. Suggested Classification," *Pub. Health Rep.* 54 (1939):1822–27.

69. On contamination of the Spencer-Parker vaccine with Q fever organisms and the hypersensitivity reaction it produced, see Richard A. Ormsbee, interview by Victoria A. Harden, Hamilton, Montana, 2 August 1985 (hereafter cited as Ormsbee interview); David B. Lackman, E. John Bell, J. Frederick Bell, and Edgar G. Pickens, "Intradermal Sensitivity Testing in Man with a Purified Vaccine for Q Fever," *Am. J. Pub. Health* 52 (1962):87–93; J. Frederick Bell, David B. Lackman, Armon Meis, and W. J. Hadlow, "Recurrent Reaction at Site of Q Fever Vaccination in a Sensitized Person," *Military Medicine* 129 (1964):591–95. Robert N. Philip noted in a personal communication to the author, 16 February 1988, that the possibility of contamination was a major compelling factor in the search for a better method of spotted fever vaccine preparation.

70. E. H. Derrick, " 'Q' Fever, a New Fever Entity: Clinical Features, Diagnosis, and Laboratory Investigation," *Medical Journal of Australia* 2 (1937):281–99; F. M. Burnet and M. Freeman, "Experimental Studies on the Virus of 'Q' Fever," ibid. 2 (1937):299–305; R. E. Dyer, "Filter-Passing Infectious Agent Isolated from Ticks. Human Infection," *Pub. Health Rep.* 53 (1938):2277–82; R. E. Dyer, "Similarity of Australian 'Q' Fever and a Disease Caused by an Infectious Agent Isolated from Ticks in Montana," *Pub. Health Rep.* 54 (1939):1229–37; H. R. Cox, "*Rickettsia diaporica* and American Q Fever," *Am. J. Trop. Med.* 20 (1940):463–69; F. M. Burnet and M. Freeman, "Studies of X Strain (Dyer) of *Rickettsia burnetii*; Chorioallantoic Membrane Infections," *Journal of Immunology* 40 (1941):405–19; C. B. Philip, "Com-

ments on Name of Q Fever Organism," *Pub. Health Rep.* 63 (1948):58. For a recent historical account of the discovery of Q fever, see Jospeh E. McDade, "Historical Aspects of Q Fever," forthcoming. I am grateful to Dr. McDade for providing me with a preprint.

71. Expansion of laboratory facilities, for example, had been authorized in 1931 by the appropriations act accompanying the purchase of the laboratory by the U.S. Public Health Service. Begun in April 1933, the new unit was designed specifically to separate vaccine production from other operations because of the hazards involved. The laboratory also benefited from New Deal expenditures under the Public Works Administration by the addition of officers' quarters and outbuildings. See RML, *Annual Report*, 1934.

72. Ibid., 2.

73. RML, Monthly Reports, December 1934, 3; April 1935, 3; and May 1935, 3; Cumming to B. K. Wheeler, 19 July 1934, file 1975–85, "Hamilton—Spotted Fever Laboratory," box 159, "Domestic Stations," PHS Records.

74. RML, Monthly Report, February 1934, 12–17; "Wood Tick Season Is Here: Residents Must Be Careful," *Spokane* [Wash.] *Press*, 19 March 1935, attached to RML, Monthly Report, March 1935, n.p.; letters in file 1975–85, "Hamilton—Spotted Fever Laboratory," box 159, "Domestic Stations," PHS Records.

75. J. H. Rosenberg to Director, Spotted Fever Laboratory, 12 March 1934; and Mefford to Director, Spotted Fever Laboratory, 25 March 1934, attached to RML, Monthly Report, March 1934.

76. RML, Monthly Report, March 1935, 4.

77. Expressions of this philosophy are in Cooley to Cogswell, 28 November 1927, vol. "W. F. Cogswell, A. H. McCray, T. D. Tuttle," CC; "U.S. Government Spotted Fever Vaccine Available for Nevada Residents," *Nevada Stockgrower*, May 1929, 14, clipping in RML Scrapbook "1919–1931."

78. Baker to Wheeler, 20 March 1935; and Parker to Surgeon General, 13 April 1935, file 1975–85, "Hamilton—Spotted Fever Laboratory," box 159, "Domestic Stations," PHS Records; 1940s newspaper notices of free vaccine clinics in Ravalli County in RML Scrapbooks.

79. RML, Monthly Report, March 1934.

80. Thompson to Parker, 25 April 1934, file 1960–62, "Hamilton—Spotted Fever," box 159, "Domestic Stations," PHS Records.

81. RML, *Annual Report*, 1933, 5.

82. RML, Monthly Report, March 1935, 2; RML, *Annual Reports*, 1936, 3; and 1937, 4.

Chapter Nine: Dr. Cox's Versatile Egg

1. Personal communications to the author.

2. E. N. Wilmer, ed., *Cells and Tissues in Culture: Methods, Biology and Physiology* (New York: Academic Press, 1965), 1–17; A. M. Harvey, "Johns Hopkins—The Birthplace of Tissue Culture: The Story of Ross G. Harrison, Warren H. Lewis, and George O. Gey," *Johns Hopkins Medical Journal* 136 (1975):142–49; Frederick B. Bang, "History of Tissue Culture at Johns Hopkins," *Bull. Hist. Med.* 51 (1977):516–37.

3. S. B. Wolbach and M. J. Schlesinger, "The Cultivation of the Microorganisms of Rocky Mountain Spotted Fever (*Dermacentroxenus rickettsi*) and

of Typhus (*Rickettsia prowazeki*) in Tissue Plasma Cultures," *J. Med. Res.* 44 (1923):231–56.

4. Alice Miles Woodruff and Ernest W. Goodpasture, "The Susceptibility of the Chorio-Allantoic Membrane of Chick Embryos to Infection with the Fowl-pox Virus," *Am. J. Pathol.* 7 (1931):209–22. For a chronology of major papers on cultivation of other organisms by this method, see B. John Buddingh, "Chick-Embryo Technics," in Thomas M. Rivers, ed., *Viral and Rickettsial Infections of Man*, 2d ed. (Philadelphia: J. B. Lippincott Co., 1952), 109–25, esp. table 8, p. 110.

5. For biographical information on Bengtson, see Barry, *Notable Contributions* (see chap. 5, n. 75), 9–12; "Ida Albertina Bengston [*sic*]," in Elizabeth Moot O'Hearn, *Profiles of Pioneer Women Scientists* (Washington, D.C.: Acropolis Books, 1985), 119–24; obituary by Alice C. Evans, *Journal of the Washington Academy of Sciences* 43 (1953):238–40.

6. Ida A. Bengtson and R. E. Dyer, "Cultivation of the Virus of Rocky Mountain Spotted Fever in the Developing Chick Embryo," *Pub. Health Rep.* 50 (1935):1489–98; Ralph D. Lillie, "Histologic Reaction to the Virus of Rocky Mountain Spotted Fever in Chick Embryos," ibid., 1498–1501.

7. P. K. Olitsky and J. E. McCartney, "Experimental Studies on the Etiology of Typhus Fever. V. Survival of the Virus in Collodion Sacs Implanted Intra-Abdominally in Guinea Pigs," *J. Exp. Med.* 38 (1928):691; Clara Nigg and Karl Landsteiner, "Studies on Cultivation of Typhus Fever Rickettsia in Presence of Live Tissue," ibid. 55 (1932):563–76; Henry Pinkerton and G. M. Haas, "Spotted Fever. I. Intranuclear Rickettsiae in Spotted Fever Studied in Tissue Culture," ibid. 56 (1932):151–56; Ida A. Bengtson, "Cultivation of the Rickettsiae of Rocky Mountain Spotted Fever in Vitro," *Pub. Health Rep.* 52 (1937):1329–35; Ida A. Bengtson, "Immunizing Properties of Formolized Rocky Mountain Spotted Fever Rickettsiae Cultivated in Modified Maitland Media," *Pub. Health Rep.* 52 (1937):1696–1702 (quotation from p. 1702).

8. *An Act to Provide for the General Welfare by Establishing a System of Federal Old-Age Benefits, and by Enabling the Several States to Make More Adequate Provision for Aged Persons, Blind Persons, Dependent and Crippled Children, Maternal and Child Welfare, Public Health, and the Administration of Their Unemployment Compensation Laws; To Establish a Social Security Board; To Raise Revenue; and for Other Purposes*, 14 August 1935, 49 *Stat. L.* 531. See esp. Title VI, "Public Health Work," 634–35.

9. Attachment to Parker to Thompson, 21 March 1935, file 0425, "Hamilton—Spotted Fever Laboratory," box 159, "Domestic Stations," PHS Records.

10. Harden, *Inventing the NIH* (see chap. 3, n. 35), 170–73.

11. RML, Monthly Report, February 1936, 1. Officially, the date of this name change was recorded as 1937, when the NIH was reorganized. See National Institute of Allergy and Infectious Diseases, *Intramural Contributions, 1887–1987*, ed. Harriet R. Greenwald and Victoria A. Harden (Bethesda, Md.: National Institute of Allergy and Infectious Diseases, 1987), 4 (hereafter cited as NIAID, *Intramural Contributions, 1887–1987*).

12. For biographical information on Cox, see "Herald R. Cox," *American Men and Women of Science*, 16th ed., ed. Jacques Cattell Press, *Physical and Biological Sciences*, vol. 2 (New York: R. R. Bowker, 1986), 414; "Herald R. Cox," *World Who's Who in Science: A Biographical Dictionary of Notable*

Scientists from Antiquity to the Present, ed. Allen G. Debus (Chicago: Marquis-Who's Who, 1968), 381; "Noted Researcher Dies in Hamilton," Daily Missoulian, 19 August 1986, 6. Cox died 17 August 1986.

13. The virologist was Thomas Rivers, cited in Benison, Tom Rivers (see chap. 6, n. 56), 251–52; RML, Monthly Reports, May 1936, 13; and June 1936, 10.

14. H. R. Cox, "Reminiscences," in Willy Burgdorfer and Robert L. Anacker, eds., Rickettsiae and Rickettsial Diseases (New York: Academic Press, 1981), 11–15 (quotations from pp. 11–12).

15. Ibid., 13. When Cox made this discovery, the identity of Nine Mile fever and Q fever had not been established.

16. H. R. Cox, "Use of Yolk Sac of Developing Chick Embryo as Medium for Growing Rickettsiae of Rocky Mountain Spotted Fever and Typhus Groups," Pub. Health Rep. 53 (1938):2241–47; idem, "Rocky Mountain Spotted Fever: Protective Value for Guinea Pigs of Vaccine Prepared from Rickettsiae Cultivated in Embryonic Chick Tissues," ibid. 54 (1939):1070–77; H. R. Cox and E. John Bell, "The Cultivation of Rickettsia diaporica in Tissue Culture and in the Tissues of Developing Chick Embryos," ibid., 2171–78; H. R. Cox and E. John Bell, "Epidemic and Endemic Typhus: Protective Value for Guinea Pigs of Vaccines Prepared from Infected Tissues of the Developing Chick Embryo," ibid. 55 (1940):110–15; H. R. Cox, "Cultivation of Rickettsiae of the Rocky Mountain Spotted Fever, Typhus, and Q Fever Groups in the Embryonic Tissues of Developing Chicks," Science 94 (1941):399–403 (quotation from p. 401).

17. Hans Zinsser, Florence K. Fitzpatrick, and Hsi Wei, "A Study of Rickettsiae Grown on Agar-Tissue Cultures," J. Exp. Med. 69 (1939):179–90; Florence K. Fitzpatrick, "Vaccination against Spotted Fever with Agar-Tissue Cultures," Proceedings of the Society for Experimental Biology and Medicine 42 (1939):219–20.

18. RML, Annual Report, 1939, 1; Cox, "Rocky Mountain Spotted Fever: Protective Value for Guinea Pigs," 1070–77; Timothy J. Kurotchkin and Ralph W. G. Wycoff, "Immunizing Value of Rickettsial Vaccines," Proc. Soc. Exp. Biol. Med. 46 (1941):223–28.

19. RML, Annual Report, 1940, 1–2; J. D. Ratcliff, "Bite of Death," Collier's, 28 March 1942, 15, 42–43.

20. "U.S. Public Health Service Orientation Course for Personnel to Serve in Health and Sanitation Activities in Connection with National Defense," Pub. Health Rep. 56 (1941):662–63.

21. Hartwin A. Schulze, "Typhus on the Western Front in World War II," Military Surgeon 101 (1947):489–98 (quotation from p. 490).

22. For biographical information on Topping, see Norman Topping, oral history interview by Harlan Phillips, 24 April 1964, in George Rosen, Transcripts of Oral History Project, 1962–64, NLM (hereafter cited as Topping oral history); American Men of Science, 11th ed., ed. Jacques Cattell Press, Physical and Biological Sciences, vol. St-Z (New York: R. R. Bowker Co., 1967), 5441; Norman Topping, with Gordon Cohn, Recollections (Los Angeles: University of Southern California, 1990). I am grateful to Dr. Topping and to Mr. Cohn for making available a copy of this book in manuscript.

23. Eugene P. Campbell and Walter H. Ketchum, "Rocky Mountain Spotted Fever: An Analysis of Seven Cases, Including One Laboratory Infection," New

England J. Med. 223 (1940):540–43 (Topping's case is discussed on p. 540). Dr. Campbell kindly provided me with a copy of his personal records of Topping's illness.

24. Rudolf Weigl, "Untersuchungen und Experimente an Fleckfieberläusen. Die Technik der Rickettsia-Forschung," *Beiträge zur Klinik der Infektionskrankheiten und zer Immunitatsforschung* 8 (1920):353–76; idem, "Die Methoden der aktiven Fleckfieber-Immunisierung," *Bulletin International de l'Académie Polonaise des Sciences et des Lettres, Classe de Médecine,* July 1930, 25–62; Peter K. Olitsky, "Hans Zinsser and His Studies on Typhus Fever," *JAMA* 116 (1941):907–12 (Weigl's vaccine is discussed on pp. 909, 911).

25. Hans Zinsser and M. Ruiz Castaneda, "Studies on Typhus Fever. V. Active Immunization against Typhus Fever with Formalinized Virus," *J. Exp. Med.* 53 (1931):325–31; idem, "A Note of Improvement in the Method of Vaccine Production with Rickettsiae of Mexican Typhus Fever," *J. Immunol.* 21 (1931):403–7; idem, "A Method of Obtaining Large Amounts of *Rickettsia provaceki* [*sic*] by X-ray Radiation of Rats," *Proc. Soc. Exp. Biol. Med.* 29 (1932):840–44; idem, "Studies on Typhus Fever. IX. On the Serum Reaction of Mexican and European Typhus Rickettsia," *J. Exp. Med.* 56 (1932):455–67; M. Ruiz Castaneda, "Experimental Pneumonia Produced by Typhus Rickettsiae," *Am. J. Pathol.* 15 (1939):467–76.

26. Paul Durand and Paul Giroud, "Essais de vaccination contre le typhus historique au moyen de rickettsias tuées par le formol (souches pulmonaires)," *Compt. rend. Acad. d. sc.* 210 (1940):493–96; Norman H. Topping and Charles C. Shepard, "The Rickettsiae," in *Annual Review of Microbiology* 1 (1947):333–50 (quotation from p. 334).

27. James Craigie, "Application and Control of Ethyl-Ether-Water Interface Effects to the Separation of Rickettsiae from Yolk Sac Suspensions," *Canadian Journal of Research* 23 (1945):104–14. Because of wartime censorship, Craigie's method was submitted in 1942 to the Associate Committee on Medical Research of the National Research Council of Canada, which had supported the work financially, as a confidential document for restricted distribution in mimeographed form. It was not published openly until January 1945.

28. E. John Bell, interview by Victoria A. Harden, Hamilton, Montana, 5 August 1985, 4, NIAID files, NIH Historical Office; Norman H. Topping, Ida A. Bengtson, and M. J. Shear, "Studies of Typhus Fever Vaccines," in "Studies of Typhus Fever," U.S. National Institute of Health *Bulletin* no. 183 (1945):1–24; Ida A. Bengtson, Norman H. Topping, and Richard G. Henderson, "Epidemic Typhus: Demonstration of a Substance Lethal for Mice in the Yolk Sac of Eggs Infected with *Rickettsia prowazeki*," U.S. National Institute of Health *Bulletin* no. 183 (1945):25–29; Richard G. Henderson, "Notes on the Mouse Test with Typhus Vaccine," U.S. National Institute of Health *Bulletin* no. 183 (1945):33–35; Harry Plotz, Report on Contributions from the Division of Virus and Rickettsial Diseases, Army Medical School, on the Development of the Typhus Vaccine, 18 January 1946. In 1940 toxic activity associated with the organism of murine typhus had been demonstrated, and subsequently it was discovered in yolk sac tissue infected with spotted fever and boutonneuse fever. See E. Gildemeister and E. Haagen, "Fleckfieberstudien. I. Mitteilung: Nachweis eines Toxins in Rickettsien-Eikulturen (*Rickettsia mooseri*)," *Deutsche med. Wchnschr.* 66 (1940):878–80, Eng.

trans. in Hahon, *Selected Papers* (see chap. 6, n. 26), 213–20; J. E. Smadel, E. B. Jackson, B. L. Bennett, and F. L. Rights, "A Toxic Substance Associated with the Gilliam Strain of *R. orientalis*," *Proc. Soc. Exp. Biol. Med.* 62 (1964):138–40; E. J. Bell and E. G. Pickens, "A Toxic Substance Associated with the Rickettsias of the Spotted Fever Group," *J. Immunol.* 70 (1953):461–72.

29. Norman H. Topping, "Notes on the Preparation of Epidemic Typhus Vaccine," 30–32. In a personal communication to the author, 2 September 1988, Norman H. Topping commented that by the time the vaccine was in production, "it had been so modified by Craigie and by us at the NIH that other than the hen's egg it had no resemblance to that described by Cox."

30. "Bolivia Experimenting with Dr. Herold [*sic*] Cox' Vaccine, May Save Millions of Lives," *Missoula Sentinel*, 4 September 1941, clipping in RML Scrapbook "1941–1942"; Topping "Recollections."

31. "Active Immunization against Typhus," *JAMA* 119 (1942):500–501; Ratcliff, "Bite of Death," 43.

32. RML, Monthly Reports, February 1942, 3; and March 1942, 1; "Immunization and Multiple Antigens," *JAMA* 128 (1945):613; "Eyes of Nation on Typhus Lab," *Spokesman Review* (Spokane, Wash.), 29 March 1942, clipping in RML Scrapbook "1942–   "; Ratcliff, "Bite of Death," 15ff.; J. Kobler, "Blitz Plague: Will Typhus Shape the Course of War?" *Saturday Evening Post* 215 (22 August 1942):26ff. George D. Brigham, a Yale-trained bacteriologist, assumed Cox's post as head of the RML's typhus unit. See "Typhus Expert to Valley Lab from Southland," *Daily Missoulian*, 29 November 1942, clipping in RML Scrapbook "1941–1942."

33. Production of yellow fever vaccine at the RML came about somewhat by chance. Before the war the U.S. Public Health Service had sent Mason V. Hargett, an officer trained in tropical diseases, to the Rockefeller Foundation headquarters in Brazil in order to learn methods of vaccine production that, it was hoped, would allow the Service to manufacture a limited amount for its own use. In October 1940, Hargett established a vaccine production unit with his assistant, Harry Burruss, at the RML—a site chosen because of the absence of *Aedes egypti* mosquitoes. Hargett's research convinced him that the vaccine could be improved by removing the human serum added as a stabilizer, and he subsequently developed an "aqueous-base" vaccine. After a 1942 outbreak of jaundice among military personnel that was traced to contaminated serum used in the Rockefeller Foundation's yellow fever vaccine, the U.S. military requested that Hargett produce all subsequent yellow fever vaccine using his modified method. See M. V. Hargett, H. W. Burruss, and A. Donovan, "Aqueous Base Yellow Fever Vaccine," *Pub. Health Rep.* 58 (1943):505–12; Mason V. Hargett, interview by Victoria A. Harden, Hamilton, Montana, 2 August 1985; and Harry Burruss, interview by Harden, Gaithersburg, Maryland, 17 April 1986, NIAID files, NIH Historical Office (copies also in NLM).

34. RML, Monthly Report, December 1941, 9–10.

35. Glen M. Kohls, "Rocky Mountain Spotted Fever," in Medical Department, U.S. Army, *Preventive Medicine in World War II*, vol. 7, *Communicable Diseases: Arthropodborne Diseases Other Than Malaria* (Washington, D.C.: Government Printing Office, 1964), 349–56.

36. "Workman's Compensation Acts: Death from Rocky Mountain Spotted Fever Caused by Bite of Wood Tick Allegedly Received in Course of Employment," *JAMA* 121 (1943):149–50.

37. Executive Order no. 9285, "Establishing the United States of America Typhus Commission," *Federal Register* 7 (no. 253, December 1942):10899; Stanhope Bayne-Jones oral history memoir (Harlan Phillips, interviewer), 5 vols., NLM, 3:641–46 (quotation from p. 644) (hereafter cited as Bayne-Jones oral history); Stanhope Bayne-Jones, "The United States of America Typhus Commission," *Army Medical Bulletin* 68 (1943):4–15; Stanhope Bayne-Jones, "Typhus Fevers," in Medical Department, U.S. Army, *Preventive Medicine in World War II*, vol. 7, *Communicable Diseases: Arthropodborne Diseases Other Than Malaria*, 175–274.

38. Material from the journal and personal files of Eugene P. Campbell, Chevy Chase, Maryland. Included in this material is the draft of an oral history prepared by Campbell with his colleague at the Institute of Inter-American Affairs, James Williams, which will be placed in the Columbia University oral history collection with other institute materials. Campbell also noted that the reference work on typhus in Guatemala used by the U.S. physicians was George C. Shattuck, *A Medical Survey of the Republic of Guatemala* (Washington, D.C.: Carnegie Institution of Washington, 1938), which cited Hans Zinsser on "Mexican typhus." This again reflects how misleading the phrase *Mexican typhus* had become, implying that typhus in Mexico was exclusively murine.

39. Topping oral history, 10; Bayne-Jones oral history, 653; Arthur P. Long, "The Army Immunization Program," in Medical Department, U.S. Army, *Preventive Medicine in World War II*, vol. 3, *Personal Health Measures and Immunization* (Washington, D.C.: Government Printing Office, 1955), 271–72, 319–23; Bayne-Jones, "Typhus Fevers," 238–39.

40. Bayne-Jones, "Typhus Fevers," table 33, p. 180. Many other publications refer to 64 as the total number of typhus cases during the war, citing Joseph F. Sadusk, Jr., "Typhus Fever in the United States Army Following Immunization," *JAMA* 133 (1947):1192–99. Bayne-Jones notes that his figure of 104 cases was based on data revised through October 1960.

41. C. H. Stuart-Harris, "Discussion on the Control of Rickettsial Infections," *Proc. R. Soc. Med.* 38 (1945):511–18; A. Sachs, "Typhus Fever in Iran and Iraq, 1942–43: A Report on 2,859 Cases," *J. Royal Army Med. Corps* 86 (1946):87–108; A. G. Gilliam, "Efficacy of Cox-Type Vaccine in the Prevention of Naturally Acquired Louse-Borne Typhus Fever," *Am. J. Hyg.* 44 (1946):401–10; Herman Gold and Florence K. Fitzpatrick, "Typhus Fever in a Previously Vaccinated Laboratory Worker," *JAMA* 119 (1942):1415–17; N. H. Topping, "Typhus Fever: A Note of the Severity of the Disease among Unvaccinated and Vaccinated Laboratory Personnel at the National Institute of Health," *Am. J. Trop. Med.* 24 (1944):57–62; R. S. Ecke, A. G. Gilliam, J. C. Snyder, Andrew Yeomans, C. J. Zarafonetis, and E. S. Murray, "The Effect of Cox-Type Vaccine on Louse-Borne Typhus Fever: An Account of 61 Cases of Naturally Occurring Typhus Fever in Patients Who Had Previously Received One or More Injections of Cox-Type Vaccine," *Am. J. Trop. Med.* 25 (1945):447–62.

42. H. L. Haller and S. J. Cristol, "The Development of New Insecticides," in *Advances in Military Medicine* (Boston: Little, Brown & Co., 1948), 2:621–

26; William A. Hardenbergh, "Control of Insects," and "The Research Background of Insect and Rodent Control," in Medical Department, U.S. Army, *Preventive Medicine in World War II,* vol. 2, *Environmental Hygiene* (Washington, D.C.: Government Printing Office, 1955), 231–32, 251–69. For a personal account of this work and remarks about the Audubon Society's warning, see Ormsbee interview (see chap. 8, n. 69), 11–12.

43. Bayne-Jones oral history, 649–50; Schulze, "Typhus on the Western Front in World War II," 491.

44. "Typhus in Naples," Rockefeller Foundation *Review* (1944):33–36 (quotation from p. 35). See also Charles M. Wheeler, "Control of Typhus in Italy 1943–1944 by Use of DDT," *Am. J. Pub. Health* 36 (1946):119–29; Bayne-Jones, "Typhus Fevers," 217–31.

45. These events were discussed in chap. 8.

46. F. L. Kelly, "Weil-Felix Reaction in Rocky Mountain Spotted Fever," *J. Inf. Dis.* 32 (1923):223–25; A. L. Kerlee and R. R. Spencer, "Rocky Mountain Spotted Fever: A Preliminary Report on the Weil-Felix Reaction," *Pub. Health Rep.* 44 (1929):179–82. The development of the Weil-Felix reaction was discussed in chap. 6.

47. R. R. Spencer and K. F. Maxcy, "The Weil-Felix Reaction in Endemic Typhus Fever and in Rocky Mountain Spotted Fever," *Pub. Health Rep.* 45 (1930):440–46.

48. "Weil-Felix Reaction in Typhus Fever," abstract in *JAMA* 90 (1928):331. Kenneth F. Maxcy, however, noted that rabbits inoculated with a patient's blood early in the illness could later be tested for the development of Weil-Felix agglutinins. Not only would this procedure confirm the diagnosis if the patient died, but it was also useful for small laboratories that lacked facilities to maintain large supplies of guinea pigs for protection tests or direct isolation of the organism. K. F. Maxcy, "The Weil-Felix Reaction of the Rabbit in the Diagnosis of Rocky Mountain Spotted Fever (Eastern Type)," *J. Inf. Dis.* 58 (1936):288–92.

49. Spencer and Maxcy, "The Weil-Felix Reaction," 441.

50. L. F. Badger, "Laboratory Diagnosis of Endemic Typhus and Rocky Mountain Spotted Fever," *Am. J. Pub. Health* 23 (1933):19–27; idem, "The Laboratory Diagnosis of Endemic Typhus and Rocky Mountain Spotted Fever with Special Reference to Cross-Immunity Tests," *Am. J. Trop. Med.* 13 (1933):179–90 (quotation from p. 179).

51. Henry Pinkerton and George M. Hass, "Spotted Fever. I. Intranuclear Rickettsiae in Spotted Fever Studied in Tissue Culture," *J. Exp. Med.* 56 (1932):151–56; idem, "Spotted Fever. III. The Identification of Dermacentroxenus rickettsi and Its Differentiation from Non-Pathogenic Rickettsiae in Ticks," ibid. 66 (1937):729–39.

52. Jules Bordet and Octave Gengou, "Sur l'existence de substances sensibilisatrices dans la plupart des sérum antimicrobiens," *Annales de l'Institut Pasteur* 15 (1901):289–302; Bordet, "Sur la mode d'action des sérums cytolytiques et sur l'unité de l'alexine dans un même sérum," ibid. 303–18; Debra Jan Bibel, *Milestones in Immunology: A Historical Exploration* (Madison, Wis.: Science Tech Publishers, 1988), 268–71.

53. Benjamin F. Davis and William F. Petersen, "Complement Deviation in Rocky Mountain Spotted Fever," *J. Inf. Dis.* 8 (1911):330–38; idem, "Unfinished Experiments of Dr. Howard T. Ricketts on Rocky Mountain Spotted

Fever," in Ricketts, *Contributions to Medical Science* (see chap. 4, n. 10), 409–18.

54. See citations to this work in Ida A. Bengtson and Norman H. Topping, "Complement-Fixation in Rickettsial Diseases," *Am. J. Pub. Health* 32 (1942):48–58, esp. the bibliography, p. 58.

55. M. Ruiz Castaneda, "Studies on the Mechanism in Typhus Fever; Complement-Fixation in Typhus Fever," *J. Immunol.* 31 (1936):285–91.

56. Other types of diagnostic tests were also investigated, several of which will be discussed in chap. 11. In one of the earliest of these studies, Florence K. Fitzpatrick and Bettylee Hampil, researchers at the Sharp and Dohme pharmaceutical house, reported that antibodies in rabbits inoculated with typhus and spotted fever antigens appeared earlier and persisted longer than did antibodies to *B. proteus*. More importantly, the sequence of appearance of the antibodies was always the same. See Florence K. Fitzpatrick and Bettylee Hampil, "Immunological Reactions in Rickettsial Diseases with Special Reference to the Time of Appearance of Antibodies," *Am. J. Pub. Health* 31 (1941):1301–5.

57. Bengtson and Topping, "Complement-Fixation in Rickettsial Diseases," 49; Ida A. Bengtson, "Applications of Complement-Fixation Test in Study of Rickettsial Diseases," *Am. J. Pub. Health* 35 (1945):701–7. Recent advances in immunology help to explain the differences between the Weil-Felix and the complement fixation tests. Weil-Felix antibodies are of the IgM class, which provide one of the earliest responses of the body to invasion by foreign organisms. These antibodies, however, do not persist for long periods of time. This may explain why the Weil-Felix test provided an earlier indication of rickettsial infection in a higher percentage of cases tested by Bengtson and Topping. Moreover, in the case of Brill's disease, IgM antibodies are not reformulated during recrudescence of the epidemic typhus infection. Because of this, a fourfold rise in Weil-Felix titer may be used to identify a new infection with *R. prowazeki* and to rule out Brill's disease.

The complement fixation text, in contrast, responds more efficiently to antibodies of the IgG class. These antibodies appear later than do IgM antibodies, but they persist longer, which explains why the complement fixation reaction responded over a longer period of time than did the Weil-Felix. See R. N. Philip, C. A. Casper, J. N. McCormack, D. J. Sexton, L. A. Thomas, R. L. Anacker, W. Burgdorfer, and S. Vick, "A Comparison of Serologic Methods for Diagnosis of Rocky Mountain Spotted Fever," *American Journal of Epidemiology* 105 (1977):56–67.

58. Harry Plotz and Kenneth Wertman, "The Use of the Complement Fixation Test in Rocky Mountain Spotted Fever," *Science* 95 (1942):441–42; Harry Plotz, K. Wertman, and B. L. Bennett, "Identification of Rickettsial Agents Isolated in Guinea Pigs by Means of Specific Complement Fixation," *Proc. Soc. Exp. Biol. Med.* 61 (1946):76–81.

59. Joseph E. Smadel, "The Practitioner and the Virus Diagnostic Laboratory," *JAMA* 136 (1948):1079–81 (quotation from p. 1080).

60. David B. Lackman, interview by Victoria A. Harden, Helena, Montana, 12 August 1985, 10–11, NIAID files, NIH Historical Office; James van der Scheer, Emil Bohnel, and Herald R. Cox, "Diagnostic Antigens for Epidemic Typhus, Murine Typhus and Rocky Mountain Spotted Fever," *J. Immunol.* 56 (1947):365–75.

61. Berton Roueché, "The Alerting of Mr. Pomeranz," *New Yorker,* 30 August 1947, 28ff; Robert J. Huebner, P. Stamps, and Charles Armstrong, "Rickettsialpox—A Newly Recognized Rickettsial Disease. I. Isolation of the Etiological Agent," *Pub. Health Rep.* 61 (1946):1605–14; Morris Greenberg, Ottavio Pellitteri, Irving F. Klein, and Robert J. Huebner, "Rickettsialpox—A Newly Recognized Rickettsial Disease. II. Clinical Observations," *JAMA* 133 (1947):901–6; Morris Greenberg, Ottavio Pellitteri, and William L. Jellison, "Rickettsialpox—A Newly Recognized Rickettsial Disease. III. Epidemiology," *Am. J. Pub. Health* 37 (1947):860–68; Robert J. Huebner, William L. Jellison, and Charles Pomerantz, "Rickettsialpox—A Newly Recognized Rickettsial Disease. IV. Isolation of a Rickettsia Apparently Identical with the Causative Agent of Rickettsialpox from *Allodermanyssus sanguineus,* a Rodent Mite," *Pub. Health Rep.* 61 (1946):1677–82; Robert J. Huebner, William L. Jellison, and Charles Armstrong, "Rickettsialpox—A Newly Recognized Rickettsial Disease. V. Recovery of *Rickettsia akari* from a House Mouse (*Mus musculus*)," *Pub. Health Rep.* 62 (1947):777–80; H. M. Rose, "The Clinical Manifestations and Laboratory Diagnosis of Rickettsialpox," *Annals of Internal Medicine* 31 (1949):871–83; L. N. Sussman, "Kew Gardens' Spotted Fever," *New York Medicine* 2 (1946):27–28; "Rickettsialpox: A New Rickettsial Disease," *JAMA* 137 (1948):384–85. For a later review of rickettsialpox, see David B. Lackman, "A Review of Information on Rickettsialpox in the United States," *Clinical Pediatrics* 2 (1963):296–301.

62. J. C. Woodland, M. M. McDowell, and J. T. Richards, "Bullis Fever (Lone Star Fever—Tick Fever)," *JAMA* 122 (1943):1156–60; "The Rickettsial Etiology of Bullis Fever," ibid. 124 (1944):926; William L. Jellison, interview by Victoria A. Harden, Hamilton, Montana, 3 August 1985, NIAID files, NIH Historical Office. In a personal communication to the author, 12 February 1988, David B. Lackman observed that clinical findings among patients as well as tests made at the RML indicated that Bullis fever was really Q fever. Other investigators disagreed, however, and the issue was never settled.

Chapter Ten: Spotted Fever Therapy, from Sage Tea to Tetracycline

1. William Osler, "Teaching and Thinking: The Two Functions of a Medical School," *Montreal Medical Journal* 23 (1895):561–72 (quotation from p. 568).

2. Contrast this with the social, political, and medical response to cholera in the nineteenth century. See Charles E. Rosenberg, *The Cholera Years: The United States in 1832, 1849, and 1866* (Chicago: University of Chicago Press, 1962).

3. The people of the Bitterroot, for example, pressed early investigators for some medical treatment for the disease and, as pointed out in chap. 4, welcomed Howard Taylor Ricketts's experimental antiserum. In 1911, Thomas B. McClintic also noted the fervor for an effective therapy. "From the view point of the inhabitants of the Bitter Root Valley, the treatment of spotted fever ranks in importance second only to the eradication of the disease. Their desire is for a remedy with which human cases of the disease may be successfully treated." See McClintic, "Investigations and Tick Eradication," 747, cited in chap. 5, n. 33.

4. McClintic, "Investigations and Tick Eradication," 748.

5. Ibid., 747–54 (quotations from p. 754).

6. Wolbach to Chairmen of the State Boards of Entomology and Health, 18 January 1918, vol. "Professors at Various Universities," CC; R. R. Spencer, "Annual Report of Rocky Mountain Spotted Fever Investigations," [1923], file 1266, box 119, Central File, 1897–1923, PHS Records.

7. H. P. Greeley, "Mercurochrome-220 Soluble in Rocky Mountain Spotted Fever," *JAMA* 83 (1924):1506–7.

8. Parker to Robert A. Cooley, 11 April 1926; and Cooley to Parker, 16 April 1926, vol. "R. R. Parker, 1926–1931," CC; L. C. Fisher, "Chemotherapy of Experimental Spotted Fever," *Proc. Soc. Exp. Biol. Med.* 29 (1932):633–35 (quotations from pp. 633–34). Laboratory research on spotted fever occasionally produced a bizarre episode that seemed to stand common sense on its head. In the late 1920s it was discovered that an induced fever had a beneficial effect on the course of syphilis, and therapeutically infecting syphilis patients with malaria was popular for a period. Rocky Mountain spotted fever, of course, similarly produced a high fever. Exploiting this line of research, European researchers inoculated rabbits with both syphilis and spotted fever. They reported that the temperature rise resulting from this spotted fever "therapy" for syphilis "exerted a curative influence on the syphilitic infection." There is no evidence, however, that virulent spotted fever was ever employed in treating human victims of syphilis. See "Fever Treatment of Experimental Syphilis," abstract in *JAMA* 89 (1927):417.

9. The best accounts of patent medicines and medical quackery in American history are Young, *Toadstool Millionaires* (see chap. 3, n. 51); and idem, *The Medical Messiahs: A Social History of Health Quackery in the Twentieth Century* (Princeton, N.J.: Princeton University Press, 1967). His analysis of the appeal of patent medicines and of quackery provided a framework for examining unorthodox spotted fever therapies.

10. "Makes a New Vaccine: Dr. Fox Finds Medicine Which Abrupts Tick Fever in Five Days," clipping dated 1916 in RML Scrapbook "1919–1931."

11. Elam to Parker, 18 December 1937, file "Cures for Spotted Fever (Letters offering to sell information)," RML Research Records.

12. See correspondence and handbills dated April and May 1932 in file "Cures for Spotted Fever (Letters offering to sell information)," RML Research Records.

13. J. J. Scott to Reserch Labritory [*sic*], [postmark 18 September 1938] file "Freak Letters," RML Research Records.

14. Lizzie W. Sonyer [spelling unclear] to State Board of Health, Cheyenne, Wyoming, 28 August 1926, file "Freak Letters," RML Research Records.

15. Cited in speech given by R. R. Parker "about 1940," and prepared for him by Hilda Holly from letters in file "Freak Letters," RML Research Records.

16. Turnquist to Ludwik Anigstein, 5 June 1944, file "Cures for Spotted Fever (Letters offering to sell information)," RML Research Records; L. W. Hartman to W. M. Cobleigh, 25 July 1921; and Cooley to Hartman, 15 November 1921, box 10, folder E2, "Tick Control—General Correspondence, 1918–1928," ZEA.

17. Mrs. Charles H. Purkis to A. E. Lien, 7 May 1946, file "Cures for Spotted Fever (Letters offering to sell information)," RML Research Records.

18. Cited in speech given by R. R. Parker "about 1940," and prepared for him by Hilda Holly from letters in file "Freak Letters," RML Research Records.

19. Parker to A. E. Lien, 14 May 1946, file "Cures for Spotted Fever (Letters offering to sell information)," RML Research Records.

20. Cited in speech given by R. R. Parker "about 1940," and prepared for him by Hilda Holly from letters in file "Freak Letters," RML Research Records.

21. Cooper to Parker, 14 July 1936, file "Freak Letters," RML Research Records.

22. Cooper to Parker, 25 July 1936, file "Freak Letters," RML Research Records.

23. Sproat to Parker, 26 February 1941, file "Cures for Spotted Fever (Letters offering to sell information)," RML Research Records.

24. My brief account of the sulfa drugs follows Harry F. Dowling, *Fighting Infection: Conquests of the Twentieth Century* (Cambridge, Mass.: Harvard University Press, 1977), 105–24.

25. "Hope of Curing Tuberculosis, Influenza, and Leprosy," *Science* 80 (1939):8. For popular response to the sulfa drugs, see also J. Stafford, "Prontosil Steals the Show at Major Medical Convention," *Science* 85 (1937):9–10; "Gonorrhea Cured in 3 Days by Sulfanilamide," *Science Newsletter* 32 (1937):388; E. W. Murtfeldt, "King of Drugs," *Popular Science* 134 (1939):63 ff.; "Killer Killed; Sulfapyridine Acts on All 32 Types of Pneumonia," *Time* 33 (1939):28.

26. Norman H. Topping, "Experimental Rocky Mountain Spotted Fever and Endemic Typhus Treated with Prontosil or Sulfapyridine," *Pub. Health Rep.* 54 (1939):1143–47; Edward A. Steinhaus and R. R. Parker, "Experimental Rocky Mountain Spotted Fever: Results of Treatment with Certain Drugs," *Pub. Health Rep.* 58 (1943):351–52; RML, Monthly Report, January 1942, 3.

27. Norman H. Topping, "Rocky Mountain Spotted Fever: Further Experience in the Therapeutic Use of Immune Rabbit Serum," *Pub. Health Rep.* 58 (1943):757–74 (quotation from p. 763). As recently as 1977, moreover, a professor of pediatrics at Mount Sinai School of Medicine in New York, felt it necessary to write a letter to the editor of the *Journal of Pediatrics* in which he reminded his colleagues of the danger of sulfonamides in rickettsial diseases. See Alex J. Steigman, "Rocky Mountain Spotted Fever and the Avoidance of Sulfonamides," *Journal of Pediatrics* 91 (1977):163–64.

28. "Green Light," *Seattle* [Wash.] *Star*, 10 April 1937, clipping in RML Scrapbook "1932–1940"; Clive Hirschorn, *The Warner Bros. Story* (New York: Crown Publishers, 1979), 172.

29. Nick Kramis, interview by Victoria A. Harden, Hamilton, Montana, 7 August 1985, NIAID files, NIH Historical Office (hereafter cited as Kramis interview); Ormsbee interview (see chap. 8, n. 69).

30. See numerous clippings in all RML Scrapbooks.

31. Kramis interview; many news clippings about civic clubs viewing this film, RML Scrapbooks; letters of permission to show film in file "R. R. Parker," box 91, "O-P," file 1650, "General Records of the National Institute of Health, 1930–1948," NIH Records, Record Group 443, National Archives and Records Administration, Washington, D.C. (hereafter cited as NIH Records). Copies of this film and of a later Kramis film entitled "The Story of Rocky Mountain Spotted Fever" are at NLM.

32. R. R. Parker, "Tick-Borne Diseases of Man in Montana and Methods of Prevention" (see chap. 8, n. 67) (quotation from p. 12).

33. RML, *Annual Report*, 1935, 3.

34. Samuel F. Harby, "Tick Talk," *Hygeia* 22 (1944):440–41.

35. George E. Baker, "Rocky Mountain Spotted Fever with Reference to Recognition, Prevention, and Treatment," *Rocky Mountain Medical Journal* 35 (1938):36–43 (quotations from pp. 40–41).

36. Norman H. Topping, "Rocky Mountain Spotted Fever: Treatment of Infected Laboratory Animals with Immune Rabbit Serum," *Pub. Health Rep.* 55 (1940):41–46. At about the same time, Timothy J. Kurotchkin, J. van der Scheer, and Ralph W. G. Wyckoff at Lederle Laboratories also reported the results of their work using Cox's infected yolk sac material to develop an antiserum. Adapting the chemical procedures used in purifying antipneumococcal rabbit serum, they stated that the toxic and allergic reactions of egg proteins could be avoided. This applied research at the NIH and at Lederle Laboratories was supplemented by more basic studies on how the immune serum protected. Ludwik Anigstein and his colleagues at the University of Texas Medical Branch in Galveston studied the production of local immunity at the site of subcutaneous or intradermal inoculation of immune serum as a step toward their goal of producing general immunity. See Timothy J. Kurotchkin, J. van der Scheer, and Ralph W. G. Wyckoff, "Refined Hyperimmune Rickettsial Sera," *Proc. Soc. Exp. Biol. Med.* 45 (1950):323; Ludwik Anigstein, Madero N. Bader, and Gerald Young, "Protective Effect of Separate Inoculation of Spotted Fever Virus and Immune Serum by Intradermal Route," *Science* 98 (1943):285–86; Ludwik Anigstein, Madero N. Bader, Gerald Young, and Dorothea Neubauer, "Protection against Spotted Fever by Specific Immune Serum Inoculated Intradermally at the Site of Infection," *J. Immunol.* 48 (1944):69–77; Ludwik Anigstein, Dorothy Whitney, and Joe Beninson, "Inhibition of Typhus and Spotted Fever by Intradermal Inoculation of Antiorgan or Certain Normal Sera," *Proc. Soc. Exp. Biol. Med.* 67 (1948):73–74.

37. Norman H. Topping, "Rocky Mountain Spotted Fever: Further Experience in the Therapeutic Use of Immune Rabbit Serum," *Pub. Health Rep.* 58 (1943):757–74; news release, file "R. R. Parker," box 91, "O-P," file 1650, "General Records of the National Institute of Health, 1930–1948," NIH Records. Efficacy figures are from the latter document.

38. Parker to Rolla E. Dyer, 10 June 1941, Notebook "R.M.S.F.—Laboratory Infections—Book I," R. R. Parker Notebooks, RML Research Records.

39. Parker to Lewis R. Thompson, 26 May 1941, Notebook "R.M.S.F.—Laboratory Infections—Book I," R. R. Parker Notebooks, RML Research Records.

40. J. Frederick Bell, interview by Victoria A. Harden, Hamilton, Montana, 6 August 1985, NIAID files, NIH Historical Office (hereafter cited as J. F. Bell interview).

41. Hospital records, telegrams, press clippings, and internal correspondence about this case are in Notebook "R.M.S.F.—Laboratory Infections—Book I," R. R. Parker Notebooks, RML Research Records; J. F. Bell interview.

42. For a review of the work on a typhus antiserum and a report of the work of the Typhus Commission's test of its efficacy, see Andrew Yeomans, J. C. Snyder, and A. G. Gilliam, "The Effects of Concentrated Hyperimmune Rabbit Serum in Louse Borne Typhus," *JAMA* 129 (1945):19–24.

43. James J. Sapero and Fred A. Butler, "Highlights on Epidemic Diseases Occurring in Military Forces: In the Early Phases of the War in the South Pacific," ibid. 127 (1945):502–6 (quotations from p. 502).

44. Morbidity and mortality figures are from Theodore E. Woodward, *Introduction to the History of the Armed Forces Medical Unit in Kuala Lumpur, Malaya, and the Armed Forces Research Institute of Medical Sciences (AFRIMS) in Bangkok, Thailand,* privately printed, n.d., 2. See also James B. Moe and Carl E. Pedersen, "The Impact of Rickettsial Diseases on Military Operations," *Military Med.* 145 (1980):780–85; Joseph F. Sadusk, Jr., "Typhus Fever in the United States Army Following Immunization," *JAMA* 133 (1947):1192–99; C. B. Philip, "Tsutsugamushi Disease (Scrub Typhus) in World War II," *J. Parasitology* 34 (1948):169–91; C. B. Philip, "Scrub Typhus and Scrub Itch," in Medical Department, U.S. Army, *Preventive Medicine in World War II,* vol. 7, *Communicable Diseases: Arthropodborne Diseases Other Than Malaria* (see chap. 9, n. 35), 275–347; C. J. D. Zarafonetis and M. P. Baker, "Scrub Typhus," in Medical Department, U.S. Army, *Internal Medicine in World War II,* vol. 2 (Washington, D.C.: Government Printing Office, 1963), 111–42. I am indebted to Margaret Pittman for bringing Dr. Woodward's recent work to my attention and to Dr. Woodward for providing a copy for the NIAID files, NIH Historical Office.

45. The deaths of Sugata and Nishibe are noted in Parker to Cohn, 7 October 1941, Notebook "R.M.S.F.—Laboratory Infections—Book I," R. R. Parker Notebooks, RML Research Records.

46. See a discussion of this in chap. 6.

47. Bayne-Jones oral history, 3:677 (see chap. 9, n. 37); F. G. Blake, K. F. Maxcy, J. F. Sadusk, Jr., G. M. Kohls, and E. J. Bell, "Studies on Tsutsugamushi Disease (Scrub Typhus, Mite-Borne Typhus) in New Guinea and Adjacent Islands: Epidemiology, Clinical Observations, and Etiology in the Dobadura Area," *Am. J. Hyg.* 41 (1945):243–73; G. M. Kohls, C. A. Armburst, E. N. Irons, and C. B. Philip, "Studies on Tsutsugamushi Disease (Scrub Typhus, Mite-Borne Typhus) in New Guinea and Adjacent Islands: Further Observations on Epidemiology and Etiology," *Am. J. Hyg.* 41 (1945): 374–99; C. B. Philip and G. M. Kohls, "Studies on Tsutsugamushi Disease (Scrub Typhus, Mite-Borne Typhus) in New Guinea and Adjacent Islands: Tsutsugamushi Disease with High Endemicity on a Small South Sea Island," *Am. J. Hyg.* 42 (1945):195–202; C. B. Philip, T. E. Woodward, and R. R. Sullivan, "Tsutsugamushi Disease (Scrub or Mite-Borne Typhus) in the Philippine Islands During American Reoccupation in 1944–45," *Am. J. Trop. Med.* 26 (1946):229–42. When the disease was identified in Burma, Thomas T. Mackie and A. G. Gilliam studied it at a laboratory established on the Irrawaddy River.

48. Posters in NLM collection; "Protection against Scrub Typhus Mite," *JAMA* 128 (1945):519; A. H. Madden, A. W. Lindquist, and E. F. Kipling, "Test of Repellents against Chiggers," *J. Econ. Entomol.* 37 (1944):283–86; R. C. Bushland, "New Guinea Field Tests of Uniforms Impregnated with Miticides to Develop Laundry-Resistant Clothing Treatments for Preventing Scrub Typhus," *Am. J. Hyg.* 43 (1946):230–47; R. N. McCulloch, "Studies in the Control of Scrub Typhus," *Med. J. Australia* 1 (1946):717–38.

49. Norman H. Topping, "Tsutsugamushi Disease (Scrub Typhus): Effects of Immune Rabbit Serum in Experimentally Infected Mice," *Pub. Health Rep.*

60 (1945):1215–20; "Vaccine for Scrub Typhus," *Army & Navy Journal*, 27 March 1948, clipping in RML Scrapbook "1942– ." The danger of research on tsutsugamushi was underscored by the five investigators who lost their lives to laboratory-acquired infections. They were Dora Lush of the Walter and Eliza Hall Institute, Melbourne, Victoria, Australia; Richard G. Henderson of the NIH Division of Infectious Diseases; Philip Leroy Jones, a laboratory technician at the RML; David J. Hein of Lederle Laboratories; and Jewel E. Roberts, a pathologist in the U.S. Army Medical Corps. Henderson's assistant, Leroy A. Shelbaker, also contracted the disease and barely escaped death. Among researchers in the war zone, A. G. Gilliam suffered the disease and lent his name to one of the standard laboratory strains of tsutsugamushi. See Philip, "Tsutsugamushi in World War II," 188; "Names of Heroes of Science Belong on Honor Roll: Philip Leroy Jones Cited," *Daily Missoulian*, 3 June 1945, clipping in RML Scrapbook "1943–1948." The "Gilliam" strain of tsutsugamushi was established by Norman Topping from a guinea pig inoculated with Gilliam's blood; Norman H. Topping, personal communication to the author, 2 September 1988. It is referred to in J. E. Smadel, E. B. Jackson, B. L. Bennett, and F. L. Rights, "A Toxic Substance Associated with the Gilliam Strain of *R. orientalis*," *Proc. Soc. Exp. Biol. Med.* 62 (1946):138–40.

50. Richard A. Ormsbee, "Q Fever Rickettsia," in Horsfall and Tamm, eds., *Viral and Rickettsial Infections of Man*, 4th ed. (see chap. 1, n. 7), 1144–63, esp. 1144–45. See also the following series of papers on Mediterranean Q fever: F. C. Robbins and C. Ragan, " 'Q' Fever in Mediterranean Area: Report of Its Occurrence in Allied Troops: Clinical Features of the Disease," *Am. J. Hyg.* 44 (1946):6–22; F. C. Robbins, R. L. Gauld, and F. B. Warner, " 'Q' Fever in Mediterranean Area: Report of Its Occurrence in Allied Troops: Epidemiology," *Am. J. Hyg.* 44 (1946):23–50; F. C. Robbins, R. Rustigan, M. J. Snyder, and J. E. Smadel, " 'Q' Fever in Mediterranean Area: Report of Its Occurrence in Allied Troops: Etiological Agent," *Am. J. Hyg.* 44 (1946):51–63; F. C. Robbins and R. Rustigan, " 'Q' Fever in Mediterranean Area: Report of Its Occurrence in Allied Troops: Laboratory Outbreak," *Am. J. Hyg.* 44 (1946):64–71.

51. T. E. Woodward and E. F. Bland, "Clinical Observations in Typhus Fever with Special Reference to the Cardiovascular System," *JAMA* 126 (1944):287–93 (quotations from p. 287).

52. G. T. Harrell, W. Venning and W. A. Wolff, "The Treatment of Rocky Mountain Spotted Fever," ibid., 929–34. See also idem, "The Treatment of Rocky Mountain Spotted Fever, with Particular Reference to Intravenous Fluids. A New Approach to Basic Supportive Therapy," ibid., 929–34; G. T. Harrell, W. A. Wolff, W. Venning, and J. B. Reinhard, "The Prevention and Control of Disturbances of Protein Metabolism in Rocky Mountain Spotted Fever," *Southern Medical Journal* 39 (1946):551–57.

53. On the development of penicillin see Dowling, *Fighting Infection*, 125–57; A. N. Richards, "Production of Penicillin in the United States (1941–1946)," *Nature* 201 (1964):441–45; H. W. Florey, "Steps Leading to the Therapeutic Application of Microbial Antagonisms," *British Medical Bulletin* 4 (1946):248–58; André Maurois, *The Life of Sir Alexander Fleming, Discoverer of Penicillin*, trans. Gerard Hopkins (New York: E. P. Dutton, 1959); Lennard Bickel, *Rise Up to Life: A Biography of Howard Walter Florey, Who Gave Penicillin to the World* (New York: Charles Scribner's Sons, 1972);

W. H. Helfand, H. B. Woodruff, K. M. H. Coleman, and D. L. Cowen, "Wartime Industrial Development of Penicillin in the United States," in John Parascandola, ed. *The History of Antibiotics: A Symposium* (Madison: University of Wisconsin Press, 1980), 31–56.

54. F. K. Fitzpatrick, "Penicillin in Experimental Spotted Fever," *Science* 102 (1945):96–97.

55. Hans Zinsser and E. B. Schoenbach, "Studies on Physiological Conditions Prevailing in Tissue Cultures," *J. Exp. Med.* 66 (1937):207–27.

56. J. C. Snyder, John Maier, and C. R. Anderson, Report to the Division of Medical Sciences (Washington, D.C.: National Research Council, 26 December 1942). Because of wartime censorship, rickettsial investigators at universities were not apprised of these findings. Thus in 1944 independent publications appeared on the rickettsiostatic action of PABA, both on infected yolk sacs and in typhus-infected mice, and of toluidine blue, a thiazine dye used in bacteriological stains, on typhus-infected mice. See O. L. Peterson, "Therapeutic Effects of Forbisen and of Toluidine Blue on Experimental Typhus," *Proc. Soc. Exp. Biol. Med.* 55 (1944):155–57. Donald Greiff, Henry Pinkerton, and Vicente Moragues, "Effect of Enzyme Inhibitors and Activators on the Multiplication of Typhus Rickettsiae: I. Penicillin, Para-Aminobenzoic Acid, Sodium Fluoride, and Vitamins of the B Group," *J. Exp. Med.* 80 (1944):561–74; "Chemotherapy of Murine Typhus," *JAMA* 125 (1944):633.

57. Their report was later published. See H. L. Hamilton, Harry Plotz, and J. E. Smadel, "Effect of p-Aminobenzoic Acid on the Growth of Typhus Rickettsiae in the Yolk Sac of the Infected Chick Embryo," *Proc. Soc. Exp. Biol. Med.* 58 (1945):255–62.

58. Andrew Yeomans, J. C. Snyder, E. S. Murray, C. J. D. Zarafonetis, and R. S. Ecke, "The Therapeutic Effect of Para-Aminobenzoic Acid in Louse Borne Typhus Fever," *JAMA* 126 (1944):349–56; see also correction to this article, ibid., 581; "Progress in the Treatment of Typhus Fever and of Rocky Mountain Spotted Fever," ibid., 964; Ludwik Anigstein and M. N. Bader, "Para-Aminobenzoic Acid—Its Effectiveness in Spotted Fever in Guinea Pigs," *Science* 101 (1945):591–92; H. M. Rose, R. B. Duane, and E. E. Fischel, "The Treatment of Spotted Fever with Para-Aminobenzoic Acid," *JAMA* 129 (1945):1160–61.

59. "Drug Cures Tick Fever When Rabbit Serum Fails," *JAMA* 131 (1946):1364; L. B. Flinn, J. W. Howard, C. W. Todd, and E. G. Scott, "Para-Aminobenzoic Acid Treatment of Rocky Mountain Spotted Fever," ibid. 132 (1946):911–14 (quotation from p. 914).

60. S. F. Ravenel, "Para-Aminobenzoic Acid Therapy of Rocky Mountain Spotted Fever: Outline of a Comprehensive Plan of Treatment with Report of Five Cases," ibid. 133 (1947):989–94. Broad spectrum antibiotics, described later in this chapter, are also rickettsiostatic, suppressing the growth of rickettsiae until the body's own immune defenses can be marshalled.

61. Dowling, *Fighting Infection*, 179. My discussion of the development of the broad-spectrum antibiotics follows ibid., 174–84. For other general surveys of this work, see idem, "History of the Broad Spectrum Antibiotics," *Antibiotics Annual*, 1958–1959 (New York: Medical Encyclopedia, 1959), 39–44; and idem, *Medicines for Man: The Development, Regulation, and Use of Prescription Drugs* (New York: Alfred A. Knopf, 1970).

62. J. Ehrlich, Q. R. Bartz, R. M. Smith, D. A. Joslyn, and P. R. Burkholder, "Chloromycetin, a New Antibiotic from a Soil Actinomycete," *Science* 106

(1947):417. A few months later a second group of researchers at the University of Illinois obtained the same antibiotic from a fungus grown on the farm of the Illinois Agricultural Experiment Station in Urbana, Illinois. See H. E. Carter, D. Gottlieb, and H. W. Anderson, "Chloromycetin and Streptothricin," *Science* 107 (1948):113; Dowling, *Fighting Infection*, 308, n. 15.

63. Ehrlich, Bartz, Smith, Joslyn, and Burkholder, "Chloromycetin," 417.

64. Woodward, *History of the Armed Forces Medical Unit in Kuala Lumpur and the AFRIMS in Bangkok*, 2.

65. J. E. Smadel and E. B. Jackson, "Chloromycetin, an Antibiotic with Chemotherapeutic Activity in Experimental Rickettsial and Viral Infections," *Science* 106 (1947):418–19.

66. Dowling, *Fighting Infection*, 179–80; W. H. Mohrhoff and W. D. Mogerman, "Chloromycetin: Another Weapon for the Doctor's Arsenal," *Process Industries Quarterly* 12, no. 1 (1949):2–14; H. L. Ley, Jr., and J. E. Smadel, "Antibiotic Therapy of Rickettsial Diseases," *Antibiotics and Chemotherapy* 4 (1954):792–802; "Scrub Typhus Research Unit Returns to Malaya," *JAMA* 139 (1949):1088. During these tests, Smadel and Cornelius B. Philip contracted scrub typhus. In Philip's case, according to his son, Robert N. Philip, he was intentionally exposed to infected mites in a field test of the prophylactic efficacy of chloramphenicol. Both men returned to the United States shortly thereafter. Because they had not developed active immunity, each suffered a bout with the disease. Both recovered. See David B. Lackman, "Immunotherapy, Immunoprophylaxis, Chemotherapy and Antibiotic Therapy: The Way It Was," manuscript, copy in NIAID files, NIH Historical Office; Robert N. Philip, personal communication to the author, 16 February 1988.

67. M. C. Pincoffs, E. G. Guy, L. M. Lister, T. E. Woodward, and J. E. Smadel, "The Treatment of Rocky Mountain Spotted Fever with Chloromycetin," *Ann. Int. Med.* 29 (1948):656–63; M. J. Carson, L. F. Gowen, and F. R. Cochrane, "Rocky Mountain Spotted Fever Treated with Chloromycetin: Report of Two Cases," *J. Pediatrics* 35 (1949):232–34; J. D. Ratcliff, "Greatest Drug Since Penicillin," *Collier's* 123 (5 February 1949):26ff. See also "Chloromycetin Claimed to be Effective in Rocky Mountain Spotted Fever Treatment," *Am. J. Pub. Health* 38 (1948):1733; "Introducing Chloromycetin," *Newsweek* 30 (17 November 1947):54; "First Artificially Made Miracle Drug: Chloramphenicol," *Science Digest* 26 (July 1949):51.

68. S. Ross, E. B. Schoenbach, F. G. Burke, M. S. Bryer, E. C. Rice, and J. A. Washington, "Aureomycin Therapy of Rocky Mountain Spotted Fever," *JAMA* 138 (1948):1213–16.

69. On the development of the tetracyclines, see Dowling, *Fighting Infection*, 180–83.

70. See, for example, Alan Gregg, "The Essential Need of Fundamental Research for Social Programs," *Science* 101 (1945):257–59.

71. Charles V. Kidd, "American Universities and Federal Research Funds," manuscript, National Institutes of Health, 1957, 288, copy in NIH Historical Office.

72. Lawrence K. Frank, "Research after the War," *Science* 101 (1945):433–34.

73. For a discussion of these developments, see J. Merton England, *A Patron for Pure Science: The National Science Foundation's Formative Years, 1945–57* (Washington, D.C.: Government Printing Office, 1982); G. Burroughs Mider, "The Federal Impact on Biomedical Research," in John Z. Bowers and

Elizabeth F. Purcell, eds., *Advances in American Medicine: Essays at the Bicentennial*, 2 vols. (New York: Josiah Macy, Jr., Foundation, 1976) 2:806–71; Daniel M. Fox, "The Politics of the NIH Extramural Program, 1937–1950," *J. Hist. Med. Allied Sci.* 42 (1987):447–66.

74. U.S. President's Scientific Research Board, *Science and Public Policy: A Report to the President*, by John R. Steelman, 5 vols. (Washington, D.C.: Government Printing Office, 1947); see esp. vol. 5, *The Nation's Medical Research*, 8, for definitions of basic and applied research.

75. For a chronology of these events, see U.S. National Institutes of Health, *NIH Almanac, 1986* (Washington, D.C.: U.S. Department of Health and Human Services, NIH Publication no. 86–5, 1986), esp. 3–18; NIAID, *Intramural Contributions, 1887–1987* (see chap. 9, n. 11), 3–7.

76. "Spotted Fever Vaccine Distribution Discontinued," *JAMA* 140 (1949):337; "Malone, Tick Vaccine Maker, Honored at Retirement Party," *Ravalli Republican*, 3 July 1958; and "Earl Malone Retires from Work at Lab after 34 Years on Job," *Western News*, 3 July 1958, clippings in RML Scrapbook "1942– ."

77. My discussion of this is taken from a transcript of a conference held at the RML, 13–14 January 1949, in Notebook "Haas Conference—1949," R. R. Parker Notebooks, RML Research Records.

78. Ibid., 11.

79. "Rocky Mountain Laboratory Head Dies at 61," *Daily Missoulian*, 5 September 1949; "Dr. R. R. Parker, 61, Laboratory Director and Noted Scientist, Dies Unexpectedly; Funeral Services Set for 2 P.M. Friday," n.d.; and "Noted Tick Fever Expert Succumbs," 4 September 1949, clippings in RML Scrapbook "1949– ."

80. Russell M. Wilder, "The Rickettsial Diseases: Discovery and Conquest," *Arch. Pathol.* 49 (1950):479–89 (quotation from p. 489).

Chapter Eleven: Spotted Fever after Antibiotics

1. J. E. McCroan, R. L. Ramsey, W. J. Murphy, and L. S. Dick, "The Status of Rocky Mountain Spotted Fever in the Southeastern United States," *Pub. Health Rep.* 70 (1955):319–25; J. E. Smadel, "Status of the Rickettsioses in the United States," *Ann. Int. Med.* 51 (1959):421–35.

2. Although related tick-borne rickettsioses exist in other parts of the world, *Rickettsia rickettsii* has never been isolated outside the western hemisphere.

3. The occurrence of Rocky Mountain spotted fever in São Paulo and Minas Gerais, Brazil, was discussed in chap. 8. Spotted fever was first reported from the state of Rio de Janeiro, Brazil, in 1941. See J. Tostes and G. Bretz, "Sobre uma rickettsioses observada em zona rural do Estado do Rio de Janeiro," *Brasil Méd.* 55 (1941):789–94.

4. R. J. Gibbons, "Survey of Rocky Mountain Spotted Fever and Sylvatic Plague in Western Canada During 1938," *Canadian Journal of Public Health* 30 (1939):184–87; M. R. Bow and J. H. Brown, "Rocky Mountain Spotted Fever in Alberta, 1935–1950," ibid. 43 (1952):109–15.

5. F. A. Humphreys and A. G. Campbell, "Plague, Rocky Mountain Spotted Fever, and Tularaemia Surveys in Canada," ibid. 38 (1947):124–30. A 1964 serological study in the Ottawa, Ontario, area demonstrated spotted fever antibodies in wild animals and in humans, even though no cases had been

reported from eastern Canada. See V. F. Newhouse, J. A. McKiel, and W. Burgdorfer, "California Encephalitis, Colorado Tick Fever and Rocky Mountain Spotted Fever in Eastern Canada: Serological Evidence," ibid. 55 (1964):257–61.

6. G. E. Davis, "Experimental Transmission of the Rickettsiae of the Spotted Fevers of Brazil, Colombia, and the United States by the Argasid Tick *Ornithodoros nicollei*," *Pub. Health Rep.* 58 (1943):1742–44.

7. M. E. Bustamante and G. Varela, "Una nueve rickettsiosis en México. Existencia de la fiebre manchada americana en los Estados de Sinaloa y Sonora," *Revista del Instituto de Salubridad y Enfermedades Tropicales* 4 (1943):189–210 (hereafter cited as *Rev. Inst. de Sal. y Enf. Tropicales*); idem, "Características de la fiebre manchada de las Montañas rocosas en Sonora y Sinaloa, México," ibid. 5 (1944):129–36; idem, "Aislamiento de Una Cepa de Fiebre Manchada Idéntica a la de las Montañas Rocosas en Sinaloa, México," *Bol. Offic. San. Panam.* 23 (1944):117–18.

8. M. E. Bustamante and G. Varela, "Distribucion de las Rickettsiasis en México," *Rev. Inst. de Sal. y Enf. Tropicales* 8 (1947):3–14; M. E. Bustamante, G. Varela, and C. Orbiz-Marcotte, "II. Estudios de fiebre manchada en la Laguna," ibid. 7 (1946):39–48; M. E. Bustamante and G. Varela, "III. Estudios de fiebre manchada en México. Hallazgo del *Amblyomma cajennese* naturalmente infectado en Vera Cruz," ibid. 7 (1946):75–78; R. Silva-Goytia and A. Elizondo, "Estudios sobre Fiebre Manchada en México. I. Clasificación de Cepas," *Medicina Revista Mexicana* 32 (1952):217–21; R. Silva-Goytia and A. Elizondo, "Estudios sobre Fiebre Manchada en México. II. Parásitos hematófagos encontrados naturalmente infectados," *Med. Rev. Mexicana* 32 (1952):278–82; R. Silva-Goytia, H. Vasquez Campos, and A. Elizondo, "Estudios sobre Fiebre Manchada en México. V. Incidencia de anticuerpos específicos para *Dermacentroxenus rickettsi* en grupos ocupacionales de diversas áreas geográficas," *Med. Rev. Mexicana* 33 (1953):425–35.

9. E. C. de Rodaniche and A. Rodaniche, "Spotted Fever in Panama: Isolation of the Etiologic Agent from a Fatal Case," *Am. J. Trop. Med.* 30 (1950):511–17; C. Calero, J. M. Nuñez, and R. Silva-Goytia, "Rocky Mountain Spotted Fever in Panama: Report of Two Cases," *American Journal of Tropical Medicine and Hygiene* 1 (1952):631–36; E. C. de Rodaniche, "Natural Infection of the Tick, *Amblyomma cajennese*, with *Rickettsia rickettsii* in Panama," *Am. J. Trop. Med. Hyg.* 2 (1953):696–99 (quotation from p. 698). In 1976, Rocky Mountain spotted fever was also reported from Costa Rica. See L. G. Fuentes, "Primer caso de fiebre de las Montañas Rocosas en Costa Rica, América Central," *Revista Latinoamericana de Microbiologia* 21 (1979):167–72; J. Tosi, "Mapa ecológico (República de Costa Rica): Según la clasificación de zonas de Vida del mundo de L. R. Holdridge." Centro Cientifico Tropical, de San José, Costa Rica (Mapa); L. Fuentes, "Ecological Study of Rocky Mountain Spotted Fever in Costa Rica," *Am. J. Trop. Med. Hyg.* 35 (1986):192–96.

10. Bustamante and Varela, "Distribucion de las Rickettsiasis en México," 14; A. Vallejo-Freire, "Spotted Fever in Mexico: Immunological Relationship between the Virus of the Rickettsiosis Observed in Sonora and Sinaloa, Mexico, and Other Spotted Fever Viruses," *Mem. Inst. Butantan* 19 (1946):159–80; W. M. Kelsey and G. T. Harrell, "Management of Tick Typhus (Rocky Mountain Spotted Fever) in Children," *JAMA* 137 (1948):1356–61.

11. In contrast, Rocky Mountain spotted fever was conspicuously not a topic of general press interest in this period. Between 1952 and 1963, the *Reader's Guide to Periodical Literature* carried no entries for articles about the disease.

12. C. L. Williams, "The Control of Murine Typhus with DDT," *Military Surgeon* 104 (1949):163–67; "Control of Murine Typhus with DDT," *JAMA* 140 (1949):878; McCroan, Ramsey, Murphy, and Dick, "Status of Rocky Mountain Spotted Fever in the Southeastern United States," 323–24; J. E. McCroan, Jr., and R. L. Ramsey, "DDT Dusting as a Control Measure for the American Dog Tick, the Vector of Rocky Mountain Spotted Fever in Georgia," *Journal of the Medical Association of Georgia* 36 (1947):242–44; "Speech by Dr. Heitor P. Fróes," in Whitlock, ed., *Proceedings of the Fourth International Congress on Tropical Medicine and Malaria* (see chap. 8, n. 27), 19.

13. Rachel Carson, *Silent Spring* (Boston: Houghton Mifflin Co., 1962), 268–69. See also A. W. A. Brown, *Insecticide Resistance in Arthropods*, World Health Organization Monograph Series no. 38 (Geneva: World Health Organization, 1958); A. W. A. Brown, "The Challenge of Insecticide Resistance," *Bulletin of the Entomological Society of America* 7 (1961):6–19.

14. McCroan, Ramsey, Murphy, and Dick, "Status of Rocky Mountain Spotted Fever in the Southeastern United States," 321; D. B. Lackman and R. K. Gerloff, "The Effect of Antibiotic Therapy upon Diagnostic, Serologic Tests for Rocky Mountain Spotted Fever," *Public Health Laboratory* 11 (1953):97–99.

15. Mary Barber and Lawrence P. Garrod, *Antibiotic and Chemotherapy* (Edinburgh: E. & S. Livingstone, 1963), 116–28 (quotation from p. 123); "Dangerous Drugs?" *Newsweek* 41 (12 January 1953):74; "Drugs Are Dangerous, Too," *Time* 60 (25 August 1952):59; "Chloromycetin Dangers Investigated After Death," *Science Newsletter* 62 (19 July 1952):43; "Chloromycetin Problem," *Scientific American* 189 (September 1952):72ff.; "Danger in Miracles," *Newsweek* 53 (18 May 1959):106.

16. R. Milch, D. Rall, and J. Tobie, "Bone Localization of the Tetracyclines," *J. Nat. Cancer Inst.* 191 (1957):87–91.

17. I. S. Wallman and H. B. Hilton, "Teeth Pigmented by Tetracycline," *Lancet* 1 (1962):827–29; idem, "Prematurity, Tetracycline, and Oxytetracycline in Tooth Development," ibid. 2 (1962):720–21; C. J. Witkop, Jr., and R. O. Wolf, "Hypoplasia and Intrinsic Staining of Enamel Following Tetracycline Therapy," *JAMA* 185 (1963):1008–11 (quotation from p. 1008). Thanks are due to the staff of the public information office of the National Institute of Dental Research for alerting me to these early papers.

18. "Prescribing of Tetracycline to Children," *JAMA* 238 (1977):579.

19. Kidd, "American Universities and Federal Research Funds" (see chap. 10, n. 71), 283. See also his table 41, p. 284, for amounts expended.

20. Dowling, *Fighting Infection* (see chap. 10, n. 24), 248; Dorland J. Davis, interview by Victoria A. Harden, Bethesda, Maryland, 27 February 1985, NIAID files, NIH Historical Office.

21. The apocryphal story has no single origin—I have heard it told by a variety of people on different occasions. Another version is noted in Sheldon G. Cohen and William R. Duncan, "Immunology and NIAID (1887–1970)," in NIAID, *Intramural Contributions, 1887–1987* (see chap. 9, n. 11), 96.

22. U.S. President's NIH Study Committee, *Biomedical Science and Its Administration: A Study of the National Institutes of Health* (Washington, D.C.: Government Printing Office, 1965), 153–57.

23. P. B. Beeson, "Infectious Diseases (Microbiology)," in Bowers and Purcell, eds., *Advances in American Medicine* (see chap. 10, n. 73), 1:136–40 (quotation from p. 136). My discussion of the Commission on Rickettsial Diseases was guided by conversations with Charles L. Wisseman, Jr., on 5 November 1987 and on 24 March 1988. Dr. Wisseman is preparing a much needed history of the commission, which he headed between 1960 and 1973. The figures for awards are taken from the conversation with Dr. Wisseman and from Joseph E. Smadel, "Remarks of Director, Commission on Rickettsial Diseases, at Semiannual Meeting of Armed Forces Epidemiological Board," 9 December 1957, copy in NIAID files, NIH Historical Office.

24. My totals, from *NIH Almanac, 1983*, 130.

25. My discussion of these centers was initially guided by Richard A. Ormsbee in a personal communication, 10 March 1986.

26. My discussion of rickettsial grants is taken from yearly NIH grants publications and data bases, 1947–present. See Note on Sources for specific titles. John P. Fox was funded for research on typhus from 1952 through 1961 at Tulane University and later at the Public Health Research Institute of New York City; H. J. Wisniewski of the Milwaukee Health Department received small grants to survey the epidemiology of rickettsial diseases in the Milwaukee, Wisconsin, area; Harry B. Harding and Opal E. Hepler of Northwestern University School of Medicine in Chicago were funded between 1953 and 1960 for immunologic studies including serologic tests for rickettsial diseases; microbiologists Freeman A. Weiss and Trygve O. Berge received support for the preservation and expansion of the rickettsial registry at the American Type Culture Collection, now at Rockville, Maryland; Richard B. Loomis of the California State College at Long Beach was funded for research on chigger mites, the vectors of scrub typhus; Robert Traub of the University of Maryland School of Medicine was supported for research on fleas, the vectors of murine typhus; Traub and colleague Charles L. Wisseman, Jr., studied the ecology and vectors of rickettsial infections in West Pakistan through the University of Maryland's International Center. For Rocky Mountain spotted fever as an individual topic of study, the picture was bleak during the 1950s. One lone grant of $3,742 was awarded to D. E. Beck at Brigham Young University in Provo, Utah, for research on parasitic arthropods related to spotted fever.

27. V. K. Zworykin, J. Hillier, and A. W. Vance, "An Electron Microscope for Practical Laboratory Service," *Transactions of the American Institute of Electrical Engineers* 60 (1941):157–61; V. K. Zworykin and J. Hillier, "A Compact High Resolving Power Electron Microscope," *Journal of Applied Physics* 14 (1943):658–83.

28. S. Mudd and T. F. Anderson, "Pathogenic Bacteria, Rickettsias, and Viruses as Shown by the Electron Microscope: Their Relationships to Immunity and Chemotherapy. I. Morphology," *JAMA* 126 (1944):561–70 (quotation from p. 561); S. Mudd, "Pathogenic Bacteria, Rickettsias, and Viruses as Shown by the Electron Microscope: Their Relationships to Immunity and Chemotherapy. II. Relationships to Immunity," ibid. 632–39 (quotation from pp. 632–33).

29. H. Plotz, J. E. Smadel, T. F. Anderson, and L. A. Chambers, "Morphological Structure of Rickettsiae," *J. Exp. Med.* 77 (1943):355–58.

30. Ibid., 357. Spencer and Parker's finding of invisible forms of rickettsiae was discussed in chap. 7. Copy of their paper with marginal note in NIAID files, NIH Historical Office. Lucille Jamieson Weiss of the Lilly Research Laboratories in Indianapolis also published electron micrographs of typhus rickettsiae, which showed the small forms dividing, an indication that they were indeed living organisms. See L. J. Weiss, "Electron Micrographs of Rickettsiae of Typhus Fever," *J. Immunol.* 47 (1943):353–57. In a personal communication to the author, 30 November 1988, David H. Walker cautioned that the electron micrographs did not constitute proof that these small forms were rickettsiae and noted that they would have to be purified free of classic forms and then demonstrated to be infective.

31. Mudd, "Pathogenic Bacteria, Rickettsias, and Viruses. II. Relationships to Immunity," 633.

32. M. Ruiz Castaneda and Roberto Silva-Goytia of the Public Health Service and the Department of Medical Research, General Hospital, Mexico City, for example, found antigenic similarities between typhus and spotted fever to be considerably greater than expected. Their studies indicated that deficiency in one important immune factor might explain the failure of total cross-protection in guinea pigs. See M. Ruiz Castaneda and R. Silva-Goytia, "Immunological Relationship between Spotted Fever and Exanthematic Typhus," *J. Immunol.* 42 (1941):1–14. For confirmation of this work in the United States, see H. Plotz, B. Bennett, K. Wertman, and M. Snyder, "Cross-Reacting Typhus Antibodies in Rocky Mountain Spotted Fever," *Proc. Soc. Exp. Biol. Med.* 57 (1944):336–39.

33. A. Pijper and C. G. Crocker, "Rickettsioses of South Africa," *South African Medical Journal* 12 (1938):613–30 (quotation from p. 614).

34. H. Plotz, R. L. Reagan, and K. Wertman, "Differentiation between Fievre Boutonneuse and Rocky Mountain Spotted Fever by Means of Complement Fixation," *Proc. Soc. Exp. Biol. Med.* 55 (1944):173–76; D. B. Lackman and E. G. Pickens, "Antigenic Types in the Rocky Mountain Spotted Fever Group of Rickettsiae," *Bacteriological Proceedings* 3 (1953):219; F. M. Bozeman, J. W. Humphries, J. M. Campbell, and P. L. O'Hara, "Laboratory Studies of the Spotted Fever Group of Rickettsiae," in *Symposium on the Spotted Fever Group*, Walter Reed Army Institute of Research Medical Science Publication no. 7 (Washington, D.C.: Government Printing Office, 1960), 7–11; E. J. Bell and H. G. Stoenner, "Immunologic Relationships Among the Spotted Fever Group of Rickettsias Determined by Toxin Neutralization Tests in Mice with Convalescent Animal Serums," *J. Immunol.* 84 (1961):737–46; H. G. Stoenner, D. B. Lackman, and E. J. Bell, "Factors Affecting the Growth of Rickettsias of the Spotted Fever Group in Fertile Hens' Eggs," *J. Inf. Dis.* 110 (1962):121–28; E. G. Pickens, E. J. Bell, D. B. Lackman, and W. Burgdorfer, "Use of Mouse Serum in Identification and Serologic Classification of *Rickettsia akari* and *Rickettsia australis*," *J. Immunol.* 94 (1965):883–89.

35. R. R. Parker, G. M. Kohls, G. W. Cox, and G. E. Davis, "Observations on an Infectious Agent from *Amblyomma maculatum*," *Pub. Health Rep.* 54 (1939):1482–84; D. B. Lackman, R. R. Parker, and R. K. Gerloff, "Serological Characteristics of a Pathogenic Rickettsia Occurring in *Amblyomma maculatum*," ibid. 64 (1949):1342–49.

36. D. B. Lackman, E. J. Bell, H. G. Stoenner, and E. G. Pickens, "The Rocky Mountain Spotted Fever Group of Rickettsias," *Health Laboratory*

Science 2 (1965):135–41. Surprisingly, toxin neutralization tests revealed that *R. parkeri* was closely related to *Rickettsia conorii*, which caused boutonneuse fever.

37. *Rickettsia montana* was originally designated Eastern Montana agent. See E. J. Bell, G. M. Kohls, H. G. Stoenner, and D. B. Lackman, "Nonpathogenic Rickettsias Related to the Spotted Fever Group Isolated from Ticks, *Dermacentor variabilis* and *Dermacentor andersoni* from Eastern Montana," *J. Immunol.* 90 (1963):770–81; Lackman, Bell, Stoenner, and Pickens, "Rocky Mountain Spotted Fever Group of Rickettsias," 137. The Western Montana U strain of *R. rickettsii* was found to be similar to but not identical with *R. montana* in the production of antibodies. See W. H. Price, "The Epidemiology of Rocky Mountain Spotted Fever. I. The Characterization of Strain Virulence of *Rickettsia rickettsii*," *Am. J. Hyg.* 58 (1953):248–68.

38. Lackman, Bell, Stoenner, and Pickens, "Rocky Mountain Spotted Fever Group of Rickettsias," 138; P. F. Zdrodovskii and H. M. Golinevich, *The Rickettsial Diseases*, trans. B. Haigh (New York: Pergamon, 1960). Mild clinical symptoms of North Asian tick typhus and an eschar at the site of the tick bite initially indicated that *Rickettsia sibirica* might be related to boutonneuse fever. A strong cross-reaction with *Rickettsia rickettsii* in the toxin-neutralization test, however, demonstrated that instead its antigens were more like those of the Rocky Mountain spotted fever organism. Cornelius B. Philip suggested that the ecology of the North Asian organism was more comparable to the ecology of *R. rickettsii* than to that of *R. conorii*. See E. J. Bell and H. G. Stoenner, "Immunologic Relationships Among the Spotted Fever Group of Rickettsias Determined by Toxin Neutralization Tests in Mice with Convalescent Animal Serums," *J. Immunol.* 84 (1960):171–82; C. B. Philip, "Some Epidemiological Considerations in Rocky Mountain Spotted Fever," *Pub. Health Rep.* 74 (1959):595–600. For more recent research on this disease, see Fan Ming-yuan, David H. Walker, Yu Shu-rong, and Liu Qing-huai, "Epidemiology and Ecology of Rickettsial Diseases in the People's Republic of China," *Reviews of Infectious Diseases* 9 (1987):823–40; Jia Gang Wang and David H. Walker, "Identification of Spotted Fever Group Rickettsiae from Human and Tick Sources in the People's Republic of China," *J. Inf. Dis.* 156 (1987):665–69; and Fan Ming-yuan, David H. Walker, Liu Qing-huai, Li Han, Bai Hai-chun, Zhang Jia-Ke, Brenda Lenz, and Cai Hong, "Rickettsial and Serologic Evidence for Prevalent Spotted Fever Rickettsiosis in Inner Mongolia," *Am. J. Trop. Med. Hyg.* 36 (1987):615–20.

39. In 1951 investigators at the RML reported that neither *R. australis* nor *R. akari* provided any immunity to guinea pigs against challenge with Rocky Mountain spotted fever. All the other spotted fever group organisms provided some measure of protection, although not complete. See D. B. Lackman and R. R. Parker, "The Serological Characterization of North Queensland Tick Typhus," *Pub. Health Rep.* 63 (1948):1624–28; R. R. Parker, E. G. Pickens, D. B. Lackman, E. J. Bell, and F. B. Thrailkill, "Isolation and Characterization of Rocky Mountain Spotted Fever Rickettsiae from the Rabbit Tick *Haemaphysalis leporis-palustris* Packard," ibid. 66 (1951):455–63; Pickens, Bell, Lackman, and Burgdorfer, "Use of Mouse Serum in Identification and Serologic Classification of *Rickettsia akari* and *Rickettsia australis*," 883–89. For additional information on Queensland tick typhus, see H. R. Cox, "The Spotted Fever Group," in Thomas M. Rivers and Frank L. Horsfall, Jr., eds., *Viral*

and Rickettsial Infections of Man, 3d ed. (Philadelphia: J. B. Lippincott, 1959), 856–58.

40. Lackman, Bell, Stoenner, and Pickens, "Rocky Mountain Spotted Fever Group of Rickettsias," 140. Their grouping was confirmed in 1978 by yet another RML group using a technique called microimmunofluorescence, which exploited the ability to "tag" particular antigens on the organisms with material that fluoresced. See R. N. Philip, E. A. Casper, W. Burgdorfer, R. K. Gerloff, L. E. Hughes, and E. J. Bell, "Serologic Typing of Rickettsiae of the Spotted Fever Group by Microimmunofluorescence," *J. Immunol.* 121 (1978):1961–68. During this study, moreover, Philip and his colleagues identified a new nonpathogenic, tick-borne rickettsial species, which they named *R. bellii* after E. John Bell. The new organism was distinct from both the spotted fever group and the typhus group rickettsiae. See R. N. Philip, E. A. Casper, R. L. Anacker, J. Cory, S. F. Hayes, W. Burgdorfer, and C. E. Yunker, "*Rickettsia bellii* sp. Nov.: A Tick-Borne Rickettsia, Widely Distributed in the United States, That Is Distinct from the Spotted Fever and Typhus Biogroups," *International Journal of Systematic Bacteriology* 33 (1983):94–106.

41. R. L. Anacker, T. F. McCaul, W. Burgdorfer, R. K. Gerloff, "Properties of Selected Rickettsiae of the Spotted Fever Group," *Infection and Immunity* 27 (1980):468–74; W. F. Myers and C. L. Wisseman, Jr., "The Taxonomic Relationship of *Rickettsia canada* to the Typhus and Spotted Fever Groups of the Genus *Rickettsia*," in Burgdorfer and Anacker, eds., *Rickettsiae and Rickettsial Diseases* (see chap. 9, n. 14), 313–25; C. L. Wisseman, "Some Biological Properties of Rickettsiae Pathogenic for Man," in Burgdorfer and Anacker, eds., *Rickettsiae and Rickettsial Diseases*, 298; Charles L. Wisseman, Jr., personal communication to the author about unpublished data, 24 March 1988. An alternative grouping for the spotted fever group rickettsiae suggested by this work is:

A—*R. rickettsii, R. conorii* and other organisms, not yet fully characterized, recovered from victims of spotted fever group rickettsial disease in Israel, India, and elsewhere

B—*R. sibirica* and *R. montana*

C—*R. australis* and *R. akari*

42. N. H. Topping, R. Helig, and V. R. Naidu, "A Note on the Rickettsioses in India," *Pub. Health Rep.* 58 (1943):1208–10; D. R. Seaton and M. G. P. Stoker, "A Serological Analysis of Typhus Cases in India by Weil-Felix, Rickettsial Agglutination, and Complement-Fixation Tests," *Annals of Tropical Medicine* 40 (1946):347–57; S. L. Kalra, "Natural History of Typhus Fevers in India," *Indian Journal of Medical Sciences* 6 (1952):569–75; R. G. Robertson, C. L. Wisseman, Jr., and R. Traub, "Tick-borne Rickettsia of the Spotted Fever Group in West Pakistan. I. Isolation of Strains from Ticks in Different Habitats," *Am. J. Epidemiol.* 92 (1970):382–94; R. G. Robertson and C. L. Wisseman, "Tick-borne Rickettsiae of the Spotted Fever Group in West Pakistan. II. Serological Classification of Isolates from West Pakistan and Thailand: Evidence for Two New Species," *Am. J. Epidemiol.* 97 (1973):55–64; S. Stephen, H. L. Rao, and K. N. Achyutha Rao, "Serological Evidence of Infection by Spotted Fever Group Rickettsiae in Karnataka State," *Indian Journal of Medical Research* 72 (1980):352–54.

43. F. Mahara, K. Koga, S. Sawada, T. Taniguchi, F. Shigemi, T. Suto, Y. Tsubio, A. Ooya, H. Koyama, T. Uchiyama, et al., "The First Report of

the Rickettsial Infections of Spotted Fever Group in Japan: Three Clinical Cases" (in Japanese), *Kansenshogaku Zasshi* 59 (1985):1165–71. I am grateful to Dr. Yoichiro Ito for translating this paper for me. See also a report of spotted fever group infections in Kyushu in S. Yamamoto, N. Kawabata, T. Uchiyama, and T. Uchida, "Evidence for Infection Caused by Spotted Fever Group Rickettsia in Kyushu, Japan," *Japanese Journal of Medical Science and Biology* 40 (1987):75–78.

44. D. Beytout, "Rickettsioses diagnostiquée par microagglutination de Janvier à Juin 1963 à Saigon," *Bull. Soc. Path. Exotique* 57 (1964):257–63; N. J. Marchette, "Rickettsioses (Tick Typhus, Q Fever, Urban Typhus) in Malaya," *Journal of Medical Entomology* 2 (1966):339–71; R. Brezina, P. Ac, J. Rehacek, and M. Majerska, "Two Strains of Rickettsiae of Rocky Mountain Spotted Fever Group Recovered from *Dermacentor marginatus* Ticks in Czechoslovakia: Results of Preliminary Serological Identification," *Acta Virologica* 13 (1969):142–45; J. Rehacek, R. Brezina, P. Ac, M. Zupancicova, and E. Kovacova, "Contribution to the Natural Focality of Rickettsiae Belonging to the Rocky Mountain Spotted Fever (RMSF) Group in Slovakia," *Folia Parasitologica* 19 (1972):41–52. On the present status of rickettsial nomenclature, see R. N. Philip, "Some Comments about the Systematics of Rickettsiae," in "Festschrift for Cornelius Becker Philip"(special issue), *Myia* 3 (1985):209–17.

45. On spotted fever group rickettsioses in Africa since World War II, see A. D. Charters, "Tick Typhus in Abyssinia," *Transactions of the Royal Society of Medicine and Hygiene* 39 (1946):335–42; G. W. A. Dick and E. A. A. Lewis, "A Rickettsial Disease in East Africa Transmitted by Ticks (*Rhipicephalus simus* and *Haemaphysalis leachi*)," ibid. 41 (1947):295–326; G. M. Findlay and G. T. L. Archer, "The Occurrence of Tick-Borne Typhus in West Africa," ibid. 41 (1948):815–18; P. Giroud, "Les Rickettsioses en Afrique équatoriale," *Bulletin of the World Health Organization* 4 (1951):535–46; P. Le Gac, P. Giroud, and C. Lemaigre, "La Forêt équatoriale doit-elle être considérée comme une zone endémique des rickettsioses? Comportment des pygmées de la Lobaye, Oubangui-Chari (A.E.F.) vis-à-vis des antigènes des typhus épidémique, murin, de la fièvre boutonneuse, et de la fièvre Q," *Bull. Soc. Path. Exotique* 45 (1952):599–602; R. B. Heisch, R. McPhee, and L. R. Rickman, "The Epidemiology of Tick-Typhus in Nairobi," *East African Medical Journal* 34 (1957):459–77; R. Kirk, "Rickettsial Infections in the Sudan Republic," *J. Trop. Med. Hyg.* 62 (1959):279–84; J. Jadin, "Les Rickettsioses en Afrique centrale," *Bull. Soc. Path. Exotique* 56 (1963):571–86; H. Hoogstraal, "Ticks in Relation to Human Diseases Caused by *Rickettsia* Species," *Annual Review of Entomology* 12 (1967):377–420; F. Weyer, "Progresses in Ecology and Epidemiology of Rickettsioses," *Acta Tropica* 35 (1978):5–21.

46. W. Burgdorfer, A. Aeschlimann, O. Peter, S. F. Hayes, and R. N. Philip, "*Ixodes ricinus*: Vector of a Hitherto Undescribed Spotted Fever Group Agent in Switzerland," *Acta Tropica* 36 (1979):357–67; W. Burgdorfer, S. F. Hayes, L. A. Thomas, and J. L. Lancaster, Jr., "A New Spotted Fever Group Rickettsia from the Lone Star Tick, *Amblyomma americanum*," in Burgdorfer and Anacker, eds., *Rickettsiae and Rickettsial Diseases*, 595–602. The Swiss organism has been named *Rickettsia helvetica*.

47. Gerard J. Tortora, Berdell R. Funke, and Christine L. Case, *Microbiology: An Introduction*, 2d ed. (Menlo Park, Calif.: Benjamin/Cummings

Publishing Co., 1986), chaps. 9, 12; H. Ris and J. P. Fox, "The Cytology of Rickettsiae," *J. Exp. Med.* 89 (1949):681–86.

48. M. R. Bovarnick and J. C. Snyder, "Respiration of Typhus Rickettsiae," *J. Exp. Med.* 89 (1949):561–65; C. L. Wisseman, Jr., E. B. Jackson, F. E. Hahn, A. C. Ley, and J. E. Smadel, "Metabolic Studies of Rickettsiae. I. The Effects of Antimicrobial Substances and Enzyme Inhibitors on the Oxidation of Glutamate by Purified Rickettsiae," *J. Immunol.* 67 (1951):123–36; A. Karp, "An Immunological Purification of Typhus Rickettsiae," *Journal of Bacteriology* 67 (1954):450–55; C. L. Wisseman, Jr., F. E. Hahn, E. B. Jackson, F. M. Bozeman, and J. E. Smadel, "Metabolic Studies of Rickettsiae. II. Studies on the Pathway of Glutamate Oxidation by Purified Suspensions of *Rickettsia mooseri*," *J. Immunol.* 68 (1952):251–64; R. A. Ormsbee and M. G. Peacock, "Metabolic Activity in *Coxiella burnetii*," *J. Bacteriol.* 88 (1964):1205–10; M. R. Bovarnick and J. C. Miller, "Oxidation and Transamination of Glutamate by Typhus Rickettsiae," *Journal of Biological Chemistry* 184 (1950):661–76; M. R. Bovarnick, "Phosphorylation Accompanying the Oxidation of Glutamate by the Madrid E Strain of Typhus Rickettsiae," *J. Biol. Chem.* 220 (1956):353–61; D. Paretsky, C. M. Downs, R. A. Consigli, and B. K. Joyce, "Studies on the Physiology of Rickettsiae. I. Some Enzyme Systems of *Coxiella burnetii*," *J. Inf. Dis.* 103 (1958):6–11.

49. Z. A. Cohn, F. M. Bozeman, J. M. Campbell, J. W. Humphries, and T. K. Sawyer, "Study on the Growth of Rickettsiae. V. Penetration of *Rickettsia tsutsugamushi* into Mammalian Cells in Vitro," *J. Exp. Med.* 109 (1959):271–92; H. H. Winkler and E. T. Miller, "Immediate Cytotoxicity and Phospholipase A: The Role of Phospholipase A in the Interaction of *R. prowazekii* and L-Cells," in Burgdorfer and Anacker, eds., *Rickettsiae and Rickettsial Diseases*, 327–33.

50. M. Schaecter, F. M. Bozeman, and J. E. Smadel, "Study on the Growth of Rickettsiae. II. Morphologic Observations of Living Rickettsiae in Tissue Culture Cells," *Virology* 3 (1957):160–72; C. L. Wisseman, Jr., E. A. Edlinger, A. D. Waddell, and M. R. Jones, "Infection Cycle of *Rickettsia rickettsii* in Chicken Embryo and L-929 Cells in Culture," *Infect. Immun.* 14 (1976):1052–64; D. H. Walker and B. G. Cain, "The Rickettsial Plaque: Evidence for Direct Cytopathic Effect of *Rickettsia rickettsii*," *Laboratory Investigation* 43 (1980):388–96; D. J. Silverman, C. L. Wisseman, Jr., and A. Waddell, "Envelopment and Escape of *Rickettsia rickettsii* from Host Membranes," in Burgdorfer and Anacker, eds., *Rickettsiae and Rickettsial Diseases*, 241–53; D. H. Walker, W. T. Firth, and C. S. Edgell, "Human Endothelial Cell Culture Plaques Induced by *Rickettsia rickettsii*," *Infect. Immun.* 37 (1982):301–6. In contrast to the spotted fever organism, *R. prowazekii*, the agent of epidemic typhus, was shown to be released only by bursting the host cell after massive intracellular accumulation. See C. L. Wisseman, Jr., and A. D. Waddell, "*In Vitro* Studies of Rickettsia-Host Cell Interactions: Intracellular Growth Cycle of Virulent and Attenuated *Rickettsia prowazekii* in Chicken Embryo Cells in Slide Chamber Cultures," *Infect. Immun.* 11 (1975):1391–1401.

51. R. A. Ormsbee, "Rickettsiae (as Organisms)," *Ann. Rev. Microbiol.* 23 (1969):275–92 (quotation from p. 287); Wisseman, "Some Biological Properties of Rickettsiae Pathogenic for Man," 293–311 (quotations from p. 293).

52. The perception that rickettsial diseases posed no threat doubtless contributed to this, for young researchers were drawn to areas viewed as pressing problems. As early as 1957, Joseph E. Smadel had remarked that, barring

atomic warfare, the rickettsial diseases in the United States "really presented no serious problems." See J. E. Smadel, "Remarks of Director, Commission on Rickettsial Diseases, at semiannual meeting of Armed Forces Epidemiological Board," 9 December 1957, copy in NIAID Public Information Office.

53. Minutes of Meeting of Board of Scientific Counselors, National Institute of Allergy and Infectious Diseases, National Institutes of Health, Bethesda, Maryland, 7 and 8 December 1967, RML Director's Files (see chap. 8, n. 60). Although no specific attribution for this remark is given in the minutes, the speaker was probably the scientific director of NIAID, John R. Seal.

54. R. A. Ormsbee, in "Rickettsial Diseases—A Public Health Problem?" *J. Inf. Dis.* 127 (1973):325–27, noted only two rickettsial grants in 1971. In U.S., National Institutes of Health, Division of Research Grants, *Research Grants Index, Fiscal Year 1971* (Washington, D.C.: Government Printing Office, [1972]), I found five that might be considered rickettsial grants, although that classification could be disputed depending upon the emphasis of the study.

55. Charles L. Wisseman, Jr., personal communication to the author, 24 March 1988; T. E. Woodward, "A Historical Account of the Rickettsial Diseases with a Discussion of Unsolved Problems," *J. Inf. Dis.* 127 (1973):583–94 (quotations from p. 593); Ormsbee, "Rickettsial Diseases—A Public Health Problem?" 326.

56. J. R. Seal, "The United States Public Health Service and Rickettsial Diseases, Past, Present, Future," in Burgdorfer and Anacker, eds., *Rickettsiae and Rickettsial Diseases*, 6.

57. My discussion of this debate is based on ibid., 6; Minutes of the Meetings of the Board of Scientific Counselors of the National Institute of Allergy and Infectious Diseases, 1955–1981, and numerous interviews with scientists and administrators at NIAID. The minutes are held by the institute in Bethesda, Maryland, and in Hamilton, Montana; the interviews are in the NIAID files, NIH Historical Office.

58. The acrimony generated by this debate reflects how difficult the process of reaching consensus about research priorities can be. Since the late 1970s, when NIAID discontinued support for medical entomology, the number of medical entomologists in the United States has continued to dwindle, as witnessed by a May 1988 policy paper in *Science* on the dangers of losing competence in arthropod systematics. See J. H. Oliver, Jr., "Crisis in Biosystematics of Arthropods," *Science* 240 (1988):967. Lists of grants and contracts for rickettsial research may be obtained from the Division of Research Grants, National Institutes of Health, Bethesda, Maryland. Those for 1979 are listed in Burgdorfer and Anacker, eds., *Rickettsiae and Rickettsial Diseases*, 7–8. Acknowledgements of support from NIAID are listed in most of the published papers in the field.

59. Ormsbee, "Rickettsial Diseases—A Public Health Problem?" 326–27. Richard A. Ormsbee noted in a personal communication to the author, 25 February 1988, that the eastern bloc rickettsial research program, especially on Q fever, was stimulated during the late 1960s by the Slovak Academy of Sciences, particularly by D. Blaskovii. Three researchers from his Laboratory of Virology in Bratislava—Rudolf Brezina, Jan Kazán, and Steve Schramek—were permitted by the Czechoslovak authorities to visit the RML, the U.S. Naval Medical Research Laboratories, and the University of Maryland School of Medicine to study rickettsial research methods.

60. Smadel, "Status of the Rickettsioses in the United States," 424; E. L. Atwood, J. T. Lamb, R. Sonnenshine, and D. E. Sonnenshine, "A Contribution to the Epidemiology of Rocky Mountain Spotted Fever in the Eastern United States," *Am. J. Trop. Med. Hyg.* 14 (1965):831–37; M. A. W. Hattwick, "Rocky Mountain Spotted Fever in the United States, 1920–1970," *J. Inf. Dis.* 124 (1971):112–14; L. J. D'Angelo, W. G. Winkler, and D. J. Bregman, "Rocky Mountain Spotted Fever in the United States, 1975–1977," *J. Inf. Dis.* 138 (1978):273–76. This increase merited attention in the *British Medical Journal*, even though spotted fever did not occur in the British Isles. See "Rocky Mountain Spotted Fever," *British Medical Journal* 2 (1978):651.

61. M. A. W. Hattwick, R. J. O'Brien, and B. F. Hanson, "Rocky Mountain Spotted Fever: Epidemiology of an Increasing Problem," *Ann. Int. Med.* 84 (1976):732–39.

62. W. Burgdorfer, "Tick-Borne Diseases in the United States: Rocky Mountain Spotted Fever and Colorado Tick Fever: A Review," *Acta Tropica* 34 (1977):103–26 (quotations from pp. 113–14).

63. The reasons for women's apparent advantage in resisting spotted fever remain an unexplored area of research. David H. Walker noted in a personal communication to the author, 30 November 1988, that "questions of host defenses and resistance seem to be key to understanding differences in morbidity and mortality among different individuals."

64. Hattwick, O'Brien, and Hanson, "Rocky Mountain Spotted Fever: Epidemiology of an Increasing Problem," 738.

65. "Rocky Mountain Spotted Fever—United States, 1985," *JAMA* 255 (1986):2861, 2867; D. B. Fishbein, J. E. Kaplan, K. W. Bernard, and W. G. Winkler, "Surveillance of Rocky Mountain Spotted Fever, United States, 1981–1983," *Morbidity and Mortality Weekly Report, CDC Surveillance Summaries* 33 (1984):15SS–18SS. In 1983 a group from the Butantan Institute in São Paulo, Brazil, noted that a presumptive case of spotted fever had been reported in 1979 but that accurate information was not available for the country as a whole. See D. A. Portari Mancini, E. M. Mendes Nascimento, V. Rosa Tavares, and M. Adelino Soares, "A ocorréncia de riquetsioses do grupo *Rickettsia rickettsii*," *Revista de Saúde pública* 17 (1983):493–99.

66. V. Scaffidi, "Attuale espansione endemo-epidemica della febre bottonosa in Italia," *Minerva Medica* 72 (1981):2063–70 (quotations from Eng. summary).

67. A. Gutman, H. Schreiber, and R. Taragan, "An Outbreak of Tick Typhus in the Coastal Plain of Israel: 13 Cases from the Sharon Area," *Trans. Royal Soc. Trop. Med. Hyg.* 67 (1973):112–21; H. Schulchynska, R. Dagan, F. Schlaefer, and A. Keynan, "Spotted Fever in the Negev," *Harefuah* 102 (1982):317–19 (in Hebrew with Eng. summary); V. Scaffidi, "Contemporaneità della recente espansione endemo-epidemica della febbre bottonosa in Italia ed in Israele," *Giornale di Malattie Infettive e Parassitarie* 34 (1982):677–81.

68. F. Segura and B. Font, "Resurgence of Mediterranean Spotted Fever in Spain," *Lancet* 2 (1982):280.

69. For citations to this work, see the bibliography in D. H. Walker, J. I. Herrero-Herrero, R. R. Beltrán, A. Bullón-Sopelana, and A. Ramos-Hidalgo, "The Pathology of Fatal Mediterranean Spotted Fever," *American Journal of Clinical Pathology* 87 (1987):669–72.

70. S. Mansueto, G. Vitale, M. D. Miceli, G. Tringlai, P. Quartararo, D. M. Picone, and C. Occhino, "A Sero-epidemiological Survey of Asymptomatic Cases of Boutonneuse Fever in Western Sicily," *Trans. Royal Soc. Trop. Med. Hyg.* 78 (1984):16–18; S. Mansueto, G. Vitale, M. Bentivegna, G. Tringali, and R. DiLeo, "Persistence of Antibodies to *Rickettsia conorii* after an Acute Attack of Boutonneuse Fever," *J. Inf. Dis.* 151 (1985):377. For research on the role of dogs in tick-borne rickettsioses, see W. W. C. Topley and G. S. Wilson, *The Principles of Bacteriology and Immunity,* 2d ed. (Baltimore: William Wood & Co., 1936), 1461; L. F. Badger, "Rocky Mountain Spotted Fever: Susceptibility of Dog and Sheep to Virus," *Pub. Health Rep.* 48 (1933):791–95; C. C. Shepard and N. H. Topping, "Rocky Mountain Spotted Fever: A Study of Complement Fixation in the Serum of Certain Dogs," *J. Inf. Dis.* 78 (1946):63–68; K. P. Keenan, W. C. Buhles, Jr., D. L. Huxsoll, R. G. Williams, P. K. Hildebrandt, J. M. Campbell, and E. H. Stephenson, "Pathogenesis of Infection with *Rickettsia rickettsii* in the Dog: A Disease Model for Rocky Mountain Spotted Fever," *J. Inf. Dis.* 135 (1977):911–17; S. Mansueto and G. Vitale, "Antibodies to *Rickettsia conorii* in Dogs in Western Sicily," *Trans. Royal Soc. Trop. Med. Hyg.* 78 (1984):681–82; G. Tringali, V. Intonazzo, A. M. Perna, S. Mansueto, G. Vitale, and D. H. Walker, "Epidemiology of Boutonneuse Fever in Western Sicily: Distribution and Prevalence of Spotted Fever Group Rickettsial Infection in Dog Ticks (*Rhipicephalus sanguineus*)," *Am. J. Epidemiol.* 123 (1986):721–27; E. B. Breitschwerdt, D. H. Walker, M. G. Levy, W. Burgdorfer, W. T. Corbett, S. A. Hurlbert, M. E. Stebbins, B. C. Curtis, and D. A. Allen, "Clinical Hematologic, and Humoral Immune Response in Female Dogs Inoculated with *Rickettsia rickettsii* and *Rickettsia montana*," *American Journal of Veterinary Research* 49 (1988):70–76.

71. Centers for Disease Control, "Fatal Rocky Mountain Spotted Fever — Georgia," *Morbidity and Mortality Weekly Report* 26 (1977):84; "Spotted Fever Kills 2 at Disease Center," n.d., clipping in personal scrapbook of David B. Lackman, Helena, Montana, copy in NIAID files, NIH Historical Office.

72. In 1979 a group of rickettsiologists met at Fort Deposit, Maryland, to discuss formation of a new professional group. The American Society of Rickettsiology and Rickettsial Diseases was officially organized in 1980 at a meeting held at the RML. I am grateful to David H. Walker for providing information about the evolution of this organization.

Chapter Twelve: Mysteries Explained, Mysteries Remaining

1. Dowling, *Fighting Infection* (see chap. 10, n. 24), 248.

2. Florman and Hafkenschiel, "The Eastern Variety of Rocky Mountain Spotted Fever" (see chap. 8, n. 41), 123–33; J. T. Aquilina, F. Rosenberg, and R. L. Wuertz, "Nodal Tachycardia in a Case of Rocky Mountain Spotted Fever," *American Heart Journal* 43 (1952):755–60; J. K. Aikawa and G. T. Harrell, "Effect of Cortisone Acetate on Experimental Rocky Mountain Spotted Fever in the Guinea Pig," *Proc. Soc. Exp. Biol. Med.* 82 (1953):698–701; H. S. Moore, "Electrocardiograms in Tick Typhus," *East African Med. J.* 40 (1963):618–22; C. W. Phillips, G. T. Kimbrough, J. A. Weaver, and A. L. Tucker, "Rocky Mountain Spotted Fever with Thrombocytopenia," *Southern Med. J.* 53 (1960):867–69; C. E. Mengel and C. Trygstad, "Thrombocytopenia

in Rocky Mountain Spotted Fever," *JAMA* 183 (1963):886; J. W. Trigg, Jr., "Hypofibrinogenemia in Rocky Mountain Spotted Fever," *New England J. Med.* 270 (1964):1042–44; W. D. Bradford and D. B. Hackel, "Myocardial Involvement in Rocky Mountain Spotted Fever," *Arch. Pathol. Lab. Med.* 102 (1978):357–59; D. H. Walker, C. E. Paletta, and B. G. Cain, "Pathogenesis of Myocarditis in Rocky Mountain Spotted Fever," *Arch. Pathol. Lab. Med.* 104 (1980):171–74.

3. Louis Berlin, "Rocky Mountain Spotted Fever," letter to the editor and response, *JAMA* 134 (1947):1580.

4. Major studies on spotted fever's neurological manifestations include G. B. Hassin, "Cerebral Changes in Rocky Mountain Spotted Fever," *Archives of Neurology and Psychiatry* 44 (1940):1290–95; M. Scheinker, "Histologic Observations on the Changes in the Brain in Rocky Mountain Spotted Fever," *Arch. Pathol.* 35 (1943):583–89; "Neurologic Sequelae of Rocky Mountain Spotted Fever," abstract in *JAMA* 141 (1949):1017; R. E. Haynes, D. Y. Sanders, and H. G. Cramblett, "Rocky Mountain Spotted Fever in Children," *J. Pediatrics* 76 (1970):685–93; and E. W. Massey, T. Thamse, C. E. Coffey, and H. A. Gallis, "Neurologic Complications of Rocky Mountain Spotted Fever," *South. Med. J.* 78 (1985):1288–90, 1303.

5. M. J. Rosenblum, R. L. Masland, and G. T. Harrell, "Residual Effects of Rickettsial Disease on the Central Nervous System: Results of Neurologic Examinations and Electroencephalograms Following Rocky Mountain Spotted Fever," *Arch. Int. Med.* 90 (1952):444–55 (quotation from p. 444).

6. A. E. Davis, Jr., and W. D. Bradford, "Abdominal Pain Resembling Acute Appendicitis in Rocky Mountain Spotted Fever," *JAMA* 247 (1982):2811–12. See also M. B. Randall and D. H. Walker, "Rocky Mountain Spotted Fever: Gastrointestinal and Pancreatic Lesions and Rickettsial Infection," *Arch. Pathol. Lab. Med.* 108 (1984):963–67; D. H. Walker, H. R. Lesesne, V. A. Varma, and W. C. Thacker, "Rocky Mountain Spotted Fever Mimicking Acute Cholecystitis," *Arch. Int. Med.* 145 (1985):2194–96.

7. D. H. Walker, "Rickettsial Diseases: An Update," in Guido Majno, Ramzi S. Cotran, and Nathan Kaufman, eds., *Current Topics in Inflammation and Infection*, International Academy of Pathology, Monographs in Pathology no. 23 (Baltimore: Williams & Wilkins, 1982), 188–204.

8. G. T. Harrell, "Rocky Mountain Spotted Fever," *Medicine* 28 (1949):333–69; Jerry K. Aikawa, *Rocky Mountain Spotted Fever* (Springfield, Ill.: Charles C. Thomas, 1966). The bibliography in Aikawa's book contains most citations to the large body of studies conducted by Harrell, Aikawa, and their colleagues. Aikawa suggested that the disease should be called *rickettsial spotted fever.* See p. 118.

9. D. H. Walker, H. N. Kirkman, and P. H. Wittenberg, "Genetic States Possibly Associated with Enhanced Severity of Rocky Mountain Spotted Fever," in Burgdorfer and Anacker, eds., *Rickettsiae and Rickettsial Diseases* (see chap. 9, n. 14), 621–30 (quotation from p. 629); D. H. Walker, H. K. Hawkins, and P. Hudson, "Fulminant Rocky Mountain Spotted Fever: Its Pathologic Characteristics Associated with Glucose-6-Phosphate Dehydrogenase Deficiency," *Arch. Pathol. Lab. Med.* 107 (1983):121–25. Glucose-6-phosphate dehydrogenase deficiency is a genetic condition that apparently evolved like the sickle-cell trait by providing its carriers with some protection against malaria. See Kimberly Weiss, "The Role of Rickettsioses in History,"

in David H. Walker, ed., *Biology of Rickettsial Diseases*, 2 vols. (Boca Raton, Fla.: CRC Press, 1988), 1:12–13.

10. T. H. Maugh II, "Rickettsiae: A New Vaccine for Rocky Mountain Spotted Fever," *Science* 201 (1978):604.

11. L. J. D'Angelo and W. G. Winkler, "Rocky Mountain Spotted Fever," *New England J. Med.* 298 (1978):54; J. E. Johnson III, and P. J. Kadull, "Rocky Mountain Spotted Fever Acquired in a Laboratory," ibid. 277 (1967):842–47; F. M. Calia, P. J. Bartelloni, and R. W. McKinney, "Rocky Mountain Spotted Fever: Laboratory Infection in a Vaccinated Individual," *JAMA* 211 (1970):2012–14; D. J. Sexton, H. A. Gallis, J. R. McRae, and T. R. Cate, "Possible Needle-Associated Rocky Mountain Spotted Fever," *New England J. Med.* 292 (1975):645; C. N. Oster, D. S. Burke, R. H. Kenyon, M. S. Ascher, P. Harber, and C. E. Pedersen, Jr., "Laboratory-Acquired Rocky Mountain Spotted Fever: The Hazard of Aerosol Transmission," *New England J. Med.* 297 (1977):859–63.

12. H. L. DuPont, R. B. Hornick, A. T. Dawkins, G. G. Heiner, I. B. Fabrikant, C. L. Wisseman, Jr., and T. E. Woodward, "Rocky Mountain Spotted Fever: A Comparative Study of the Active Immunity Induced by Inactivated and Viable Pathogenic *Rickettsia rickettsii*," *J. Inf. Dis.* 128 (1973):340–44.

13. R. R. Parker and E. A. Steinhaus, "Rocky Mountain Spotted Fever: Duration of Potency of Tick-Tissue Vaccine," *Pub. Health Rep.* 58 (1943):230–32; "Minimum Requirements: Rocky Mountain Spotted Fever Vaccine Prepared from Infected Membranes of the Embryonated Chicken Egg," mimeo., National Institute of Health, Bethesda, Maryland, 13 August 1945; D. B. Lackman and R. R. Parker, "Comparison of the Immunogenic and Anaphylactogenic Properties of Rocky Mountain Spotted Fever Vaccines Prepared from Infected Yolk Sacs and from Infected Tick Tissue," *Am. J. Pub. Health* 38 (1948):1402–4; E. J. Bell and H. G. Stoenner, "Spotted Fever Vaccine: Potency Assay by Direct Challenge of Vaccinated Mice with Toxin of *Rickettsia rickettsii*," *J. Immunol.* 87 (1961):737–46.

14. R. H. Kenyon, W. M. Acree, G. G. Wright, and F. W. Melchoir, Jr., "Preparation of Vaccines for Rocky Mountain Spotted Fever from Rickettsiae Propagated in Cell Culture," *J. Inf. Dis.* 125 (1972):146–52; R. H. Kenyon and C. E. Pedersen, Jr., "Preparation of Rocky Mountain Spotted Fever Vaccine Suitable for Human Immunization," *Journal of Clinical Microbiology* 1 (1975):500–503; R. H. Kenyon, L. St. C. Sammons, and C. E. Pedersen, "Comparison of Three Rocky Mountain Spotted Fever Vaccines," *J. Clin. Microbiol.* 2 (1975):300–304; M. S. Ascher, C. N. Oster, P. I. Harber, R. H. Kenyon, and C. E. Pedersen, "Initial Clinical Evaluation of a New Rocky Mountain Spotted Fever Vaccine of Tissue Culture Origin," *J. Inf. Dis.* 138 (1978):217–21.

15. Augerson to Krause, 9 November 1976, cited in Robert Edelman, chief, Clinical Studies Branch, Microbiology and Infectious Diseases Program, National Institute of Allergy and Infectious Diseases, to Deputy Director, NIAID, memorandum, 16 November 1976, file "RMSF," files of the Microbiology and Infectious Diseases Program, NIAID (hereafter cited as MIDP files, NIAID).

16. "Rocky Mountain Spotted Fever in Children: The Case for Immunization," remarks by Samuel L. Katz, M.D., to the Microbiology and Infectious

Diseases Advisory Committee of the National Institute of Allergy and Infectious Diseases, 30 October 1978, file "RMSF—Volunteer Study," MIDP files, NIAID.

17. Chief, Development and Applications Branch, MIDP, NIAID, to Executive Officer, NIAID, draft memorandum, 14 November 1978, file "RMSF," MIDP files, NIAID.

18. John R. Seal, NIAID deputy director, to Director, MIDP, memorandum, 25 April 1979, file "RMSF—Volunteer Study," MIDP files, NIAID. The U.S. Food and Drug Administration regulates the procedures under which investigational new drugs are developed and tested. The process is explained in lay terminology in U.S. Food and Drug Administration, *From Test Tube to Patient: New Drug Development in the United States,* an *FDA Consumer* special report, HHS Publication no. (FDA) 88-3168 (Washington, D.C., 1988).

19. C. M. Wilfert, E. Austin, V. Dickinson, K. Kleeman, J. L. Hicks, J. N. MacCormack, R. L. Anacker, E. A. Casper, and R. N. Philip, "The Incidence of Rocky Mountain Spotted Fever as Described by Prospective Epidemiologic Survelliance and the Assessment of Persistence of Antibodies to *R. rickettsii* by Indirect Hemagglutination and Microimmunofluorescence Tests," in Burgdorfer and Anacker, eds., *Rickettsiae and Rickettsial Diseases,* 179–89; J. D. Folds, D. H. Walker, B. C. Hegarty, D. Banasiak, and J. V. Lange, "Rocky Mountain Spotted Fever Vaccine in an Animal Model," *J. Clin. Microbiol.* 18 (1983):321–26.

20. M. L. Clements, C. L. Wisseman, Jr., T. E. Woodward, P. Fiset, J. S. Dumler, W. McNamee, R. E. Black, J. Rooney, T. P. Hughes, and M. M. Levine, "Reactogenicity, Immunogenicity, and Efficacy of a Chick Embryo Cell-Derived Vaccine for Rocky Mountain Spotted Fever," *J. Inf. Dis.* 148 (1983):922–30 (quotation from p. 922).

21. U.S. Department of Health, Education, and Welfare, Food and Drug Administration, "Review of Rocky Mountain Spotted Fever (RMSF) Vaccine," pp. 25736–37 in "Viral and Rickettsial Vaccines: Proposed Implementation of Efficacy Review," *Federal Register* 45 (1980):25652–25758.

22. Ibid., 25737; DuPont et al., "Rocky Mountain Spotted Fever: A Comparative Study," 343; Clements et al., "Reactogenicity, Immunogenicity, and Efficacy," 929.

23. My discussion of this follows Tortora, Funke, and Case, *Microbiology: An Introduction* (see chap. 11, n. 47), 438. See also D. H. Walker and F. W. Henderson, "Effect of Immunosuppression on *Rickettsia rickettsii* Infection in Guinea Pigs," *Infect. Immun.* 20 (1978):221–27; R. H. Kenyon and C. E. Pedersen, Jr., "Immune Responses to *Rickettsia akari* Infection in Congenitally Athymic Nude Mice," *Infect. Immun.* 28 (1980):310–13; L. N. Kokorin, E. A. Kabanova, E. A. Shirokova, G. E. Abrosimova, N. N. Rybkina, and V. I. Pushkareva, "Role of T-Lymphocytes in *Rickettsia conorii* infection," *Acta Virol.* 26 (1982):91–97; Han Li, T. R. Jerrells, G. L. Spitalny, and D. H. Walker, "Gamma Interferon as a Crucial Host Defense Against *Rickettsia conorii* in Vivo," *Infect. Immun.* 55 (1987):1252–55.

24. For an overview and bibliography of recent work on rickettsial vaccines see D. H. Walker, "Role of the Composition of Rickettsiae in Rickettsial Immunity: Typhus and Spotted Fever Groups," in Walker, ed., *Biology of Rickettsial Diseases* 2:101–9.

25. Hui Min Feng, C. Kirkman, and D. H. Walker, "Radioimmunoprecipitation of [I^{35}S] Methionine-Radiolabeled Proteins of *Rickettsia conorii* and

Rickettsia rickettsii," *J. Inf. Dis.* 154 (1986):717–21 (quotation from p. 717); R. L. Anacker, R. N. Philip, J. C. Williams, R. H. List, R. E. Mann, "Biochemical and Immunochemical Analysis of *Rickettsia rickettsii* Strains of Various Degrees of Virulence," *Infect. Immun.* 44 (1984):559–64; J. V. Lange and D. H. Walker, "Production and Characterization of Monoclonal Antibodies to *Rickettsia rickettsii,*" *Infect. Immun.* 46 (1984):289–94; R. L. Anacker, R. H. List, R. E. Mann, S. F. Hayes, and L. A. Thomas, "Characterization of Monoclonal Antibodies Protecting Mice against *Rickettsia rickettsii,*" *J. Inf. Dis.* 151 (1985):1052–60; R. L. Anacker, R. H. List, R. E. Mann, and D. L. Wiedbrauk, "Antigenic Heterogeneity in High- and Low-virulence Strains of *Rickettsia rickettsii* Revealed by Monoclonal Antibodies," *Infect. Immun.* 51 (1986):653–60; D. H. Walker, P. Hanff, and B. Hegarty, "Analysis of Protein Antigens of *Rickettsia rickettsii* and *Rickettsia conorii* by Western Immunoblotting," in J. J. Kazar, ed., *Rickettsiae and Rickettsial Diseases: Proceedings of the IIIrd International Symposium* (Bratislava: Publishing House of the Slovak Academy of Sciences, 1985), 92–98; J. C. Williams, D. H. Walker, M. G. Peacock, S. T. Stewart, "Humoral Immune Response to Rocky Mountain Spotted Fever in Experimentally Infected Guinea Pigs: Immunoprecipitation of Lactoperoxidase ^{125}I-labeled Proteins and Detection of Soluble Antigens of *Rickettsia rickettsii,*" *Infect. Immun.* 52 (1986):120–27; H. M. Feng, D. H. Walker, and J. G. Wang, "Analysis of T-Cell-Dependent and -Independent Antigens of *Rickettsia conorii* with Monoclonal Antibodies," *Infect. Immun.* 55 (1987):7–15; H. Li, B. Lenz, and D. H. Walker, "Protective Monoclonal Antibodies Recognize Heat-Labile Epitopes on Surface Proteins of Spotted Fever Group Rickettsiae," *Infect. Immun.* 56 (1988):2587–93; Robert L. Anacker, interview by Victoria A. Harden, Hamilton, Montana, 26 October 1984, NIAID Files, NIH Historical Office.

26. G. A. McDonald, R. L. Anacker, and K. Garjian, "Cloned Gene of *Rickettsia rickettsii* Surface Antigen: Candidate Vaccine for Rocky Mountain Spotted Fever," *Science* 235 (1987):83–84.

27. C. C. Shepard, M. A. Redus, T. Tzianabos, and D. T. Warfield, "Recent Experience with the Complement Fixation Test in the Laboratory Diagnosis of Rickettsial Diseases in the United States," *J. Clin. Microbiol.* 4 (1976):277–83 (quotation from p. 283).

28. M. A. W. Hattwick, H. Retailliau, R. J. O'Brien, M. Slutzker, R. E. Fontaine, and B. Hanson, "Fatal Rocky Mountain Spotted Fever," *JAMA* 240 (1978):1499–1503 (quotation from p. 1502).

29. For a survey of the most recent methods of laboratory diagnosis, see D. H. Walker and M. G. Peacock, "Laboratory Diagnosis of Rickettsial Diseases," in Walker, ed., *Biology of Rickettsial Diseases*, 2:135–55.

30. S. Chang, "A Serologically Active Erythrocyte-Sensitizing Substance from Typhus Rickettsiae. I. Isolation and Titration," *J. Immunol.* 70 (1953):212–14; S. Chang, J. C. Snyder, and E. S. Murray, "A Serologically Active Erythrocyte-Sensitizing Substance from Typhus Rickettsiae. II. Serological Properties," ibid., 215–21; S. Chang, E. S. Murray, and J. C. Snyder, "Erythrocyte-Sensitizing Substances from Rickettsiae of the Rocky Mountain Spotted Fever Group," ibid. 73 (1954):8–15; D. M. Hersey, M. C. Clovin, and C. C. Shepard, "Studies on the Serologic Diagnosis of Murine Typhus and Rocky Mountain Spotted Fever. II. Human Infections," ibid. 79 (1957):409–15.

31. A. Shirai, J. W. Dietel, and J. V. Osterman, "Indirect Hemagglutination Test for Human Antibody to Typhus and Spotted Fever Group Rickettsiae," *J. Clin. Microbiol.* 2 (1975):430–37; R. L. Anacker, R. K. Gerloff, L. A. Thomas, R. E. Mann, W. R. Brown, and W. D. Bickel, "Purification of *Rickettsia rickettsii* by Density-Gradient Zonal Centrifugation," *Canadian Journal of Microbiology* 20 (1974):1523–27; R. L. Anacker, R. K. Gerloff, L. A. Thomas, R. E. Mann, and W. D. Bickel, "Immunological Properties of *Rickettsia rickettsii* Purified by Zonal Centrifugation," *Infect. Immun.* 11 (1975):1203–9; R. L. Anacker, R. N. Philip, L. A. Thomas, and E. A. Casper, "Indirect Hemagglutination Test for Detection of Antibody to *Rickettsia rickettsii* in Sera from Humans and Common Laboratory Animals," *J. Clin. Microbiol.* 10 (1979):677–84.

32. P. Fiset, R. A. Ormsbee, R. Silberman, M. Peacock, and S. H. Spielman, "A Microagglutination Technique for Detection and Measurement of Rickettsial Antibodies," *Acta Virol.* 13 (1969):60–66; K. E. Hechemy, R. W. Stevens, and H. A. Gaafar, "Detection of *Escherichia coli* Antigens by a Latex Agglutination Test," *Applied Microbiology* 28 (1974):306–11; K. E. Hechemy, R. W. Stevens, J. Sroka and H. A. Gaafar, "Latex Test for Quantitative Determination of *Escherichia coli* Antibody," *Applied Microbiol.* 28 (1974):1073–75; K. E. Hechemy, R. W. Stevens, and H. A. Gaafar, "Antigen Distribution in a Latex Suspension and Its Relationship to Test Sensitivity," *J. Clin. Microbiol.* 4 (1976):82–86; K. E. Hechemy, R. L. Anacker, R. N. Philip, K. T. Kleeman, J. N. McCormack, S. J. Sasowski, and E. E. Michaelson, "Detection of Rocky Mountain Spotted Fever Antibodies by a Latex Agglutination Test," *J. Clin. Microbiol.* 12 (1980):144–50.

33. A. H. Coons, J. C. Snyder, F. S. Cheevers, and E. S. Murray, "Localization of Antigen in Tissue Cells. IV. Antigens of Rickettsiae and Mumps Virus," *J. Exp. Med.* 91 (1950):31–37; W. Burgdorfer and D. B. Lackman, "Identification of *Rickettsia rickettsii* in the Wood Tick, *Dermacentor andersoni*, by Means of Fluorescent Antibody," *J. Inf. Dis.* 107 (1960):241–44; W. Burgdorfer, "Evaluation of the Fluorescent Antibody Technique for the Detection of Rocky Mountain Spotted Fever Rickettsiae in Various Tissues," *Pathologie et Microbiologia* 24 (1961):27–39.

34. C. E. Pedersen, Jr., L. R. Bagley, R. H. Kenyon, L. S. Sammons, and G. T. Burger, "Demonstration of *Rickettsia rickettsii* in the Rhesus Monkey by Immune Fluorescence Microscopy," *J. Clin. Microbiol.* 2 (1975):121–25; R. N. Philip, E. A. Casper, R. A. Ormsbee, M. G. Peacock, and W. Burgdorfer, "Microimmunofluorescence Test for the Serological Study of Rocky Mountain Spotted Fever and Typhus," ibid. 3 (1976):51–61; R. D. DeShazo, J. R. Boyce, J. V. Osterman, and E. H. Stephenson, "Early Diagnosis of Rocky Mountain Spotted Fever: Use of Primary Monocyte Culture Technique," *JAMA* 235 (1976):1353–55; D. H. Walker, A. Harrison, F. Henderson, and F. A. Murphy, "Identification of *Rickettsia rickettsii* in a Guinea Pig Model by Immunofluorescent and Electron Microscopic Techniques," *Am. J. Pathol.* 86 (1977):343–58; M. L. Clements, J. S. Dumler, Paul Fiset, C. L. Wisseman, Jr., M. J. Snyder, and M. M. Levine, "Serodiagnosis of Rocky Mountain Spotted Fever: Comparison of IgM and IgG Enzyme-Linked Immunoabsorbent Assays and Indirect Fluorescent Antibody Test," *J. Inf. Dis.* 148 (1983):876–80.

35. Philip et al., "Comparison of Serologic Methods" (see chap. 9, n. 57); V. F. Newhouse, C. C. Shepard, M. D. Redus, T. Tzianabos, and J. E. McDade,

"A Comparison of the Complement Fixation, Indirect Fluorescent Antibody, and Microagglutination Tests for the Serological Diagnosis of Rickettsial Diseases," *Am. J. Trop. Med. Hyg.* 28 (1979):387–95; K. E. Hechemy, R. L. Anacker, N. L. Carlo, J. A. Fox, and H. A. Gaafar, "Absorption of *Rickettsia rickettsii* Antibodies by *Rickettsia rickettsii* Antigens in Four Diagnostic Tests," *J. Clin. Microbiol.* 17 (1983):445–49.

36. T. E. Woodward, C. E. Pedersen, Jr., C. N. Oster, L. R. Bagley, J. Romberger, and M. J. Snyder, "Prompt Confirmation of Rocky Mountain Spotted Fever. Identification of Rickettsiae in Skin Tissues," *J. Inf. Dis.* 134 (1976):297–301; D. H. Walker and B. G. Cain, "A Method for Specific Diagnosis of Rocky Mountain Spotted Fever on Fixed, Paraffin-Embedded Tissue by Immunofluorescence," ibid. 137 (1978):206–9; D. H. Walker, B. G. Cain, and P. M. Olmstead, "Laboratory Diagnosis of Rocky Mountain Spotted Fever by Immunofluorescent Demonstration of *Rickettsia rickettsii* in Cutaneous Lesions," *Am. J. Clin. Pathol.* 69 (1978):619–23; W. R. Green, D. H. Walker, and B. G. Cain, "Fatal Viscerotropic Rocky Mountain Spotted Fever: Report of a Case Diagnosed by Immunofluorescence," *American Journal of Medicine* 64 (1978):523–28; G. Fleisher, E. T. Lennette, and P. Honig, "Diagnosis of Rocky Mountain Spotted Fever by Immunofluorescent Identification of *Rickettsia rickettsii* in Skin Biopsy Tissue," *J. Pediatrics* 95 (1979):63–65.

37. Walker, "Rickettsial Diseases: An Update," 188–204; D. H. Walker, R. M. Gay, and M. Valdes-Dapena, "The Occurrence of Eschars in Rocky Mountain Spotted Fever," *Journal of the American Academy of Dermatology* 4 (1981):571–76.

38. "Virginia Chapter Campaigns against RMSF," *Double Helix*, newsletter of the National Foundation for Infectious Diseases, 1 (July 1977):4.

39. L. J. D'Angelo, D. J. Bregman, and W. G. Winkler, "Rocky Mountain Spotted Fever in the United States: Use of Age-Specific Incidence to Determine Public Health Policy for a Vector-Borne Disease," *Southern Med. J.* 75 (1982):3–5; Willy Burgdorfer, interview by Victoria A. Harden, Hamilton, Montana, 22 October 1984, NIAID files, NIH Historical Office (hereafter cited as Burgdorfer interview).

40. J. K. Miller, "Rocky Mountain Spotted Fever on Long Island," *Ann. Int. Med.* 33 (1950):1398–1406; W. Burgdorfer, "Hemolymph Test: A Technique for Detection of Rickettsiae in Ticks," *Am. J. Trop. Med. Hyg.* 19 (1970):1010–14.

41. Quotations from Burgdorfer interview. Major papers growing out of this investigation were: W. Burgdorfer, A. G. Barbour, S. F. Hayes, J. L. Benach, E. Grunwaldt, and J. P. Davis, "Lyme Disease—A Tick-Borne Spirochetosis?" *Science* 216 (1982):1317–19; E. M. Bosler, J. L. Coleman, J. L. Benach, D. A. Massey, J. P. Hanrahan, W. Burgdorfer, and A. G. Barbour, "Natural Distribution of the *Ixodes dammini* Spirochete," ibid. 220 (1983):321–22; W. Burgdorfer and J. E. Kerians, "Ticks and Lyme Disease in the United States," *Ann. Int. Med.* 99 (1983):121; A. C. Steere, R. L. Grodzicki, A. N. Kornblatt, J. E. Craft, A. G. Barbour, W. Burgdorfer, G. P. Schmid, E. Johnson, and S. E. Malawista, "The Spirochetal Etiology of Lyme Disease," *New England J. Med.* 308 (1983):733–40; J. L. Benach, E. M. Bosler, J. P. Hanrahan, J. L. Coleman, G. S. Habicht, T. F. Bast, D. J. Cameron, J. L. Ziegler, A. G. Barbour, W. Burgdorfer, R. Edelman, and R. A. Kaslow, "Spirochetes Isolated from the Blood of Two Patients with Lyme Disease," *New England J. Med.* 308 (1983):740–42; A. G. Barbour, W. Burgdorfer, E. Grunwaldt, and A. C.

Steere, "Antibodies of Patients with Lyme Disease to Components of the *Ixodes dammini* Spirochete," *Journal of Clinical Investigation* 72 (1983):504–15; and L. A. Magnarelli, J. F. Anderson, W. Burgdorfer, and W. A. Chappel, "Parasitism by *Ixodes dammini* (Acari: Ixodidae) and Antibodies to Spirochetes in Mammals and Lyme Disease Foci in Connecticut, USA," *J. Med. Entomol.* 21 (1984):52–57.

42. M. R. Bovarnik and E. G. Allen, "Reversible Inactivation of Typhus Rickettsiae. I. Inactivation by Freezing," *Gen. Physiol.* 38 (1954):169–79; idem, "Reversible Inactivation of Typhus Rickettsiae at 0°C," *J. Bacteriol.* 73 (1957):56–62; idem, "Reversible Inactivation of the Toxicity and Hemolytic Activity of Typhus Rickettsiae by Starvation," *J. Bacteriol.* 74 (1957):637–45; W. H. Price, "The Epidemiology of Rocky Mountain Spotted Fever. I. The Characterization of Strain Virulence of *Rickettsia rickettsii*," *Am. J. Hyg.* 58 (1953):248–68; W. H. Price, "Variation in '*Rickettsia rickettsii*' under Natural and Experimental Conditions," in F. W. Hartman, F. L. Horsfall, Jr., and I. G. Kidd, eds., *Dynamics of Virus and Rickettsial Infections* (New York: Blakiston Co., 1954), 164–83; J. H. Gilford and W. H. Price, "Virulent-Avirulent Conversions of *Rickettsia rickettsii* in Vitro," *Proceedings of the National Academy of Sciences* 41 (1955):870–73; E. Weiss, H. B. Rees, and J. R. Hayes, "Metabolic Activity of Purified Suspensions of *Rickettsia rickettsii*," *Nature* 213 (1967):1020–22.

43. S. F. Hayes and W. Burgdorfer, "Reactivation of *Rickettsia rickettsii* in *Dermacentor andersoni* Ticks: An Ultrastructural Analysis," *Infect. Immun.* 37 (1982):779–85. Information about current research on the reactivation phenomenon was kindly supplied by David H. Walker in a personal communication to the author, 30 November 1988.

44. J. R. Audy, "The Localization of Disease with Special Reference to the Zoonoses," *Trans. Royal Soc. Trop. Med. Hyg.* 52 (1958):308–28 (quotations from p. 309); C. A. Hoare, review of E. N. Pavlovsky, P. A. Petrishcheva, D. N. Zasukhin, and N. G. Olsufiev, eds., *Natural Nidi of Human Diseases and Regional Epidemiology. Proceedings of the Joint Conference of the USSR Ministry of Public Health, the USSR Academy of Medical Sciences, the Gamalea Institute of Epidemiology and Microbiology of the USSR Academy of Medical Sciences, Dedicated to the Seventieth Anniversary of E. N. Pavlovsky, Member, USSR Academy of Sciences, March 29–April 1, 1954* (Leningrad: State Publishing House of Medical Literature, 1955) (in Russian); D. Blaskovic, ed., *Natural Foci of Infectious Diseases. Symposium on Natural Focalization of Infections in Man, Animals and Plants, According to the Doctrine of Academician E. N. Pavlovsky* (Bratislava: Slovakian Academy of Sciences) (in Czech and Slovakian). Historian William H. McNeill has utilized an ecological perspective similar to Pavlovsky's in his interpretation of how diseases contributed to the political and economic ascendency of particular human populations. See his *Plagues and Peoples* (Garden City, N.Y.: Anchor Press/Doubleday, 1976).

45. W. Burgdorfer, S. F. Hayes, and A. J. Mavros, "Nonpathogenic Rickettsiae in *Dermacentor andersoni*: A Limiting Factor for the Distribution of *Rickettsia rickettsii*," in Burgdorfer and Anacker, eds., *Rickettsiae and Rickettsial Diseases*, 585–94 (quotation from p. 585).

46. Ibid., 592. Robert N. Philip cautions, however, that the interference phenomenon may provide only a partial explanation of why *R. rickettsii*

appears limited to the west side of the valley. "The phenomenon is probably an exceedingly complex one which still remains hypothetical even after eighty years of study," he noted in a personal communication to the author, 16 February 1988. Antigenic interference by nonpathogenic rickettsiae has also been noted by Philip and Elizabeth Casper in ticks on the west side of the valley. See R. N. Philip and E. A. Casper, "Serotypes of Spotted Fever Group Rickettsiae Isolated from *D. andersoni* (Stiles) Ticks in Western Montana," *Am. J. Trop. Med. Hyg.* 30 (1981):234–42.

47. R. R. Parker, "Transmission of Rocky Mountain Spotted Fever by the Rabbit Tick *Haemaphysalis leporis-plaustris* Packard," *Am. J. Trop. Med.* 3 (1923).39–45; R. R. Parker, C. B. Philip, and W. L. Jellison, "Rocky Mountain Spotted Fever: Potentialities of Tick Transmission in Relation to Geographical Occurrence in the United States," ibid. 13 (1933):341–79; W. L. Jellison, "The Geographical Distribution of Rocky Mountain Spotted Fever and Nuttall's Cottontail in the Western United States," *Pub. Health Rep.* 60 (1945):958–61; R. R. Parker, E. G. Pickens, D. B. Lackman, E. J. Bell, and F. B. Thrailkill, "Isolation and Characterization of Rocky Mountain Spotted Fever Rickettsiae from the Rabbit Tick *Haemaphysalis leporis-palustris* Packard," *Pub. Health Rep.* 66 (1951):455–63.

48. W. Burgdorfer, J. C. Cooney, A. J. Mavros, W. L. Jellison, and C. Maser, "The Role of Cottontail Rabbits (*Sylvilagus* spp.) in the Ecology of *Rickettsia rickettsii* in the United States," *Am. J. Trop. Med. Hyg.* 29 (1980):686–90. In a personal communication to the author, 30 November 1988, David H. Walker noted: "*H. leporis-palustris* contains a strain of *R. rickettsii* called HLP. It is genetically closely related to the strains isolated from human cases of RMSF but has never been isolated from a human. Robert L. Anacker has shown that it has unique surface antigens. Thus there is no evidence that the rabbit tick is a vector of the disease. HLP strain may or may not cause any disease in humans. It might even be a vaccine candidate. It causes a mild, nonfatal disease in guinea pigs."

49. The term *mouse* was widely used in early studies to describe rodents that are at present termed voles.

50. W. L. Jellison, "Rocky Mountain Spotted Fever: The Susceptibility of Mice," *Pub. Health Rep.* 49 (1934):363–67; D. J. Gould and M. L. Miesse, "Recovery of a Rickettsia of the Spotted Fever Group from *Microtus pennsylvanicus* from Virginia," *Proc. Soc. Exp. Biol. Med.* 85 (1954):558–61; W. Burgdorfer, V. F. Newhouse, E. G. Pickens, and D. B. Lackman, "Ecology of Rocky Mountain Spotted Fever in Western Montana. I. Isolation of *Rickettsia rickettsii* from Wild Mammals," *Am. J. Hyg.* 76 (1962):293–301; W. Burgdorfer, K. T. Friedhoff, and J. L. Lancaster, Jr., "Natural History of Tick-Borne Spotted Fever in the USA: Susceptibility of Small Mammals to Virulent *Rickettsia rickettsii*," *Bull. WHO* 35 (1966):149–53; W. Burgdorfer, "Ecology of Tick Vectors of American Spotted Fever," *Bull. WHO* 40 (1969):375–81; L. A. Magnarelli, J. F. Anderson, Willy Burgdorfer, R. N. Philip, and W. A. Chappell, "Antibodies to *Rickettsia rickettsii* in *Peromyscus leucopus* from a Focus of Rocky Mountain Spotted Fever in Connecticut," *Can. J. Microbiol.* 30 (1984):491–94.

51. R. R. Parker, "Rocky Mountain Spotted Fever: Epidemiology with Particular Reference to Distribution and Prevalence in the Western United States," *Northwest Medicine* 34 (1935):111–21 (quotations from p. 114).

52. F. J. Spencer, "Tick-Borne Disease in Virginia, 1949–1958: An Ecological Note," *Am. J. Trop. Med. Hyg.* 10 (1961):220–22.

53. V. F. Newhouse, K. Choi, R. C. Holman, S. B. Thacker, L. J. D'Angelo, and J. D. Smith, "Rocky Mountain Spotted Fever in Georgia, 1961–75: Analysis of Social and Environmental Factors Affecting Occurrence," *Pub. Health Rep.* 101 (1986):419–28; J. E. McDade and V. F. Newhouse, "Natural History of *Rickettsia rickettsii*," *Ann. Rev. Microbiol.* 40 (1986):287–309.

Note on Sources

In the study of the history of diseases, the quality of materials available is highly variable, especially when the subject spans a number of centuries. Fortunately, the archival record of Rocky Mountain spotted fever, compiled essentially within the twentieth century, is especially rich. Most early investigators of this disease were meticulous in preserving data, correspondence, and scrapbook material. Many of those who have contributed to spotted fever research since World War II are still active in the laboratory or are recently retired. Although their papers have not yet been accessioned into libraries, a number generously agreed to provide oral interviews for this project. In this bibliographic essay, I have not attempted an exhaustive listing of sources consulted. What follows is a discussion of the major categories that attempts to provide some indication of their usefulness.

Histories of Rocky Mountain Spotted Fever

Aside from medical reviews and official publications of the state of Montana, which are discussed below, the earliest survey of Rocky Mountain spotted fever is James W. Sampson, "Rocky Mountain Spotted Fever: A Review of the Literature with Some Previously Unreported Notes from a Number of Wyoming Physicians," senior thesis, University of Nebraska College of Medicine, 1936. This was followed shortly afterward by Ernest L. Berry, "A Study of Rocky Mountain Spotted Fever," M.S. in public health thesis, University of Michigan, 1940. Both are reviews of the published scientific literature by students within the medical establishment. The book that has stood for decades as the standard history of spotted fever is Esther Gaskins Price, *Fighting Spotted Fever in the Rockies* (Helena, Mont.: Naegele Printing Co., 1948). A medical writer who had previously worked for the Mayo Clinic, Price prepared her book for the Montana State Board of Entomology, and it is thus biased toward the efforts of that group. Nearly two decades later, Jerry K. Aikawa published *Rocky Mountain Spotted Fever* (Springfield, Ill.: Charles C. Thomas, 1966). A distinguished rickettsiologist, Aikawa cited Price's book as the major source for his historical interpretation but added more material on Howard Taylor Ricketts, whom he admired. The goal of Aikawa's book, however, was to educate medical students about spotted fever, hence much of the material is written in technical language.

Reviews of Rickettsial Diseases

In setting Rocky Mountain spotted fever in the context of research on rickettsial diseases, one must begin with the classic history of epidemic typhus by Hans Zinsser, *Rats, Lice, and History* (Boston: Little, Brown & Co., 1935). This book and Zinsser's *As I Remember Him: The Autobiography of R.S.*

(Boston: Little, Brown & Co., 1940) provided a lively overview of the role
of typhus in history and of the personalities of many rickettsial investigators.
Another invaluable source for a general overview of the field was Nicholas
Hahon, ed., *Selected Papers on the Pathogenic Rickettsiae* (Cambridge, Mass.:
Harvard University Press, 1968). In addition to helpful essays introducing
each scientific paper, Hahon's book provided English translations of important
foreign papers.

The successive editions of *Bergey's Manual of Determinative Bacteriology*
(Baltimore: Williams & Wilkins, various dates) also proved an indispensable
aid and a primary source for charting changes in rickettsial classification and
nomenclature. Laboratory techniques for diagnosing rickettsial diseases were
described in *Diagnostic Procedures for Viral and Rickettsial Infections* (New
York: American Public Health Association, 1964). Two general textbooks of
microbiology served as references and sources of general overviews on several
fields relating to rickettsial research. They are: Bernard D. Davis, Renato
Dulbecco, Herman N. Eisen, Harold S. Ginsberg, W. Barry Wood, and Maclyn
McCarty, *Microbiology*, 2d ed. (New York: Harper & Row, 1973); and Gerard
J. Tortora, Berdell R. Funke, and Christine L. Case, *Microbiology: An Introduction*, 2d ed. (Menlo Park, Calif.: Benjamin/Cummings Publishing Co.,
1986).

Following the change over time of scientific ideas in rickettsial research was
facilitated by a series of books. These were: *Virus and Rickettsial Diseases,
with Especial Consideration of Their Public Health Significance*, proceedings
of a symposium, Harvard School of Public Health, 12–17 June 1939 (Cambridge, Mass.: Harvard University Press, 1940); F. R. Moulton, ed., *Rickettsial
Diseases of Man*, proceedings of a symposium of the American Association
for the Advancement of Science, Boston, 26–28 December 1946 (Washington,
D.C.: American Association for the Advancement of Science, 1948); Thomas
M. Rivers, ed., *Viral and Rickettsial Infections of Man*, 2d ed. (Philadelphia:
J. B. Lippincott Co., 1952); Thomas M. Rivers and Frank L. Horsfall, Jr.,
eds., *Viral and Rickettsial Infections of Man*, 3d ed. (Philadelphia: J. B. Lip-
pincott Co., 1959); Frank L. Horsfall, Jr. and Igor Tamm, eds. *Viral and
Rickettsial Infections of Man*, 4th ed. (Philadelphia: J. B. Lippincott Co.,
1965); Willy Burgdorfer and Robert L. Anacker, eds. *Rickettsiae and Rick-
ettsial Diseases* (New York: Academic Press, 1981). A new book, published
just as work on this book was being completed, continues this trend. It is
David H. Walker, ed., *Biology of Rickettsial Diseases*, 2 vols. (Boca Raton,
Fla.: CRC Press, 1988). One additional source, which provided information
about rickettsial research from the perspective of the Soviet Union, is P. F.
Zdrodovskii and H. M. Golinevich, *The Rickettsial Diseases*, trans. B. Haigh
(New York: Pergamon, 1960).

Histories of the Bitterroot Valley

Because Rocky Mountain spotted fever is a disease of nature, its well-
documented history in the Bitterroot Valley of Montana provided an excellent
case study in how human communities deal with diseases they encounter
through an unwitting alteration of an area's ecology. Searching for evidence
of the apparently disease-free ecology of the valley during its occupation by
the Salish, or Flathead, Indians was facilitated by Peter Ronan, *History of the*

Flathead Indians (Minneapolis: Ross & Haines, 1890), a record left by an Indian agent, and by Reuben G. Thwaites, ed., *The Journals of Lewis and Clark*, 8 vols. (New York, 1905; reprint, New York: Arno Press, 1969). Because of the active interest of Ravalli County citizens in their past, the period after white settlement is copiously documented in the archives of the Ravalli County Historical Society. Two publications on Bitterroot history were helpful in following social, political, and economic developments; curiously, neither mentions Rocky Mountain spotted fever. These are Samuel Lloyd Cappious, "A History of the Bitter Root Valley to 1914," M.A. thesis, University of Washington, 1939, and Bitter Root Valley Historical Society, ed., *Bitterroot Trails*, 2 vols. (Darby, Mont.. Professional Impressions, 1982). On the history of medicine in the Bitterroot and in Montana, Paul C. Phillips, *Medicine in the Making of Montana* (Missoula: Montana State University Press, 1962) is essential and contains only minor errors. One document that proved especially helpful was Robert N. Philip's study of newspapers, "A Journalistic View of Western Montana, 1870–1910: Some Newspaper Items Relevant to the Development of the Bitter Root Valley and the Occurrence of Rocky Mountain Spotted Fever," manuscript, Ravalli County Historical Society, Hamilton, Montana, and the University of Montana, Missoula, 1984. With the care of an epidemiologist, this study documents land use patterns, population trends, transportation and industrial developments, and the broader medical context in which evidence regarding Rocky Mountain spotted fever first appeared.

Manuscripts and Official Publications—Montana

Two other archival repositories in Montana contained rich records relating to Rocky Mountain spotted fever. At the Montana State Archives in Helena, the Montana State Board of Health Records, 1908–77, Record Group 28, contained not only internal state correspondence about the disease but also an abundance of correspondence with Howard Taylor Ricketts, S. Burt Wolbach, and representatives of the U.S. Public Health Service. The Minutes of the Montana State Board of Health, 15 March 1907–21 November 1975, on microfilm, provided a record of official decisions during the period in which spotted fever research was under the aegis of the Montana State Board of Health. In addition, the state archives holds a complete collection of the monthly reports of the laboratory in Hamilton between the 1920s and World War II. Also in their collections are the following useful reports of state boards that dealt with spotted fever: Montana State Board of Health, *Biennial Reports*, 1901–13, and Montana State Board of Entomology, *Biennial Reports*, 1913–31. These published documents, of course, are also available elsewhere. Because Robert A. Cooley, who served as secretary of the Montana State Board of Entomology from 1913 to 1931, spent his academic career at the institution now called Montana State University in Bozeman, it also houses materials important to the history of spotted fever. They are a part of the Zoology and Entomology Archives in the Renne Library and contain significant information from the 1920s through the 1940s about spotted fever work in Hamilton.

At the Rocky Mountain Laboratories (RML) of the National Institute of Allergy and Infectious Diseases (NIAID), a number of key documents relating to early spotted fever research had for years been preserved as a part of its institutional memory. Concerned about the security of these materials and their availability to other scholars, NIAID administrators requested that they be evaluated and placed in appropriate archival repositories. Of those materials, two collections generated when the state of Montana was in charge of investigations were transferred to the Montana State Archives. They were the seventeen bound volumes of the correspondence of Robert A. Cooley during his tenure as secretary of the Montana State Board of Entomology and one bound typescript volume of the Minutes of the Montana State Board of Entomology. Both, of course, are a mine of information on spotted fever and should be useful also to scholars interested in the history of entomology. The disposition of additional RML materials relating to the period of federal support of spotted fever research is discussed below.

Manuscript Materials—Federal Government

U.S. Public Health Service investigations of spotted fever commenced in 1902, and the Records of the Public Health Service, held in Record Group 90 at the National Archives and Records Administration, Washington, D.C., contain much material between that date and World War II. In addition, federal records long stored at the RML have been added to the spotted fever holdings of the National Archives, accessioned as Research Records of the Rocky Mountain Laboratory, Records of the National Institutes of Health, Record Group 443. These include correspondence files of early investigators; and the notebooks of case records by state and year prepared by Ralph R. Parker. In addition to information on Rocky Mountain spotted fever, a number of these notebooks document other arthropod-borne diseases, such as tularemia and Q fever, and one contains the transcript of a conference on post World War II plans for research.

Many materials remaining at the RML were also invaluable to this history. Copies of the Rocky Mountain Laboratory *Annual Reports* were essential. Robert K. Bergman, chief of the Rocky Mountain Operations Branch, NIAID, also permitted me to examine files known as the "director's office files," which provided much background information on the history of the laboratory. A collection of seven scrapbooks that covered the period 1919–60 contained much material that did not appear in official reports and was especially useful for following news accounts of the work outside Montana. Laboratory photographer Nick Kramis rendered the historian a great service when he prepared an index to his large collection of photographs, both of which are held at the RML.

The collections of the History of Medicine Division of the National Library of Medicine (NLM) in Bethesda, Maryland, contain U.S. Public Health Service scrapbooks of clippings on diseases and on the work of the service, 1876–1914, as well as U.S. Hygienic Laboratory Registers, 1901–23. The library's large number of oral histories provide personal perspectives on the development of medical research, especially within the federal government.

The active files of NIAID, both in Bethesda, Maryland, and at the RML in Hamilton, Montana, contain materials documenting the history of the institute and its predecessor organizations in spotted fever research. The Minutes of the Board of Scientific Counselors of the National Institute of Allergy and Infectious Diseases, 1955–81, for example, record the deliberations of this policy advisory board of nonfederal scientists. Recommendations of this board helped to explain the changing focus of institute research priorities in recent decades. The files of the NIAID Microbiology and Infectious Diseases Program, moreover, contain material on the mid-1970s withdrawal of the military services from Rocky Mountain spotted fever research and its assumption in toto by NIAID. William Jordan, director of the program, and Robert Edelman, chief of its Clinical Studies Branch, kindly made these files available. The institute's Public Information Office also contains some historical materials, and, in the course of this project, I collected a vertical file of information and correspondence now held in the NIH Historical Office.

Other Manuscript Collections

The papers of Howard Taylor Ricketts, held in the Department of Special Collections, Joseph Regenstein Library, University of Chicago, proved to be a rich source of information about his research. A scrapbook, prepared by his family and deposited in selected libraries, reproduces selected papers from the larger collection and serves as a useful introduction to Ricketts's work. After his death in 1910, his associates in Chicago published a collection of scientific papers relating to his work as Howard T. Ricketts, *Contributions to Medical Science by Howard Taylor Ricketts, 1870–1910* (Chicago: University of Chicago Press, 1911). Copies of Ricketts's correspondence and reprints of his scientific papers appear in several of these collections, as well as in the records of the Montana State Board of Health. To save space, I have not attempted to cite multiple sources for each document.

The Hideyo Noguchi Papers, located in Record Group 210.3, Rockefeller University Archives, New York, contain little correspondence about Noguchi's spotted fever research. They were useful, however, for providing information about the laboratory-acquired infection of Noguchi's assistant, Stephen Molinseck, and the impact of his disease on acceptance of a rickettsial organism as the etiological agent of spotted fever.

Other collections of papers on major spotted fever researchers did not prove so useful. The Louis B. Wilson Papers at the Mayo Clinic, unfortunately, do not include manuscript materials relating to his spotted fever work. S. Burt Wolbach's spotted fever correspondence is well documented in the Montana State Board of Health Records, mentioned above. His papers at the Francis A. Countway Library, Harvard University Medical School, Boston, however, would provide a rich source for the scholar interested in epidemic typhus.

Published Sources Relating to Federal Research

For background information on the history of the U.S. Public Health Service, Ralph C. Williams, *The United States Public Health Service, 1798–1950* (Washington, D.C.: Commissioned Officers Association, 1951) is the essential starting point. My own book, *Inventing the NIH: Federal Biomedical Research Policy, 1887–1937* (Baltimore: Johns Hopkins University Press, 1986), traces the emergence of medical research within the larger framework of the U.S. Public Health Service. For the post–World War II period, Charles V. Kidd's *American Universities and Federal Research* (Cambridge, Mass.: Belknap Press, 1959) is helpful in following the change in research priorities. His 1957 manuscript by the same title, on which his book was based, contains additional information and tables. It is available in the National Institutes of Health (NIH) Historical Office.

Other official sources for federal information include: the *Annual Reports* of the Surgeon General of the U.S. Public Health Service and its predecessor agencies; U.S. *Congressional Record*, House of Representatives and Senate; and U.S. *Statutes at Large*. An overview of the major lines of infectious disease research conducted by NIAID and its predecessors is provided in National Institute of Allergy and Infectious Diseases, *Intramural Contributions, 1887–1987*, ed. Harriet R. Greenwald and Victoria A. Harden (Bethesda, Md.: National Institute of Allergy and Infectious Diseases, 1987). In addition, reference information on budgets, personnel, and leadership within the NIH may be quickly accessed through the National Institutes of Health, *NIH Almanac*, published annually (Washington, D.C.: U.S. Department of Health and Human Services).

More detailed data about NIH funding for rickettsial disease research projects is available through yearly grants publications. From 1948 to 1961, titles vary slightly and types of summary data change. The first, covering the period 1946 (when the grants program began) to 1949, is U.S. National Institutes of Health, Division of Research Grants, *Research Grants Awarded by the Public Health Service*, comp. David E. Price, suppl. 205 to the *Public Health Reports*, rev. 1948, addendum 1949. The 1948 revision of this publication also includes National Cancer Institute grants dating from 1937. In 1961 the first edition of a new format that continued through 1971 was issued. With changing years, this is idem, *Research Grants Index, Fiscal Year 1961* (Washington, D.C.: Government Printing Office). Beginning in 1972, this information was stored in a data base at the Division of Research Grants, NIH. Information on grants after 1971 came from a search of this data base for the descriptor "Rocky Mountain spotted fever and other rickettsial diseases."

Bibliographic and Periodical Sources

In the beginning of a search of the periodical literature, the tools available through the NLM are indispensable. The volumes of *Index Medicus* provide not only lists of the scientific papers on spotted fever but also a good indication of how the medical concept of the disease changed over time, as indicated by different headings under which entries were filed. Most papers published since 1966 may be accessed through computer data bases on the MEDLARS system supported by NLM. Research in the history of medicine is catalogued in the library's *Bibliography of the History of Medicine*, with papers published since 1970 also indexed in the data base HISTLINE. Especially useful in this project were such medical journals of record as the *Journal of the American Medical Association*, indexed separately, and *Science*, because they contained a wealth of editorial, news, bibliographic, and international information in addition to reports on clinical and laboratory research findings.

For amplifying and cross-checking sources, the bibliographies in early research papers and in later review papers were most useful. In 1954, David G. Cooman prepared the *Bibliography on the Rocky Mountain Spotted Fever Group of Rickettsioses*, which is available at NLM, for the U.S. Army Chemical Corps Technical Library. Information on rickettsial diseases in Africa can be accessed through K. David Patterson, comp., *Infectious Diseases in Twentieth-*

Century Africa: A Bibliography of Their Distribution and Consequences (Waltham, Mass.: African Studies Association, Crossroads Press, 1979), especially "Typhus and Other Rickettsial Infections," 195–98. Publications about ticks and tick-borne diseases are indexed in Harry Hoogstraal, *Bibliography of Ticks and Tickborne Diseases from Homer (about 800 B.C.) to 31 December 1969*, 5 vols. (Cairo: U.S. Naval Medical Research Unit No. 3, 1970). The *Reader's Guide to Periodical Literature* provided an index to the popular literature on spotted fever and on attitudes toward medicine in general in the United States. The *New York Times Index* similarly served as a source from which societal response to disease could be followed over time.

Biographical Information

Many sources proved useful for biographical information on key figures in the history of spotted fever. Jeanette Barry, comp., *Notable Contributions to Medical Research by Public Health Service Scientists: A Bibliography to 1940* (Washington, D.C.: Government Printing Office, 1960) summarized biographical and bibliographical information about the most notable federal scientists. The personnel files of deceased U.S. Public Health Service officers, located at the Federal Records Center in Saint Louis, Missouri, provided information not only about the leaders of federal research, but also about those who never achieved fame. I am indebted to the Commissioned Officers Corps staff in Rockville, Maryland, for helping me obtain copies of these records. Elizabeth Moot O'Hearn, *Profiles of Pioneer Women Scientists* (Washington, D.C.: Acropolis Books, 1985) is useful for women investigators, and Paul F. Clark, *Pioneer Microbiologists of America* (Madison: University of Wisconsin Press, 1961) contains many helpful sketches. The Library and Information Management Section of the American Medical Association kindly provided information about several early spotted fever investigators and public health figures who were not documented in published sources. Other major biographical tools included various editions of *American Men of Science* and *American Men and Women of Science* (editors and other details of publication vary; information for the relevant edition is supplied in the notes); Charles Coulston Gillispie, ed., *Dictionary of Scientific Biography*, 16 vols. (New York: Charles Scribner's Sons, 1970–80); *Dictionary of American Biography*, 20 vols., 6 suppls. (New York: Charles Scribner's Sons, 1932–80); *Who's Who in America* (Chicago: Marquis–Who's Who, various editions); Allen G. Debus, ed., *World Who's Who in Science: A Biographical Dictionary of Notable Scientists from Antiquity to the Present*, (Chicago: Marquis–Who's Who, 1968). There is, unfortunately, a paucity of biographical information about foreign scientists. Biographical dictionaries for British and German investigators are available, but it is often impossible to locate first names, let alone background information, on many other European, Latin American, and Japanese researchers.

Oral Histories and Interviews

For personal assessments of twentieth-century medical research, the oral histories in the NLM provide an excellent starting point. During the 1960s, Harlan Phillips conducted a number of oral histories that are catalogued as George Rosen, "Transcripts of Oral History Project, 1962–1964," Manu-

scripts Collection, History of Medicine Division, NLM. Among those inter-
viewed in this series are Roscoe R. Spencer, Rolla Eugene Dyer, Norman H.
Topping, and Victor H. Haas. Phillips also conducted an extensive oral history
project with Stanhope Bayne-Jones, director of the U.S.A. Typhus Commission.
Its five volumes are indexed separately at NLM. In addition, former NIH and
NLM historian Wyndham Miles interviewed a number of NIH administrators.
These interviews are now catalogued and augment the already large collection.

During the course of my research, I conducted short interviews with many
scientists connected with the RML and the NIH. These are available in the
NIAID files, NIH Historical Office. Those interviews related to research for
this book were with Robert L. Anacker, E. John Bell, J. Frederick Bell, Willy
Burgdorfer, Dorland J. Davis, Victor H. Haas, William L. Jellison, Nick
Kramis, David B. Lackman, Richard A. Ormsbee, Cornelius B. Philip, and
Robert N. Philip.

Conversations and Correspondence

As my thinking about the ideas in this book took shape, a number of people
generously offered suggestions, criticism, encouragement, and advice. Among
my historian colleagues, thanks are due to James Harvey Young, Charles
Howard Candler Professor Emeritus at Emory University; Saul Benison of the
University of Cincinnati; Robert J. T. Joy of the Uniformed Services University
of the Health Sciences; Suzanne White of the U.S. Food and Drug Administration; Caroline Hannaway and Kimberly Pelis of the Institute of the History
of Medicine, Johns Hopkins University School of Medicine. Ruth Levy Guyer,
formerly at NIAID and now on the staff of *Science*, patiently introduced me
to immunology. James Kerians, curator of the tick collection formerly at the
RML and now at the Smithsonian Institution, answered questions about tick
taxonomy; Robert Traub, curator of the flea collection at the Smithsonian,
alerted me to a photograph collection on rickettsialpox and encouraged my
efforts in a variety of other ways. As the project commenced, Jim C. Williams
of NIAID provided an overview of current rickettsial work. Charles L. Wisseman, Jr., former head of the Commission on Rickettsial Diseases of the Armed
Forces Epidemiological Board, kindly shared information about that body and
guided my understanding of recent research in rickettsiology. David H. Walker,
chairman of the Department of Pathology, University of Texas Medical Branch,
Galveston, discussed with me the larger framework in which recent research
has taken place, fine-tuned my discussion of molecular biology and immunology, and traced the lines of international collaboration in recent rickettsial
work.

History of Medicine Surveys

The history of Rocky Mountain spotted fever, of course, is embedded in
the broader context of medical history. For the general reader seeking to
understand major trends, a number of works are available. Erwin H. Ackerknecht, *A Short History of Medicine*, rev. ed. (Baltimore: Johns Hopkins
University Press, 1982) is a standard textbook on the history of medicine in
western civilization. John Duffy, *The Healers: A History of American Medicine*
(Urbana: University of Illinois Press, 1979) provides a similar overview of

medicine in the United States. An older but classic interpretative work is Richard H. Shryock, *The Development of Modern Medicine: An Interpretation of the Social and Scientific Factors Involved* (New York: Alfred A. Knopf, 1936; reprint, Madison: University of Wisconsin Press, 1979). Many other works relating to specific topics are listed in the general references.

General References

The secondary sources used in this research that should prove most useful to other scholars are: Erwin H. Ackerknecht, *Medicine in the Paris Hospital, 1794–1848* (Baltimore: Johns Hopkins Press, 1967); idem, *Rudolf Virchow: Doctor, Statesman, Anthropologist* (Madison: University of Wisconsin Press, 1953); J. R. Audy, *Red Mites and Typhus* (London: Athlone Press, 1968); Mary Barber and Lawrence P. Garrod, *Antibiotic and Chemotherapy* (Edinburgh: E. & S. Livingstone, 1963); William B. Bean, *Walter Reed: A Biography* (Charlottesville: University Press of Virginia, 1982); Saul Benison, *Tom Rivers: Reflections on a Life in Medicine and Science* (Cambridge: MIT Press, 1967); Debra Jan Bibel, *Milestones in Immunology: A Historical Exploration* (Madison, Wis.: Science Tech Publishers, 1988); Lennard Bickel, *Rise Up to Life: A Biography of Howard Walter Florey, Who Gave Penicillin to the World* (New York: Charles Scribner's Sons, 1972); John Z. Bowers and Elizabeth F. Purcell, eds., *Advances in American Medicine: Essays at the Bicentennial,* 2 vols. (New York: Josiah Macy, Jr., Foundation, 1976); Savile Bradbury, *The Evolution of the Microscope* (Oxford: Pergamon Press, 1967); Emile Brumpt, *Précis de parasitologie* (Paris: Masson et Cie., 1927); Jenks Cameron, *The Bureau of Biological Survey: Its History, Activities, and Organization,* Institute for Government Research Service Monographs of the United States Government no. 54 (Baltimore: Johns Hopkins Press, 1929); Rachel Carson, *Silent Spring* (Boston: Houghton Mifflin Co., 1962); George Clark and Frederick H. Kasten, *History of Staining,* 3d ed. (Baltimore: Williams & Wilkins, 1983); Rennie W. Doane, *Insects and Disease: A Popular Account of the Way in Which Insects May Spread or Cause Some of Our Common Diseases* (New York: Henry Holt, 1910); Harry F. Dowling, *Fighting Infection: Conquests of the Twentieth Century* (Cambridge, Mass.: Harvard University Press, 1977); Harry F. Dowling, *Medicines for Man: The Development, Regulation, and Use of Prescription Drugs* (New York: Alfred A. Knopf, 1970); Gustav Eckstein, *Noguchi* (New York: Harper, 1931); J. Merton England, *A Patron for Pure Science: The National Science Foundation's Formative Years, 1945–1957* (Washington, D.C.: Government Printing Office, 1982); John Ettling, *The Germ of Laziness: Rockefeller Philanthropy and Public Policy in the New South* (Cambridge, Mass.: Harvard University Press, 1981); Abraham Flexner, *Medical Education in the United States and Canada* (New York: Carnegie Foundation, 1910); William D. Foster, *A History of Parasitology* (Edinburgh: E. & S. Livingstone, 1965); Nicholas Hahon, ed., *Selected Papers on Virology* (Englewood Cliffs, N.J.: Prentice-Hall, 1964); Robert S. Henry, *The Armed Forces Institute of Pathology: Its First Century, 1862–1962* (Washington, D.C.: Office of the Surgeon General of the Army, 1964); William B. Herms, *Medical Entomology: With Special Reference to the Health and Well-Being of Man and Animals* (New York: Macmillan, 1939); Ronald Hilton, *The Scientific Institutions of Latin America, with Special Reference to Their Or-*

ganization and Information Facilities (Stanford: California Institute of International Studies, 1970); R. Hoeppli, *Parasites and Parasitic Infections in Early Medicine and Science* (Singapore: University of Malaya Press, 1959); Sally Smith Hughes, *The Virus: A History of the Concept* (New York: Science History Publications, 1977); Howard A. Kelly, *Walter Reed and Yellow Fever*, 3d rev. ed. (Baltimore: Norman, Remington, 1923); Robert Koch, *The Aetiology of Tuberculosis* (New York: National Tuberculosis Association, 1922); Paul de Kruif, *Men against Death* (New York: Harcourt, Brace, 1932); Erna Lesky, *The Vienna Medical School in the Nineteenth Century* (Baltimore: Johns Hopkins University Press, 1976); Esmond R. Long, *A History of American Pathology* (Springfield, Ill.: Charles C. Thomas, 1962); Esmond R. Long, *A History of Pathology* (Baltimore: Williams & Wilkins, 1928; reprint, New York: Dover, 1965); Esmond R. Long, *History of the American Society for Experimental Pathology* (Bethesda, Md.: American Society for Experimental Pathology, 1972); Kenneth M. Ludmerer, *Learning to Heal: The Development of American Medical Education* (New York: Basic Books, 1985); André Maurois, *The Life of Sir Alexander Fleming, Discoverer of Penicillin*, trans. Gerard Hopkins (New York: E. P. Dutton, 1959); William H. McNeill, *Plagues and Peoples* (Garden City, N.Y.: Anchor Press/Doubleday, 1976); Aristides A. Moll, *Aesculapius in Latin America* (Philadelphia: W. B. Saunders Co., 1944); William Osler, *The Evolution of Modern Medicine* (New Haven, Conn.: Yale University Press, 1922); Isabel R. Plesset, *Noguchi and His Patrons* (Rutherford, N.J.: Fairleigh Dickinson University Press, 1980); Mazyck P. Ravenel, ed., *A Half Century of Public Health* (New York: American Public Health Association, 1921); Henrique da Rocha Lima, *Estudos sôbre o Tifo Exantemático*, comp. Edgard de Cerqueira Falcão, with commentary by Otto G. Bier (São Paulo, Brazil, 1966); Charles E. Rosenberg, *The Cholera Years: The United States in 1832, 1849, and 1866* (Chicago: University of Chicago Press, 1962); H. Harold Scott, *A History of Tropical Medicine*, 2 vols. (London: Edward Arnold, 1939); Ray F. Smith, Thomas E. Mittler, and Carroll N. Smith, eds., *History of Entomology* (Palo Alto, Calif.: Annual Reviews, 1973); Nancy Stepan, *Beginnings of Brazilian Science: Oswaldo Cruz, Medical Research and Policy, 1890–1920* (New York: Science History Publications, 1981); *Symposium on the Spotted Fever Group*, Walter Reed Army Institute of Research Medical Science Publication no. 7 (Washington, D.C.: Government Printing Office, 1960); U.S. Army, Medical Department, *Preventive Medicine in World War II*, vol. 2, *Environmental Hygiene* (Washington, D.C.: Government Printing Office, 1955); U.S. Army, Medical Department, *Internal Medicine in World War II*, vol. 2 (Washington, D.C.: Government Printing Office, 1963); U.S. Army, Medical Department, *Preventive Medicine in World War II*, vol. 7, *Communicable Diseases: Arthropodborne Diseases Other Than Malaria* (Washington, D.C.: Government Printing Office, 1964); U.S. President's NIH Study Committee, *Biomedical Science and Its Administration: A Study of the National Institutes of Health* (Washington, D.C.: Government Printing Office, 1965); U.S. President's Scientific Research Board, *Science and Public Policy: A Report to the President*, by John R. Steelman, 5 vols. (Washington, D.C.: Government Printing Office, 1947); Gustavus A. Weber, *The Bureau of Entomology: Its History, Activities, and Organization*, Institute for Government Research, Service Monographs of the United States Government no. 60 (Washington, D.C.: Brookings Institution, 1930); Carolyn Whitlock, ed., *Proceedings of the Fourth International Congresses on Tropical Medicine and Malaria, Washington, D.C., May 10–18, 1948* (Washington, D.C.: Government Printing Office, 1948); Robert H. Wiebe, *The Search for Order, 1877–1920* (New York: Hill & Wang, 1967); E. N. Willmer, ed., *Cells and Tissues in Culture: Methods, Biology, and Physiology* (New York: Academic Press, 1965); S. Burt Wolbach, John L. Todd, and Francis W. Palfrey, *The Etiology and Pathology of Typhus* (Cambridge, Mass.: League of Red Cross Societies, Harvard University Press, 1922); Theodore E. Woodward, *Introduction to the History of the Armed Forces Medical Unit in Kuala Lumpur, Malaya, and the Armed Forces Research Institute of Medical Sciences (AFRIMS) in Bangkok, Thailand* (privately printed, n.d.); James Harvey Young, *The Toadstool Millionaires: A Social History of Patent Medicines in America before Federal Regulation* (Princeton, N.J.: Princeton University Press, 1961); James Harvey Young, *The Medical Messiahs: A Social History of Health Quackery in the Twentieth Century* (Princeton, N.J.: Princeton University Press, 1967).

Index

References to illustrations appear in italic type; tables appear underscored.

Book designed by Kachergis Book Design

Composed by Capitol Communication Systems, Inc. Sabon text and display
Printed by Thomson-Shore, Inc. on 60-lb. Spring Forge White paper and bound in
Roxite B.